Afoot & Afield

Orange County

A comprehensive hiking guide

FOURTH EDITION

T0151193

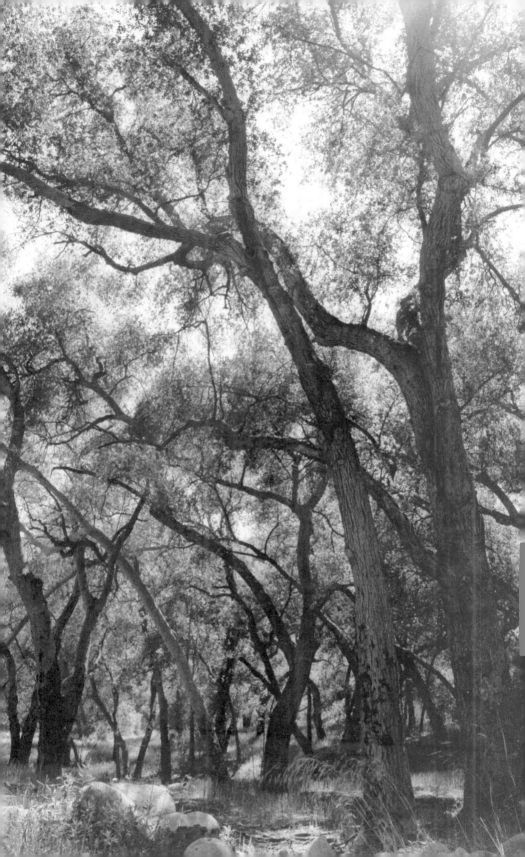

Afoot & Afield

Orange County

A comprehensive hiking guide

FOURTH EDITION

Jerry Schad and
David Money Harris

WILDERNESS PRESS ...*on the trail since 1967*

IN MEMORY OF JERRY SCHAD, 1949–2011

Afoot & Afield Orange County: A Comprehensive Hiking Guide

Fourth edition, second printing 2022

Copyright © 1988, 1996, 2006, and 2015 by Jerry Schad and David Money Harris

Editor: Laura Shauger
Project editor: Ritchey Halphen
Interior photos by Jerry Schad and David Money Harris, except where noted
Maps: Jerry Schad and David Money Harris
Cover design: Scott McGrew
Original text design: Andreas Schuller; adapted by Annie Long
Proofreader: Emily C. Beaumont
Indexer: Sylvia Coates

Library of Congress Cataloging-in-Publication Data

Schad, Jerry.
  Afoot & afield Orange County : a comprehensive hiking guide / Jerry Schad and David Money Harris.
    pages cm
  ISBN 978-0-89997-757-7 (paperback) — ISBN 0-89997-757-X — eISBN 978-0-89997-758-4
  1. Hiking--California—Orange County—Guidebooks. 2. Orange County (Calif.)—Guidebooks.
3. Natural history—California—Orange County. I. Harris, David Money. II. Title.
  GV199.42.C22O737 2015
  796.5109794'96—dc23
                        2014033607

Manufactured in the United States of America

Distributed by Publishers Group West

Published by: **WILDERNESS PRESS**
              An imprint of AdventureKEEN
              2204 First Avenue South, Suite 102
              Birmingham, AL 35233
              800-678-7006, fax 877-374-9016

Visit **wildernesspress.com** for a complete listing of our books and for ordering information.

Cover photos, clockwise from top: Dana Point tidepools (see Chapter 6), David Money Harris; Black Star Falls (see Chapter 15), Joel Robinson/Naturalist for You; descending San Juan Hill (see Chapter 7), David Money Harris

Frontispiece: Southern oak woodland, San Mateo Canyon Wilderness (see Chapter 17), Jerry Schad

SAFETY NOTICE Although Wilderness Press and the author have made every attempt to ensure that the information in this book is accurate at press time, they are not responsible for any loss, damage, injury, or inconvenience that may occur to anyone while using this book. You are responsible for your own safety and health while in the wilderness. The fact that a trail is described in this book does not mean that it will be safe for you. Be aware that trail conditions can change from day to day. Always check local conditions, and know your own limitations.

Acknowledgments

I am honored that Jerry Schad, this guide's original author, entrusted his book to my care. The dean of Southern California guidebook authors, Professor Schad originated the *Afoot & Afield* series in 1986 and wrote 16 books in all, mostly about the outdoors. His breadth of knowledge of the region's trails and natural history was unsurpassed. An accomplished athlete in enviable physical condition, he was diagnosed with kidney cancer in March 2011 and passed away six months later at age 61. I have endeavored to update this edition with recent developments and new trails while honoring his high standards. Learning about our wild places is a journey of a lifetime.

Most of the words in this book were written by Jerry, and the multitude who assisted him are recognized in the third edition.

Many more people have contributed their time and knowledge to this fourth edition. Steve Aleshire, Carroll Baldwin, Debra Clarke, Kelly Elliott, Eric Ey, Rob Hicks, Candice Hubert, Trude Hurd, Ellen Loftin, Vlesydi Loveland, Marisa O'Neil, Barbara Norton, Zachary Salazar, Jim Simkins, Ron Slimm, Jenn Starnes, and Joanne Taylor reviewed materials and provided insights. Volunteer docents of the Irvine Ranch Conservancy guided tours across the historic Irvine Ranch. Joel Robinson of Naturalist for You shared his trove of knowledge and his spectacular photographs.

Students from the Claremont Colleges and colleagues from Broadcom Corporation joined me during the fieldwork. Greg Fong, Aaron Stratton, and Avi Thaker were especially regular. My long-time climbing buddy, Craig Clarence, was excellent canyoneering company. My sons, Benjamin, Samuel, and Abraham, were my most frequent companions, hiking or mountain biking with me for 53 delightful days on the trail. This work would not have been possible without the support of my wife, Jennifer.

I would like to thank the team at Wilderness Press for making this book come together. Molly Merkle envisioned the new edition. Laura Shauger brought her outstanding editing skills to the project. Ritchey Halphen guided the book through production. The remaining errors are my own.

—*David Money Harris*
Upland, California
November 2014

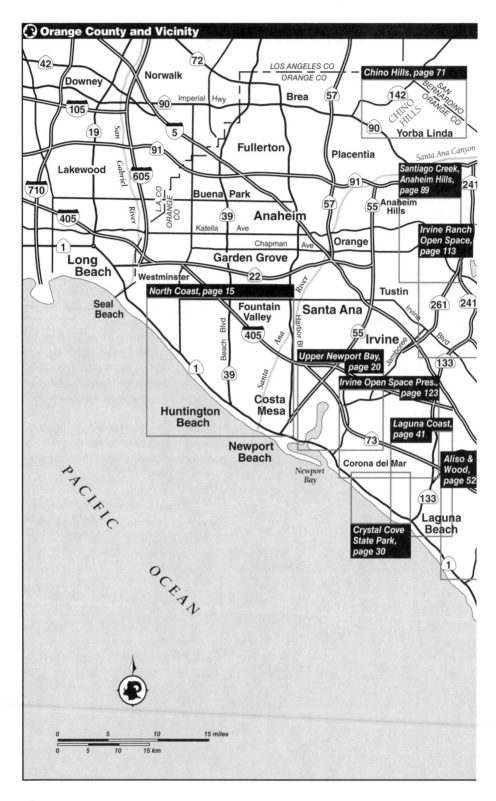

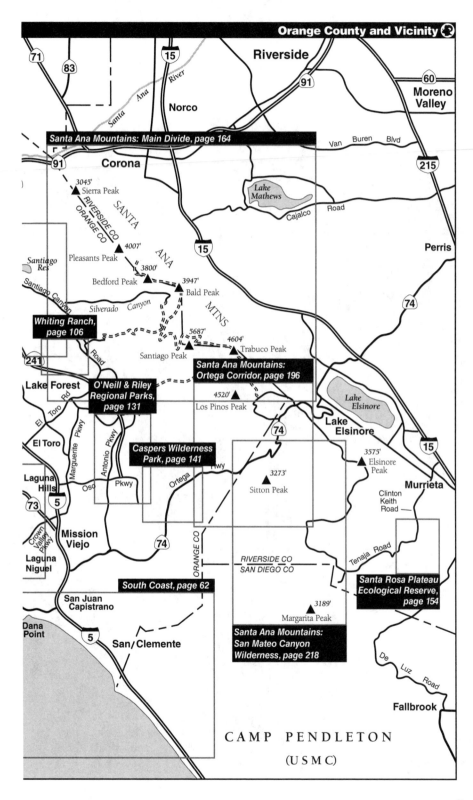

⑺₁
⑻₃
①₅ (15)
Riverside
⑼₁ (91)
⑹₀ (60)
Moreno Valley

Santa Ana *River*

Norco

Van Buren Blvd

②₁₅ (215)

Santa Ana Mountains: Main Divide, page 164

⑼₁ (91) **Corona**

3045'
▲ Sierra Peak

Lake Mathews

Cajalco Road

SANTA

RIVERSIDE CO
ORANGE CO

4007'
▲ Pleasants Peak

①₅ (15)

Perris

Santiago Res

3800'
▲ Bedford Peak

3947'
▲ Bald Peak

ANA

Santiago Canyon

Silverado *Canyon*

MTNS

⑺₄ (74)

Whiting Ranch, page 106

Road

5687'
▲ Santiago Peak

4604'
▲ Trabuco Peak

②₄₁ (241)

Lake Forest

O'Neill & Riley Regional Parks, page 131

Santa Ana Mountains: Ortega Corridor, page 196

Lake Elsinore

El Toro Rd

4520' ▲
Los Pinos Peak

Lake Elsinore

Marguerite Pkwy

Antonio Pkwy

Caspers Wilderness Park, page 141

⑺₄ (74)

3575'
▲ Elsinore Peak

①₅ (15)

El Toro

Laguna Hills

⑺₃ (73)
⑤ (5)

Oso Pkwy

Ortega Hwy

3273'
▲ Sitton Peak

Clinton Keith Road

Murrieta

Crown Valley Pkwy

Mission Viejo

⑺₄ (74)

ORANGE CO

RIVERSIDE CO
SAN DIEGO CO

Tenaja Road

Laguna Niguel

South Coast, page 62

Santa Rosa Plateau Ecological Reserve, page 154

San Juan Capistrano

3189'
▲ Margarita Peak

Dana Point

⑤ (5)

San/Clemente

Santa Ana Mountains: San Mateo Canyon Wilderness, page 218

De Luz Road

Fallbrook

C A M P   P E N D L E T O N

(U S M C)

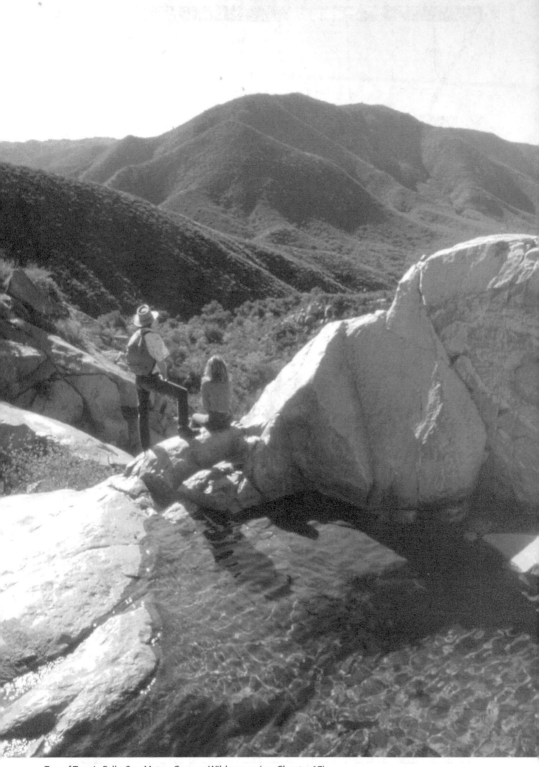

Top of Tenaja Falls, San Mateo Canyon Wilderness *(see Chapter 17)*

Contents

Preface

Hidden within or just beyond Orange County's urban sprawl lies more opportunity for the appreciation of the natural world than most county residents imagine. Barely a few hundred yards from busy highways and shimmering glass high-rises, shorebirds haunt protected estuaries and marshes. Along the southern coast, ocean swells roll in and spend themselves against lonely sands and jagged cliffs. Over the foothill country, hawks and eagles cruise in search of a furry meal. And deep within the corrugated fastness of the Santa Ana Mountains, mountain lions, deer, and coyotes roam cool, dark canyon bottoms and sun-warmed, chaparral-covered slopes.

Surrounding Orange County's densely populated coastal plain are parks, preserves, designated open spaces, and public lands totaling approximately 200,000 acres. Within this domain, intriguing pathways introduce explorers to natural landscapes ranging from the intertidal zone to oak and coniferous woodlands. Orange County boasts, either within or abutting its rather compact borders, 8 state parks and beaches, 19 regional (county) parks and wilderness areas, more than 130,000 acres of national forest, and more than 500 miles of trails and roads for hiking.

Our goal in writing this guide was to bring into sharp focus virtually every walk worth taking on still-wild public lands conveniently accessible to the average Orange Countian. The hikes range in difficulty from short strolls through selected urban parks and preserves to canyon treks in the Santa Ana Mountains that challenge any adventurer.

Because of Orange County's rather small area (782 square miles) but larger sphere of influence, a number of hikes in this book lie either partly or wholly outside the county boundaries. These are found in the following areas: Chino Hills State Park, extending into San Bernardino and Riverside Counties; Santa Rosa Plateau Ecological Reserve, in southwestern Riverside County; San Onofre State Beach, in northern San Diego County; and the entire Trabuco Ranger District of Cleveland National Forest, spilling into Riverside and San Diego Counties. (Two other units of the Cleveland Forest, the Palomar and Descanso Districts, extend farther east and south across Riverside and San Diego Counties. Those units, along with other public lands in San Diego County, are covered in *Afoot & Afield San Diego County*. For those interested in hikes in other parts of Southern California, the *Afoot & Afield* series also encompasses Los Angeles County and the Inland Empire.)

I (David) recently hiked every trip in this book. The fourth-edition fieldwork involved more than 850 miles of hiking and 10,000 miles of driving, spread across more than 100 days. For this edition, I eliminated three hikes: Laurel Spring is less interesting after the Santiago Fire, the access gate for Cold Spring Canyon is closed, and the Oak Trail Loop is less compelling than the partially overlapping Bell Canyon hike. In return, I added 40 hikes, most notably trips in Irvine Ranch, Aliso Canyon, the Santa Ana Mountains, and Chino Hills, as well as three regional trails from the foothills to the ocean.

Roads and trails can and do change. Publicly accessible open-space acreage is increasing, and new trails are being constructed and opened for public use. In the national forest, the greater demand for recreational use is leading to new regulations and new use patterns. I will continue to insert fresh updates in future printings of this edition, and a fifth edition will undoubtedly appear in the future. You can keep me apprised of recent developments and/or changes by writing to me in care of Wilderness Press at **info@wildernesspress .com.** I will appreciate your comments.

OVERVIEW OF HIKES

NUMBER	HIKE	DISTANCE (miles)	ELEVATION GAIN (feet)	TRAIL TYPE	BACKPACKING	MOUNTAIN BIKING	EQUESTRIANS	DOGS	KIDS
CHAPTER 1: NORTH COAST									
1.1	Bolsa Chica Ecological Reserve	1.6-plus	0	↺					🚶
1.2	Talbert Nature Preserve	2-plus	50	↺		⊛		🐕	🚶
CHAPTER 2: UPPER NEWPORT BAY									
2.1	Upper Newport Bay Nature Preserve	2.7	200	↺		⊛		🐕	🚶
2.2	Newport Back Bay Loop	10	300	↺		⊛		🐕	
2.3	San Joaquin Wildlife Sanctuary	2–4	0	↺					🚶
2.4	Buck Gully	5	600	↺		⊛			
CHAPTER 3: CRYSTAL COVE STATE PARK									
3.1	Corona Rock-Hop	2.4	100	↗					🚶
3.2	Crystal Cove Beaches	2–5.5	100	↺					🚶
3.3	Emerald Vista Point	4.6	800	↺	🎒	⊛	🏇		🚶
3.4	El Moro Canyon Loop	8	1,400	↺		⊛	🏇		
3.5	Deer Canyon Loop	3.6	600	↺	🎒	⊛	🏇		
CHAPTER 4: LAGUNA COAST WILDERNESS PARK									
4.1	Nix Loop	4.4	800	↺					
4.2	Laurel Canyon Loop	3.5	700	↺					🚶
4.3	Emerald Canyon	8	1,400	↗		⊛	🏇		
4.4	Big Bend Loop	3.9	1,100	↺					
4.5	Laguna Bowl Loop	4.1	950	↺		⊛	🏇		
4.6	Dilley Preserve	2.9	350	↺					🚶
CHAPTER 5: ALISO AND WOOD CANYONS WILDERNESS PARK									
5.1	Seaview Park Overlook and Aliso Summit	0.6–1.6	50–500	↗				🐕	🚶
5.2	Seaview and Badlands Trail	2.0	150	↗		⊛	🏇	🐕	🚶
5.3	Aliso Summit Trail	4.4	350	↗		⊛	🏇	🐕	🚶
5.4	Top of the World Loop	6	1,000	↺		⊛	🏇		
5.5	Aliso and Wood Canyons Loop	10	1,000	↺		⊛	🏇		
5.6	Pecten Reef via Aliso Creek	7	150	↺		⊛	🏇	🐕	
5.7	Sulphur Creek Reservoir	1.7	100	↺		⊛	🏇	🐕	🚶

OVERVIEW OF HIKES

NUMBER	HIKE	DISTANCE (miles)	ELEVATION GAIN (feet)	TRAIL TYPE	BACKPACKING	MOUNTAIN BIKING	EQUESTRIANS	DOGS	KIDS
CHAPTER 6: SOUTH COAST									
6.1	Salt Creek Trail	7	500	↗		●		🐕	👫
6.2	San Juan Creek Trail	5	150 loss	↗		●	🏇	🐕	
6.3	Dana Point Headlands	1.4	0	↗					👫
6.4	San Clemente State Beach	3.1	150	⟳					👫
6.5	San Onofre State Beach	1–6	150	⟳					👫
CHAPTER 7: CHINO HILLS STATE PARK									
7.1	Bane Rim Loop	7	1,300	⟳		●	🏇		
7.2	McLean Overlook	1.8	350	↗		●	🏇		👫
7.3	Water Canyon	3.6	300	↗					👫
7.4	Lower Aliso Canyon Loop	10	1,500	⟳		●	🏇		
7.5	Upper Aliso Canyon	3.8	700	⟳		●	🏇		👫
7.6	Hills for Everyone Trail	4.6	700	⟳					👫
7.7	Telegraph Canyon Traverse	8	650	↗		●	🏇		
7.8	Gilman Peak	8	1,400	↗		●	🏇		
7.9	San Juan Hill	7	1,600	↗		●	🏇		
7.10	Sonome Canyon	3.9	1,100	⟳		●	🏇		
7.11	Carbon Canyon Nature Trail	2.6	50	⟳		●	🏇	🐕	👫
7.12	Coal Canyon	6	600	↗					
CHAPTER 8: SANTIAGO CREEK AND ANAHEIM HILLS									
8.1	Oak Canyon Nature Center	1.5-plus	200	↗					👫
8.2	Deer Canyon Park Preserve	2.8	500	⟳		●	🏇	🐕	👫
8.3	Santiago Oaks Regional Park	0.8-plus	100	⟳		●	🏇	🐕	👫
8.4	Robbers Peak	5	1,000	⟳		●	🏇	🐕	
8.5	Weir Canyon Loop	4	700	⟳		●	🏇	🐕	👫
8.6	Irvine Regional Park	3	200	⟳		●	🏇	🐕	👫
8.7	Irvine to Santiago Loop	4.5	600	⟳		●	🏇	🐕	
8.8	El Modena Open Space	2.4	700	⟳		●	🏇	🐕	👫
8.9	Peters Canyon Regional Park	2.2-plus	200	⟳		●	🏇	🐕	👫

OVERVIEW OF HIKES

NUMBER	HIKE	DISTANCE (miles)	ELEVATION GAIN (feet)	TRAIL TYPE	BACKPACKING	MOUNTAIN BIKING	EQUESTRIANS	DOGS	KIDS
CHAPTER 9: WHITING RANCH WILDERNESS PARK									
9.1	Borrego and Red Rock Canyons	4.4	500	↗					🚶
9.2	Vista Lookout	4.8	800	↗		⊛	🏇		
9.3	Whiting Ranch Loop	6	650	↻		⊛	🏇		
9.4	Dreaded Hill	5	1,000	↻		⊛	🏇		
CHAPTER 10: IRVINE RANCH OPEN SPACE									
10.1	Limestone Canyon: The Sinks	8	500	↗		⊛	🏇		
10.2	Hicks Haul Road	3.5	400	↗		⊛			
10.3	Agua Chinon	5	800	↗		⊛	🏇		
10.4	Round Canyon	2.4	300	↗					🚶
10.5	Black Star Canyon	3–4	500	↻		⊛	🏇		🚶
10.6	Red Rock Trail	2.6	0	↗					🚶
10.7	Fremont Canyon	varies				⊛	🏇		
10.8	Weir Canyon	varies				⊛	🏇		
CHAPTER 11: IRVINE OPEN SPACE PRESERVE									
11.1	Bommer Canyon and Ridge Loop	3.2	700	↻		⊛			🚶
11.2	Big Bommer Loop	14	1,600	↻		⊛	🏇		
11.3	Quail Hill Loop	1.7	150	↻		⊛	🏇	🐕	🚶
11.4	Turtle Ridge Loop	5.5	900	↻		⊛	🏇		
CHAPTER 12: O'NEILL AND RILEY REGIONAL PARKS									
12.1	Ocean Vista Point	3.5	700	↻		⊛	🏇		🚶
12.2	Edna Spaulding Nature Trail	1	250	↻					🚶
12.3	Arroyo Trabuco	6	170	↗		⊛	🏇		
12.4	Tijeras Creek	6	300	↗		⊛	🏇		
12.5	Riley Wilderness Park	2.8	500	↻		⊛	🏇		🚶
CHAPTER 13: CASPERS WILDERNESS PARK									
13.1	Pinhead Peak	1.5	400	↗			🏇		🚶
13.2	West Ridge to Bell Canyon Loop	3.3	400	↻			🏇		🚶
13.3	East Ridge to Bell Canyon Loop	6	900	↻		⊛	🏇		

OVERVIEW OF HIKES

NUMBER	HIKE	DISTANCE (miles)	ELEVATION GAIN (feet)	TRAIL TYPE	BACKPACKING	MOUNTAIN BIKING	EQUESTRIANS	DOGS	KIDS
13.4	Oso to Juaneno Loop	9	1,400	Loop			🐴		
13.5	Hot Springs Loop	13	1,500	Loop			🐴		
13.6	Bell View Trail	8	1,000	↗		●	🐴		
CHAPTER 14: SANTA ROSA PLATEAU ECOLOGICAL RESERVE									
14.1	Granite Loop	1.6	100	Loop					👪
14.2	Punta Mesa Loop	8	650	Loop					
14.3	Wiashal Trail	6.6	1,700	↗					
14.4	Sylvan Meadows	6	500	Loop		●	🐴	🐕	
14.5	Oak Tree Loop	2.1	100	Loop					👪
14.6	Los Santos to Trans Preserve Loop	4.8	500	Loop					
14.7	Vernal Pool Trail	1.2	50	↗					👪
CHAPTER 15: SANTA ANA MOUNTAINS: MAIN DIVIDE									
15.1	Tecate Cypress Preserve	9.5	1,900	↗		●	🐴	🐕	
15.2	Tin Mine Canyon	5	700	↗		●	🐴	🐕	👪
15.3	Sierra Peak via Skyline Drive	14.5	3,200	↗		●	🐴	🐕	
15.4	North Main Divide Traverse	13.5	1,950	↗		●	🐴	🐕	
15.5	Black Star Canyon Falls	7	800	↗					
15.6	Silverado Trail to Bedford Peak	7	2,000	↗		●	🐴	🐕	
15.7	Silverado to Modjeska Peak Loop	19	4,400	Loop		●	🐴	🐕	
15.8	Harding Road to Main Divide	18.5	3,650	↗		●	🐴	🐕	
15.9	Harding Canyon	5	900	↗				🐕	
15.10	Santiago Trail	16	2,650	↗		●	🐴	🐕	
15.11	Falls Canyon	0.8	200	↗					👪
15.12	Holy Jim Falls	2.8	650	↗		●	🐴	🐕	👪
15.13	Santiago Peak via Holy Jim Trail	16	4,000	↗		●	🐴	🐕	
15.14	Indian Truck Trail	14	2,600	↗		●	🐴	🐕	
15.15	Trabuco Canyon	3.6	850	↗		●	🐴	🐕	👪
15.16	West Horsethief to Trabuco Canyon Loop	10	2,700	Loop		●	🐴	🐕	
15.17	Bell Peak	4	1,300	↗		●		🐕	
15.18	East Horsethief Trail	9	2,600	↗		●		🐕	

OVERVIEW OF HIKES

NUMBER	HIKE	DISTANCE (miles)	ELEVATION GAIN (feet)	TRAIL TYPE	BACKPACKING	MOUNTAIN BIKING	EQUESTRIANS	DOGS	KIDS
CHAPTER 16: SANTA ANA MOUNTAINS: ORTEGA CORRIDOR									
16.1	El Cariso Nature Trail	1.5	200	Loop				🐕	👪
16.2	Ortega Falls	0.5	200	Loop				🐕	👪
16.3	San Juan Loop Trail	2.1	350	Loop		🚲	🏇	🐕	👪
16.4	San Juan Trail	11.5	550	Out & back		🚲	🏇	🐕	
16.5	Chiquito Basin	3	700	Out & back		🚲	🏇	🐕	👪
16.6	Viejo Tie Loop	7	1,000	Loop		🚲	🏇	🐕	
16.7	Chiquito Trail	9	900	Out & back		🚲	🏇	🐕	
16.8	Los Pinos Ridge	10	2,500	Out & back		🚲		🐕	
16.9	Upper Hot Spring Canyon	3	450	Out & back					
16.1	Lower Hot Spring Canyon	10	1,600	Out & back					
16.11	Morgan Trail	5	300	Out & back	🎒		🏇	🐕	👪
16.12	Sitton Peak	9.5	2,150	Out & back	🎒			🐕	
16.13	Lucas Canyon	19.5	3,400	Out & back	🎒		🏇	🐕	
CHAPTER 17: SANTA ANA MOUNTAINS: SAN MATEO CANYON WILDERNESS									
17.1	Tenaja Falls	1.4	300	Out & back	🎒		🏇	🐕	👪
17.2	Tenaja Falls Traverse	8	600	Out & back	🎒		🏇	🐕	
17.3	Tenaja Canyon	7	1,300	Out & back	🎒		🏇	🐕	👪
17.4	Fishermans Camp Loop	5	550	Loop	🎒		🏇	🐕	👪
17.5	San Mateo Canyon	8	1,100	Out & back	🎒		🏇	🐕	
17.6	Bluewater Traverse	13	2,400	Out & back	🎒			🐕	
CHAPTER 18: LONG-DISTANCE TRAILS									
18.1	Santa Ana River Trail	up to 29		Point to point		🚲	🏇	🐕	
18.2	Mountains to Sea Trail	up to 18		Point to point		🚲	🏇	🐕	
18.3	Aliso Creek Trail	up to 13		Point to point		🚲	🏇	🐕	

Introducing Orange County

From the look-alike cities in the north to the newer, planned communities of the south, Orange County seems little distinguished from its colossal neighbor and economic parent, Los Angeles. But a deeper identity, rooted in geography, transcends the urban sprawl. Orange Countians are reminded of their uniqueness not so much by the human architecture of city and suburb, but rather by the blue Pacific, the green and tawny coastal hills, and the purple wall of the Santa Ana Mountains.

Out on the coastline and up along the foothills and mountains, you may discover for yourself Orange County's place in the natural world. An hour or less of driving and less than two hours' walk will take you from the frenetic city to any of several interesting natural environments, ranging from tidepools to fern-bedecked canyon streams to mountain peaks affording views stretching a hundred miles. You'll discover fascinating rock formations, rich and varied plant life, a healthy population of native animals, and a sense of peace and tranquility.

In the next few pages, you'll learn briefly about the "other" Orange County: its climate, geology, flora, and fauna. Following that, you'll find some notes about safety and courtesy on the trail and some tips on how to get the most out of this book. After perusing that material, you can dig into the heart of this book—descriptions of 124 hiking routes from the coast to the Santa Ana Mountains. Happy reading and happy hiking!

Land of Gentle Climate

A succinct summary of Orange County's climate might take the form of just two phrases: "warm and sunny" and "winter-wet, summer-dry." But some variation in climate exists across the county's width from coast to mountain crests. Without resorting to technical classification schemes, let's divide the county into two climate zones: The coastal zone, extending inland 10–15 miles across the coastal plain and low coastal foothills, is largely under the moderating influence of the Pacific Ocean. This climate is characterized by mild temperatures that are relatively stable, both daily and seasonally. Average temperatures range from the 60s to 40s (daily highs and lows in Fahrenheit) in winter to the 70s to 60s in summer. Rainfall averages about 15 inches annually. Overall this climate closely matches the classic Mediterranean climate associated with coastal areas along the Mediterranean Sea.

The inland zone, consisting of the Santa Ana Mountains and foothills, experiences somewhat more extreme daily and seasonal temperatures because it is less influenced by onshore flows of marine air. The higher summits of the Santa Ana Mountains, for example, have average temperatures in the 50s to 20s in winter, and the 80s to 50s in summer. Precipitation averages about 30 inches annually in the higher Santa Anas, which is just enough to support natural pockets of coniferous and broadleaf trees, such as pines, oaks, and maples. Almost every year, some fraction of the precipitation arrives in the form of snow, which briefly blankets the mountain slopes down to an elevation of about 3,000 feet.

Despite its reputation for a gentle climate, Orange County is occasionally subject to hot, dry winds called "Santa Ana winds" (after Santa Ana Canyon, just north of the Santa Ana Mountains). These winds occur when an air mass moves southwest from a high-pressure area over the interior United States out toward Southern California. As the air flows downward toward the coast, it compresses and becomes warm and dry. Low passes in the mountains or river valleys that act as wind gaps (such as Santa Ana Canyon) funnel these desertlike winds toward the coast. During stronger Santa Anas, common in late summer and fall, Orange County basks under warm, blue skies swept clear of every trace of pollution (except possibly smoke from wildfires). Temperatures along the coast can then reach record-high levels; the city of Orange, for example, once recorded a temperature of 119 degrees during a Santa Ana.

Rainfall in Orange County is as erratic as it is slight. On the coastal plain, the annual precipitation has ranged from merely 4 inches to a record of 32 inches. Up to 5 inches have fallen on the coastal plain in a single day, and in the Santa Ana Mountains, one storm dumped 9 inches in a single night.

By and large, Orange County's balmy, dry climate is remarkably well suited to year-round outdoor activity. Nevertheless, high temperatures, scarcity of water, and occasionally smoggy air during summer and early fall make that particular period less desirable for hiking in the inland foothills and mountains. During the other seven or eight months of the year, the weather is often ideal.

Reading the Rocks

Of California's many geomorphic (natural) provinces, Orange County claims parts of only two: the Los Angeles Basin and the Peninsular Ranges. The bulk of the county's urbanized area lies in the Los Angeles Basin, while the mostly undeveloped Santa Ana Mountains and the semideveloped San Joaquin Hills belong to the Peninsular Ranges province.

The Los Angeles Basin province extends from the base of the San Gabriel and Santa Monica Mountains (part of the Transverse Ranges province) to the north to the base of the Santa Ana Mountains and the San Joaquin Hills on the south. In a geologic context, it can be pictured as a huge, deeply folded basin filled to a depth of up to 7 miles by some volcanic material and land-laid sediments, but mostly by sediments of marine origin—sand and mud deposited on the ocean bottom from 80 million years ago to as recently as 1 million years ago.

The Los Angeles Basin area has experienced uplift during the past 1–2 million years, and as this took place, the surface of the basin accumulated a layer of terrestrial sediment shed from the surrounding hills and mountains. The basin, in fact, would

Cloud-walking, Laguna Bowl Road *(see Chapter 4)*

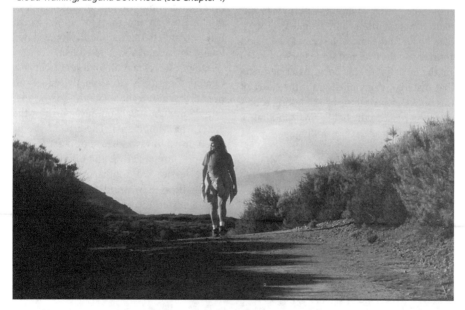

still be filling up with sediment were it not for the flood-control dams and channeled riverbeds that have largely replaced the original meandering Santa Ana, San Gabriel, and Los Angeles Rivers.

Hikers following this guidebook will discover many interesting and sometimes colorful exposures of marine sedimentary rocks in places like the Chino Hills, San Joaquin Hills, and foothills of the Santa Ana Mountains. These sediments, uplifted by a variety of geologic processes, are continuations of the formations that lie deep underground in the center of the Los Angeles Basin.

The marine sediments you will see— sandstone, siltstone, shale, and conglomerate—tend to be rather soft and easily eroded. Along the south coast, where the San Joaquin Hills meet the sea, several wave-cut "marine terraces" are identifiable on the coastal headlands. They exhibit a record of changing sea levels and gradual uplift over the past 1–2 million years. In many places, the terraces themselves are deeply cut by drainage channels—the coastal canyons— which themselves are quite recent features.

The Santa Ana Mountains, along with the San Jacinto Mountains, lie at the northwest tip of the extensive Peninsular Ranges province, stretching south toward the tip of Baja California (the province, in fact, derives its name from Baja's peninsular shape). Each range in this province possesses a core of granitic (granitelike) rock, overlain in many places by a veneer of older metamorphic rocks. Many of the Peninsular Ranges, including the Santa Anas, are raised and tilted fault blocks, typically with steep east escarpments and more gradually inclined western slopes.

As you travel through the Santa Ana Mountains (and their distinctly named subdivisions, the Elsinore and the Santa Margarita Mountains), you'll begin to piece together their geologic history. Starting at, say, Caspers Wilderness Park in the foothills and moving up toward the crest of the Santa Anas, you first pass among light-colored marine sedimentary rock formations that were pushed up and tilted by the rise of the mountains to the east. Next comes metamorphic rock of two basic kinds— metasedimentary and metavolcanic. These brown- or gray-colored rocks, roughly 200– 150 million years old, are metamorphosed (changed by heat and pressure) forms of marine sedimentary and volcanic rock that were plastered against the core of the North American continent some tens of millions of years ago. These rocks were riding on one or more of the Earth's tectonic plates, which collided with and were subducted (forced under) the western edge of the continent.

Near the crest of the Santa Ana Mountains, you find light-colored granitic rocks. Here's the reason: About 100 million years ago, when the subduction process was in full swing, much of the material on the edge of the plate being subducted melted underground and accumulated in the form of vast pools of magma. Because this magma was less dense than the surrounding materials, it rose toward the surface. Some escaped through volcanoes, but most of it remained underground long enough to slowly cool and crystallize, forming coarse-grained "plutonic" (generally granitic) rocks. Erosion then nibbled away at the overlying metamorphic rocks, finally exposing—typically in high places—the granitic rocks.

In the southern Santa Anas and throughout most of California's share of the Peninsular Ranges, this granitic rock is now well exposed. In the northern Santa Anas, however, its distribution is less extensive. The highest peaks in the range, Santiago and Modjeska Peaks (together called Old Saddleback), are still covered by older, overlying metamorphic rocks.

The granitic rocks are still rising, more than offsetting the leveling effects of erosion. Thus, although the rocks of the Santa Ana Mountains range between old and ancient, the origin of the range itself as a structural unit is quite recent.

Of more than casual interest to Orange Countians is the fact that for at least the past 10 million years, the Peninsular Ranges province (along with the present Los Angeles Basin and a wedge of coastal central California) has been drifting northwest relative to the rest of the North American continent. In a global view, this motion is seen as a lateral sliding (or rather a repeated lurching) at the interface between the largely oceanic Pacific Plate and the largely continental North American Plate. The average rate of movement in the early 21st century is about 2 inches per year—enough, if it continues, to put Orange County abreast of San Francisco 12 million years from now.

The famous San Andreas Fault (which runs about 40 miles northeast of Orange County) is the principal division between the two plates. But earth movement can also take place along splinter faults south and west of the San Andreas. One such splinter fault, the Elsinore Fault, passes along the eastern base of the Santa Ana Mountains. Horizontal and vertical movements along this fault over the past 5 million years have shifted the Santa Ana Mountains northwest relative to the adjacent landforms to the east, and have raised and tilted the whole mountain block into its characteristic west-sloping orientation. Sudden earth movements along any of these faults have been and will again be responsible for most of Southern California's devastating earthquakes.

The geologic history of Orange County is a fascinating one, and the diversity of landforms and rocks in Orange County and the Santa Ana Mountains is enough to pique the curiosity of most any amateur geologist. Refer to Appendix 2 for sources of additional information.

Native Gardens

About 800 different kinds of wild flowering plants are found within Orange County's 782 square miles, a remarkably large number considering its diminutive size among California counties.

There are two reasons for this abundance of plant species. One reason has to do with physical factors: topography, geology, soils, and climate. Countywide, the diversity of physical factors and the complex interrelationships among these factors have led to the existence of many kinds of biological habitats.

The second reason is Orange County's location between two groups of flora: a southern, drought-tolerant group, most clearly represented by various forms of cacti; and a northern group, represented by moisture-loving plants typical of California's northern and central Coast Ranges. As the climate changed, varying from cool and wet to warm and dry over the past million years or so, species from one group and then the other invaded the county. Once established, many of these species persisted in protected niches even as the climate turned unfavorable for them. Some survived unchanged; others evolved into unique forms. Some are present only in very specific habitats.

The bulk of Orange County's undeveloped land can be grouped into three general classes, which botanists often call plant communities or plant associations. In a broader sense, they are biological communities because they include animals as well as plants. These plant communities are briefly described below.

The sage scrub (or coastal sage scrub) community lies mostly below 2,000 feet in elevation and extends east from the coastline to the foothills and lower spurs of the Santa Ana Mountains. The dominant species are small shrubs, typically California sagebrush, black sage, white sage, and wild buckwheat. Two larger shrubs often found here are laurel sumac and lemonade berry, which like poison oak are members of the sumac family. Interspersed among the somewhat loosely distributed shrubs is a variety of grasses and wildflowers, green and colorful during the rainy season but dry and withered during the summer and early-fall drought.

The chaparral community is commonly found above 2,000 feet in the Santa Ana Mountains, where it cloaks the slopes like a thick-pile carpet. The dominant plants are chamise, scrub oak, manzanita, mountain mahogany, toyon, and various forms of ceanothus ("wild lilac"). These are tough, intricately branched shrubs with deep root systems that ensure their survival during the long, hot summers. Chaparral is sometimes referred to as an "elfin forest," a literal description of a mature stand. Without the benefit of a trail, travel through mature chaparral, which is typically 10–15 feet high, is almost impossible. Sage scrub and chaparral vegetation tend to intermix readily throughout the Santa Anas, the chaparral preferring shadier, north-facing slopes, and the sage scrub preferring hot, dry, south-facing slopes.

The southern oak woodland community is found in scattered locations throughout the county, from the bigger coastal canyons in the San Joaquin Hills to moist flats and canyons throughout the Santa Ana Mountains. Within the Orange County area, the indicator tree is the live oak, but sycamores may also be abundant. In the Chino Hills, native walnut trees form a major component of the southern oak woodland community. Beneath the trees, various chaparral and sage scrub plants often form a sparse understory.

Aside from these three widespread natural communities, much of the nonurbanized land in and around Orange County is given over to agriculture and grazing. Areas characterized by heavy grazing have grassy flats and bald slopes called *potreros* (pastures) supporting mostly nonnative grasses and herbs, such as wild oats, filaree, mustard, and fennel.

To a small extent, several other natural communities are found in Orange County: rocky shore, coastal strand, coastal salt marsh, freshwater marsh, riparian woodland, and coniferous forest.

The riparian (streamside) woodland community, existing in discontinuous strips along some of the bigger watercourses, is perhaps the most biologically valuable. Not only is this kind of environment essential for the continued survival of many kinds of birds and animals, it is also very appealing to the senses. Massive sycamores, cottonwoods, and live oaks and a screen of water-hugging willows are the hallmarks of the riparian woodland. Most of this habitat has already been usurped by urbanization and the development of water resources.

The coniferous (cone-bearing-tree) forest community was once more widespread in the Santa Ana Mountains. The west-side canyons were logged a century ago in connection with various short-lived mining booms; this logging and subsequent wildfires have reduced the forest to small, isolated patches that cling to the slopes of the deeper canyons. Bigcone Douglas-fir and Coulter pine are the indicator species of coniferous forest in the Santa Anas, although live oaks and other broadleaf trees are also frequently present.

A few species of plants of limited geographic extent in the county are worth noting:

Knobcone pine, somewhat widely distributed in the northern and central California Coast Ranges and the foothills of the Sierra Nevada, clings to a small toehold in the Santa Ana Mountains on the slopes of Pleasants Peak. Here, it finds the warm, dry climate and the particular kind of soil—serpentine—it thrives on.

Bigleaf maple, California bay (bay laurel), and madrone, found in the west-side canyons of the Santa Ana Mountains, are three more examples of trees at or close to the southern end of their natural range. The madrones are restricted to a tiny area in upper Trabuco Canyon.

The Tecate cypress, once widespread throughout Southern California, is now confined to small arboreal islands in San Diego County, in northern Baja California, and along the slopes of Coal and Gypsum Canyons in the northern Santa Anas (just outside the Cleveland National Forest boundary). Here, it finds the extra moisture, in the form of nocturnal fogs moving in from the coast, that it needs in order to hold onto its biological niche.

Late winter to mid-spring is the best time to appreciate the cornucopia of Orange County's native plants. Many of the showiest species—the annual wildflowers—burgeon at this time, and other plants exhibit fresh, new growth. For more information about the wildflowers, shrubs, trees, and other flora typically found in Orange County, see Appendix 2.

Creatures Great and Small

Your first sighting of an eagle, mountain lion, badger, or any other seldom-seen form of wildlife is always a memorable experience. Because of the diversity of the still-natural parts of Orange County, they are host to a healthy population of indigenous creatures, including a few rare and endangered species. If you're willing to stretch your legs a bit and spend some time in the areas favored by wild animals, you'll eventually be rewarded by some kind of close visual contact.

While doing fieldwork for an earlier edition of this book, Jerry Schad was lucky to spot a young mountain lion while hiking in the Santa Ana Mountains, and a golden eagle while driving on Interstate 5 through the hills of south county.

The most numerous large creature in Orange County is the mule deer, with a population of perhaps several hundred. These deer prefer areas of forest and chaparral, especially at higher elevations in the Santa Anas.

The mountain lion, once hunted to near-extinction in California, has made a comeback as a protected species. Perhaps two dozen lions now roam the remote canyons of the Santa Ana Mountains and foothill areas.

Counting them is difficult, since mountain lions have a large territorial range (up to 100 square miles) and are normally very secretive. Because of their wide-ranging travels, however, tracks and other signs of them are quite frequently seen.

The county's mammals also include the coyote, which has adapted to a broad range of habitats, including the margins of suburbia; the bobcat, a creature sometimes mistaken for a mountain lion, but smaller and more common and with a short bobtail rather than the lion's 3-foot tail; the gray fox; skunk; opossum; raccoon; ringtail cat; badger; and various rabbits, squirrels, bats, woodrats, and mice.

Among the more commonly seen reptiles are rattlesnakes, discussed later under "Special Hazards."

The richness of birdlife in the Orange County area is impressive, not only because of the diversity of its habitats, but also because the county lies along the Pacific Flyway route of spring–fall bird migration and serves as a wintering area for waterfowl. Several species of rare or endangered birds nest or visit, including the southern bald eagle, peregrine falcon, lightfooted clapper rail, least tern, Belding's savannah sparrow, and least Bell's vireo.

Fire Ecology

Chaparral and sage scrub have evolved to burn periodically. Many species have highly flammable resinous leaves, and many have underground root burls that survive moderately intense fire and resprout shortly afterward. Some species depend on occasional fires to reproduce, and many "fire follower" wildflowers grow only after a wildfire. Before humans impacted the area, lightning-induced fires typically burned any given acre every 30–150 years.

The arrival of humans has greatly impacted these plant communities. People and cattle have brought a number of invasive species, especially mustard and nonnative grasses. These plants grow vigorously in the spring, then die and dry up

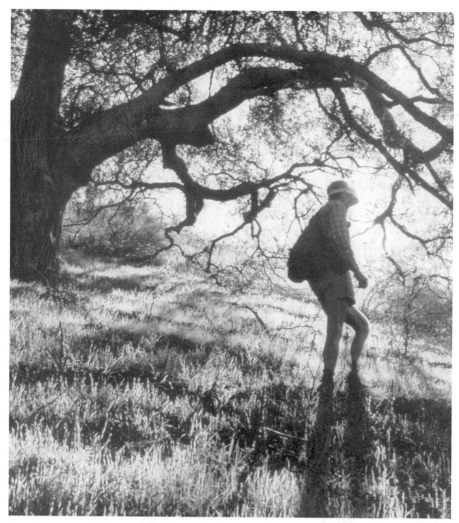

Deep inside Water Canyon, Chino Hills State Park *(see Chapter 7)*

in the summer, adding vast amounts of tinder for fires. People have also increased the frequency of ignition; downed power lines, vehicle accidents, careless smokers and campers, kids with matches, and malicious arsonists have all caused major fires in Southern California.

As a result, wildfires have become much more frequent in Southern California. In 1993, Orange County became keenly aware of its fire risk as the Ortega Fire incinerated 21,010 acres around Highway 74 and the Laguna Beach Fire swept through Laguna Canyon, burning 14,337 acres and 336 homes. From 2006 to 2008, the Sierra Fire and Santiago Fire burned major portions of the Santa Ana Mountains and western foothills, and then the Freeway Complex Fire swept across almost all of Chino Hills State Park. Fires have become so frequent in some areas that plants may not be able to reestablish themselves before the next wave arrives, threatening to cause permanent ecological changes in which the native sage scrub is replaced by even more flammable invasive weeds.

Health, Safety, and Courtesy

Good preparation is always important for any kind of recreational pursuit. Hiking Southern California's backcountry is no exception. Although most of our local environments are seldom hostile or dangerous to life and limb, hikers should be aware of some pitfalls.

Preparation and Equipment

An obvious safety requirement is being in good health. Some degree of physical conditioning is always desirable, even for those trips designated as easy or moderate. The more challenging trips (rated "moderately strenuous" or "strenuous" in difficulty) require stamina and occasionally some technical expertise. Fast walking, running, bicycling, swimming, aerobic dancing, and any similar exercise that develops both your leg muscles and the whole body's aerobic capacity are recommended as preparatory exercise.

For long trips over rough trails or cross-country terrain (there are several in this guide), the most adequate way to prepare is by practicing the activity itself. Start with easy or moderately long trips first to accustom your leg muscles to the peculiar stresses involved in walking over uneven terrain and scrambling over boulders, and to acquire a solid sense of balance. As I note later, hiking boots rather than lightweight shoes are preferred for such travel, primarily from a safety standpoint.

Because all hiking in the Orange County area is below 6,000 feet in elevation, health complications due to high altitude are rare. You may, however, notice that you lose some energy and breathe more rapidly in the higher parts of the Santa Ana Mountains.

An important aspect of preparation is choosing your equipment and supplies. The essentials you should carry with you at all times into the backcountry are the items that would allow you to survive, in a reasonably comfortable manner, one or two unscheduled nights out on the trail. It's important to note that no one ever plans to experience these nights! No one plans to get lost, injured, stuck, or pinned down by the weather. Always do a "what if" analysis for a worst-case scenario, and plan accordingly. These essential items are your safety net; keep them with you on all your hikes.

Chief among the essential items is warm clothing. Away from the coast, winter temperatures can plummet from warm at midday to subfreezing at night. Layer your clothing; it is better to take along two or more midweight outer garments than rely on a single heavy or bulky jacket. Add to this a cap, gloves, and a waterproof or water-resistant shell (a large trash bag with a hole for your head will do in a pinch), and you'll be quite prepared for all but the most severe weather experienced in the areas described in this book.

In hot, sunny weather, sun-shielding clothing is another "essential." It normally includes a sun hat and a light-colored, long-sleeved top.

Water and, to a lesser extent, food are next in importance. Because potable water isn't generally available, carry a generous supply. On a hot summer's day in the Santa Anas, you might need to drink up to a gallon of water on a 10-mile hike. You need to eat food to stave off hunger and keep your energy stores up, but it is less essential than water in a survival situation.

Down the list farther, but still "essential," are a map and compass (or a GPS unit and the know-how to use it); flashlight; fire-starting devices (examples: waterproof matches or lighter) and candle; and first-aid kit.

Items that are not always essential, but potentially very useful and convenient, include sunglasses, a pocketknife, whistle (or other signaling device), sunscreen, and toilet paper.

Every member of a hiking party should carry the essential items mentioned above because individuals or splinter groups may end up separating from the party for one reason or another. If you plan to hike solo in the backcountry, being well equipped is all-important. Be sure to check in with a park ranger, or leave your itinerary with some other responsible person. That way, if you do get stuck, help will probably come to the right place—eventually.

Special Hazards

Other than getting lost or pinned down by a rare sudden storm, you may face these three most common hazards in the foothill and mountain areas: poison oak, ticks, and rattlesnakes.

Poison oak, in bush or vine form, is common along many hillsides and canyons below 5,000 feet. It often grows thickly on the banks of streamcourses, where it seems to prefer the semishade of live and scrub oaks. Learn to recognize its distinctive three-leafed structure, and avoid touching it with your skin or clothing. Poison oak is deciduous, losing its leaves usually in summer or fall, but the bare stems harbor some of the urushiol that causes an allergic reaction in some people. If you cannot avoid contact with the poison oak plant, thick pants (such as jeans) and a long-sleeved shirt will serve as fair barriers for protecting your skin. Remove these clothes as soon as you're finished hiking, and make sure you wash them carefully afterward. Take a shower as soon as possible. And be aware that dogs can pick up the urushiol on their fur, so wash your pup when you get home if he brushed up against the plant.

Ticks can sometimes be the scourge of overgrown trails in the Santa Ana Mountains, particularly in mid-spring when they climb to the tips of shrub branches and lie in wait for warm-blooded hosts. Ticks are especially abundant along trails used by cattle, deer, and coyotes. If you can't avoid brushing up against vegetation along the trail, be sure to check for ticks frequently. Upon finding a host, a tick will usually

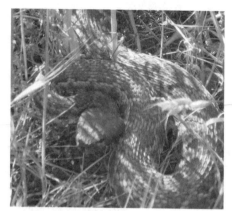

Southern Pacific rattlesnake

crawl upward some distance in search of a protected spot, where it will try to attach itself. If you're sensitive to the slightest irritation on your skin, you'll be able to intercept a tick long before it attempts to bite.

Rattlesnakes are fairly common in brushy, rocky, and streamside habitats from coast to mountains. Seldom seen in either cold or very hot weather, they favor temperatures in the 75–90°F range. Expect to see (or hear) rattlesnakes out and about in the daytime from early spring to mid-fall and at night in summer and early fall. Most rattlesnakes are every bit as interested in avoiding contact with you as you are with them. Watch carefully where you put your feet, and especially your hands, during rattlesnake season. In brushy or rocky areas where your sight is limited, try to make your presence known from afar. Tread with heavy footfalls, or use a stick to bang against rocks or bushes. Rattlesnakes will pick up the vibrations through their skin and will usually buzz (unmistakably) before you get too close for comfort.

Here are a few more safety tips: Regard most free-flowing water as unsafe for drinking without purification, excluding, of course, developed water sources within campgrounds and picnic areas. Chemical (iodine or chlorine) treatment, filtering, and ultraviolet light are the most convenient purification methods, but secondary in effectiveness to boiling. A bigger problem, of course, in this part of the world is the availability of the water itself. Many springs and watercourses in the Santa Anas are intermittent, flowing only after winter rains. Your best bet is to carry all the water you'll need on the trail.

Deer-hunting season in Cleveland National Forest occurs during mid-autumn. Although conflicts between hunters and hikers are uncommon, you may want to confine your explorations at that time of year to state and county parks, where hunting is prohibited.

Mountain lions do frequent the wilder corners of Orange County and have even been spotted on the edge of suburban neighborhoods. While recent news stories have trumpeted every instance of encounters with mountain lions, attacks on hikers or mountain bikers remain statistically rare, with one fatal attack in 2004 on a solo mountain biker at Whiting Ranch and two nonfatal attacks on children in Caspers Wilderness Park in 1986. All persons entering mountain lion country are urged to take the following precautions:

- Hike with one or more companions.
- Keep children close at hand.
- Never run from a mountain lion. Doing so may trigger its instinct to attack.
- Make yourself "large." Face the animal, maintain eye contact with it, shout, blow a whistle, and do not act fearful. Do anything to convince the animal that you are not its prey.
- Carry a hiking stick and use it, or pitch stones or other objects at the animal if it advances.

There is always some risk in leaving a vehicle unattended at a remote trailhead. Fortunately, automobile vandalism and burglary are not acute problems in the described areas. Report all theft and vandalism of personal property to park officials or the county sheriff, and report vandalism of public property to the appropriate park or forest agency.

Trail Courtesy

Whenever you travel the backcountry wilderness or a well-trodden park trail, you take on a burden of responsibility to preserve the natural environment. Aside from commonsense prohibitions against littering and vandalism, here are a few of the less obvious guidelines every hiker should be aware of.

Never cut trail switchbacks. This practice breaks down the trail tread and hastens erosion. Improve designated trails by removing branches, rocks, or other debris if you can. Report any trail damage and misplaced or broken signs to the appropriate ranger office (Cleveland National Forest has a form for this purpose).

When backpacking, be a "no trace" camper. Camp well away from water, and leave your campsite as you found it or leave it in an even more natural condition. Because of the danger of wildfire in Orange County, you cannot have open fires (campfires or barbecues) except in developed campgrounds and picnic grounds. For cooking, you can use a campstove (with the proper permit), but only in an area cleared of flammable vegetation. In the backcountry, dig a hole at least 6 inches deep and bury human waste; carry out used toilet paper in a plastic bag so that animals don't dig it up and scatter it about.

Collecting minerals, plants, animals, and historical objects without a special permit is prohibited in state and county parks and national forests. This regulation includes common things, such as pinecones, wildflowers, and lizards. Leave them for all visitors to enjoy.

It's impractical to review here all the specific rules associated with the use of public lands in the Orange County area, but you, as a visitor, are responsible for knowing them. Refer to Appendix 4 for sources of information.

Using This Book

Whether you wish to use this book as a reference tool or as a guide to read cover to cover, take a few minutes to read this section. It explains the exact meaning of the capsulized information that appears before each trip description, and it also describes the way in which trips are grouped geographically.

One way to expedite the process of finding a suitable trip, especially if you're unfamiliar with hiking opportunities in Orange County, is to turn to Appendix 1, which calls out the most highly recommended hikes. The main map of Orange County and vicinity (on pages vi and vii) shows the area that each chapter covers.

Each chapter's introduction includes any general information about the area's history, geology, plants, and wildlife not included in the trip descriptions. Important information about possible restrictions or special requirements (wilderness permits, for example) appears here too, and you should review this material before starting on a hike in a particular chapter.

At the time of this writing, most trailheads in the national forests of Southern California are signed to indicate that you must post a National Forest Adventure Pass or Interagency Annual Pass on your vehicle. You can purchase an Adventure Pass at ranger stations and some retailers but not at the trailhead, which is a significant inconvenience for casual visitors. However, according to the Federal Lands and Recreation Enhancement Act that authorized

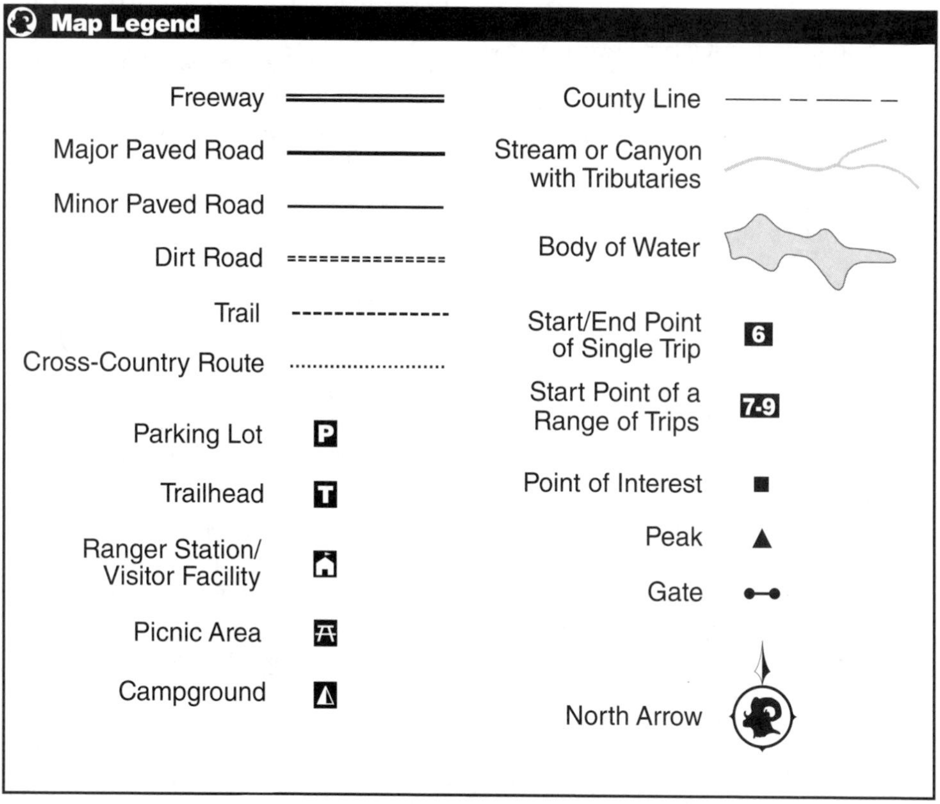

Map Legend

Freeway	══════	County Line	── ─ ── ─
Major Paved Road	──────	Stream or Canyon with Tributaries	
Minor Paved Road	─────		
Dirt Road	=============	Body of Water	
Trail	------------	Start/End Point of Single Trip	**6**
Cross-Country Route	············	Start Point of a Range of Trips	**7-9**
Parking Lot	**P**	Point of Interest	■
Trailhead	**T**	Peak	▲
Ranger Station/ Visitor Facility		Gate	●─●
Picnic Area			
Campground		North Arrow	

the Adventure Pass system, the US Forest Service is prohibited from charging a fee solely for parking. In May 2014, a US District Court ruled that the Adventure Pass is required only for visitors who use developed trailhead facilities, such as picnic tables or restrooms. If you want to simply park and hike, the Adventure Pass is not required, despite signage to the contrary. You may wish to follow the latest developments in the media.

Each chapter contains a sketch map of the locations and routes of all the hikes it describes. The boxed numbers on those maps correspond to the trip numbers and refer to the start and end points of out-and-back and loop trips. Point-to-point trips have two boxed numbers, indicating the separate start and end points. The map also shows GPS coordinates for key waypoints. A map legend is provided on the previous page.

Capsulized Information

Each trip begins with capsulized information, including distance, hiking time, elevation gain, difficulty, trail use, best times, and agency. If you are simply browsing, these summaries alone can be used as a tool to eliminate hikes that are either too difficult or too trivial for your abilities or desires.

DISTANCE

An estimate of total distance is given. Out-and-back trips show the sum of the distances of the out-and-back segments. After the trail distance, I've noted whether the trip (as described) is a loop, an out-and-back route, or a point-to-point trip, requiring a car shuttle. There is some flexibility, of course, in the way in which a hiker follows a trip. Distances beyond 5 miles are rounded off to avoid suggesting a false level of accuracy.

HIKING TIME

This figure is for the average hiker and includes only the time spent in motion. It does not include time for rest stops, lunch, etc. Fast walkers can complete the routes in perhaps 30% less time, and slower hikers

may take 50% longer. The hiker is assumed to be traveling with a light daypack. (*Important note:* Hikers carrying heavy packs could easily take twice as long, especially if they are traveling under adverse weather conditions. Remember, too, that a group's progress is limited by the pace of its slowest member or members.)

ELEVATION GAIN

The elevation gain is an estimate of the sum of all the vertical gain segments along the total length of the route (includes both ways for out-and-back trips). It is often considerably more than the net difference in elevation between the high and low points of the hike. For one-way hikes, the gain and loss are reported separately, assuming that you follow the described direction of travel.

DIFFICULTY

This overall rating takes into account the length of the trip and the nature of the terrain. The following are general definitions of the four categories:

- **Easy:** Suitable for every member of the family.
- **Moderate:** Suitable for all physically fit people.
- **Moderately strenuous:** Long length, substantial elevation gain, and/or difficult terrain. Suitable for experienced hikers only.
- **Strenuous:** Full day's hike (or overnight backpack) over a long and often difficult route. Suitable only for experienced hikers in excellent physical condition.

Each higher level represents more or less a doubling of the difficulty. On average, moderate trips are twice as hard as easy trips, moderately strenuous trips are twice as hard as moderate trips, and so on.

TRAIL USE

All trails are suitable for dayhikes. This category lists other uses for a particular trail, chosen from the following five options.

- **Backpacking:** Most trips in this book are not suitable for backpacking. Although there are several roadside campgrounds in the Orange County vicinity, trail camping is not widely permitted.
- **Cyclists:** The route, as described, is open to mountain biking. Orange County is an extremely popular mountain biking destination, and many trails see more bikers than hikers. Some of the trails are suitable only for advanced riders, so cyclists may wish to consult other sources before relying on this book to choose trails.
- **Equestrians:** The route is open to horse riders.
- **Dogs:** Allowed on the trail but must generally be on a leash no longer than 6 feet.
- **Children:** These trips are especially recommended for inquisitive children. They were chosen on the basis of their safety and ease of travel, as well as their potential for entertaining the whole family.

BEST TIMES

Nearly all the short trips in this book are passable year-round, but some of the longer trips, especially those inland, are much more rewarding when temperatures are mild and/or water is present along the trail.

AGENCY

These code letters refer to the agency or office that has jurisdiction or management over the area being hiked (for example, **CNF: TD** means "Cleveland National Forest, Trabuco District"). You can contact the agency for more information. Full names, phone numbers, and some addresses (of larger agencies) are listed in Appendix 4.

PERMIT

Any required permits or use fees are listed in this category. Some of these listings use the same acronyms as the agency listings (again, refer to Appendix 4 for the full names).

Optional or Recommended Maps

Earlier editions of this book recommended US Geological Survey 7.5-minute topographic maps for each hike. Unfortunately, most of the trails outside the Cleveland National Forest are not portrayed on the USGS maps. The *Cleveland National Forest Visitor Map* is your best option for most hikes in the Santa Ana Mountains. This large folding color relief map shows all of the trails and roads in the national forest and also covers some of the surrounding areas. You can buy it at ranger stations, through the US Forest Service website, or from local outdoor stores, or you can search for a free but obscure PDF download on the Forest Service site.

The Forest Service also produces the *San Mateo Wilderness* topographic map, your best choice for hikes in that wilderness. This map is most easily obtained at the El Cariso Visitor Center on Highway 74. The Forest Service also offers the *Cleveland National Forest Topographic Atlas* if you need topographic maps of the forest.

For other trips, your best bet is to rely on this book's sketch maps. Most Orange County Parks and Chino Hills State Park graciously offer good free park maps at the ranger stations and on their websites, but the information is similar to what you'll find in this book.

Electronic Supplements

Please visit **eTrails** (**etrails.net**) for GPS coordinates and tracks for the hikes in this book and to review hike updates and other information. iPhone and iPad users may wish to download eTrails from the App Store. The mobile app includes an Orange County guide with electronic maps for all the trips in this book, showing your position and the trails on USGS topographic base maps. It also helps with automated driving directions from your present location to the trailheads.

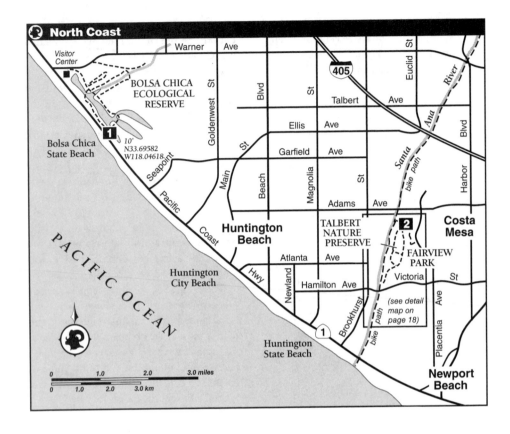

North Coast

chapter 1

North Coast

Orange County's northernmost stretch of coastline consists of a wide, sandy strand stretching through the cities of Seal Beach and Huntington Beach. Tens of thousands of people flock to these beaches on warm, sunny days, while tens of thousands more live immediately back of the coastline on low-lying land that once supported extensive saltwater and freshwater marshes.

The underlying sedimentary rocks are rich in petroleum; you're reminded of that by the sight of rocker pumps, storage tanks, and refineries. That activity, however, is waning. New housing developments are springing up, especially along the Pacific Coast Highway (Highway 1). Formerly environmentally abused wetlands and floodplains are in the process of being restored to some semblance of an original condition.

Two areas along this north stretch of coast stand out as excellent examples of ecological rehabilitation: Bolsa Chica Ecological Reserve and Talbert Nature Preserve. Both are perfect for easygoing exercise and early-morning bird- and wildlife-watching. Huntington Beach boasts of being one of the nation's best birding sites, with nearly half of all species of birds in the nation spotted there. The prevalence of hikers and bird-watchers with elaborate spotting scopes and telephoto lenses at Bolsa Chica and other nearby coastal locales attests to that.

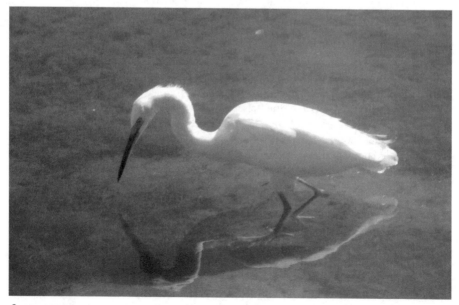

Snowy egret

| | | see map on p. 14 |

trip 1.1   Bolsa Chica Ecological Reserve

Distance	1.6-plus miles (loop)
Hiking Time	1 hour
Elevation Gain	Negligible
Difficulty	Easy
Trail Use	Good for kids
Best Times	All year
Agency	BCER

DIRECTIONS The trailhead lies on the inland side of the Pacific Coast Highway (Highway 1), 1.5 miles south of Warner Avenue, and 1.5 miles north of Seapoint Avenue in Huntington Beach.

The Bolsa Chica Ecological Reserve protects the largest saltwater marsh between Monterey Bay and the Tijuana River. Its name, Spanish for "little purse," came from a subdivided portion of an 1834 Mexican land grant. The wetlands were dammed to create a duck hunting preserve around 1895, and then they were built up for oil drilling in 1940 and for a coastal defense artillery battery during World War II. Since 1973, California has recognized the ecological significance of the wetlands and has been restoring them. In 2006, a major project was completed to remove the dam and much of the oil equipment. Birds and fish are now flourishing, making it a very popular destination for wildlife observation.

This hike makes a loop around Bolsa Chica Slough. Binoculars, spotting scopes, and/or cameras are de rigueur, of course.

First, consider paying a visit to the Bolsa Chica Interpretive Center on Warner Avenue at the Pacific Coast Highway. Visitors can also get a checklist of local birds and information about the reserve there. You could also start your hike from there, if you'd like.

From the parking lot on the PCH, a long, wooden bridge leads over some shallow stretches of tide water invaded by typical saltwater marsh plants: cordgrass, alkali heath, sea lavender, and pickleweed. Interpretive panels tell of two endangered species of birds that frequent this area: the least tern, which nests on two small, sandy islands nearby; and the Belding's savannah sparrow, a bird that can drink seawater, processing it with its hyperefficient kidneys. Early on weekend mornings, photographers use the bridge as a stable platform for their often sophisticated equipment.

On the far side of the bridge, a path goes left atop a levee, eventually encircling a segment of the slough. On the surface and the shoreline, you may spot gulls, terns, egrets, cormorants, pelicans, stilts, plovers, avocets, grebes, marsh hawks, herons, and kites. The number and diversity of birds vary with the season.

At 0.9 mile, pass the Wintersburg Channel, and then walk up to a scenic viewpoint on the lip of a nearby mesalike terrace. Gabrieleno Indians contemplated a lonely scene here centuries ago. They beheld a broad, shallow bay extending well inland, rimmed by saltwater and freshwater marshes as far as the eye could see. Later, two 155-millimeter guns were mounted here to defend Southern California's coastline during World War II.

From this viewpoint, you can add an optional 0.8-mile loop northwest to visit the Bolsa Pocket Wetlands. The Pocket Loop Trail begins along the ridge but soon splits. Make a counterclockwise loop, dropping down along the edge of the wetlands for more birding opportunities. Come back up on the ridge for views of Catalina Island beyond the oil platforms in the channel. Listen for birds nesting in the eucalyptus trees nearby.

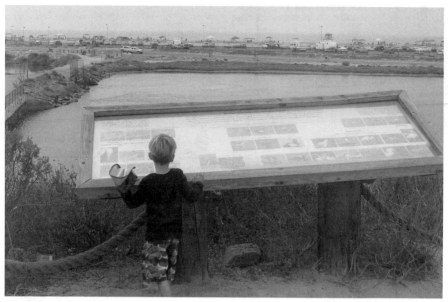

Bolsa Chica

Whether you take the pocket wetlands loop or not, the most expedient way to return is to head south across the levee and follow a mostly paved path back along the side of the Pacific Coast Highway. You can enjoy another set of views of the birds from this path. However, you'll have to endure the highway noise, so some people will prefer to retrace their steps along the quieter route by which you came.

trip 1.2 Talbert Nature Preserve

see map on next page

Distance	2-plus miles (loop)
Hiking Time	1 hour
Elevation Gain	50′
Difficulty	Easy
Trail Use	Cyclists, dogs, good for kids
Best Times	All year
Agency	OC Parks: TNP

DIRECTIONS The trip begins at Fairview Park on the western edge of the city of Costa Mesa. From the 55 Freeway, exit at Victoria Street, and pay close attention at the complex exit. Take Victoria west for 1.4 mile, then turn right on Placentia Avenue, and proceed 0.8 mile to Fairview Park on the left.

Another large restoration project has been in progress since 1993 along the floodplain just east of the channelized Santa Ana River in the city of Costa Mesa. Talbert Nature Preserve consists of two 90-acre sections, divided by busy Victoria Street: a north parcel laced with wide, smooth trails, and a south parcel still in the midst of restoration. The proposed Orange Coast River Park would be centered on Talbert and would permanently protect habitat and recreation along the lower end of the Santa Ana River.

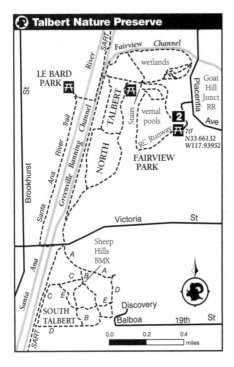

Talbert Nature Preserve

where you pass a staircase on the left and a wetlands trail on the right, continue straight to reach the signed Talbert Nature Preserve entrance on the left, 0.5 mile from the start. (The paved path itself continues west to tie-in with the Santa Ana River bike path, another way to reach Talbert's entrance if you are arriving by bicycle.)

A wide, flat, decomposed-granite path suitable for hikers, cyclists, and horses runs toward the south from the entrance for a mile, beneath the brow of a steep bluff. It then connects with a segment of paved bike path leading to Victoria Street. Short of that juncture, there are opportunities to branch west and loop back to the entrance using unimproved trails. Those alternate trails may turn muddy after significant rainfall.

Talbert Nature Preserve is an extraordinarily quiet place, screened from traffic noise by the bluff rising on the east and levees on the west, which effectively deaden the din from the surrounding cityscape.

Fairview Park has many other points of interest worthy of exploration while you are in the area. A Tongva village was once situated atop the bluff, and the countless shards of shellfish provide a reminder of their coastal lifestyle. Five rare vernal pools that fill up during spring rains can be found here. Some support fairy shrimp, which lay their eggs in the mud, and which then hatch the next year when the rainy season begins again. The shrimp can complete their life-cycle in only 16 days, growing to maturity, mating, and laying their eggs in the mud before their ephemeral ponds evaporate.

At the north end of the park, a system of ponds has been established to naturally treat water from the Greenville-Banning Channel before it enters the Santa Ana River. A mazelike trail network through the wetlands provides good views of the waterfowl and wildflowers.

The planting of native vegetation in the preserve is being guided both by remaining native vegetation on-site and by attempts to recreate plant communities similar to those that existed in this region before nearly every available acre was put to use for agriculture, housing, or industry. Several plant "zones" in the preserve, including coastal strand, native grassland, alluvial woodland, and wetland vegetation, are identified by means of trailside interpretive plaques. Thus, the preserve serves as a native botanical garden, refuge for wildlife, and educational and recreational resource.

From the restrooms near the main entrance to Fairview Park, walk a short distance west, and turn right on the asphalt bike path. Follow the path north and then west down a hill. At the base of the hill

The Harbor Soaring Society flies an impressive array of remote-control aircraft at a dirt strip on the south side of Fairview Park. On the east side of Placentia, the Orange County Model Engineers operate a miniature railroad and offer rides to the public on the third weekend of each month.

VARIATION

South Talbert Preserve is most conveniently accessed from a gate on the corner of Balboa Avenue and Discovery Drive. The section includes a major stand of willows and mulefat. Naturalists are removing invasive species, especially pampas grass, and planting native vegetation. Various 2-mile strolls are possible, and the northwest and southwest corners also connect to the Santa Ana River Trail. In the center of the preserve is the incongruous but fascinating Sheep Hills BMX course, where you may see riders testing their skills on epic jumps.

Matalija poppies resemble fried eggs.

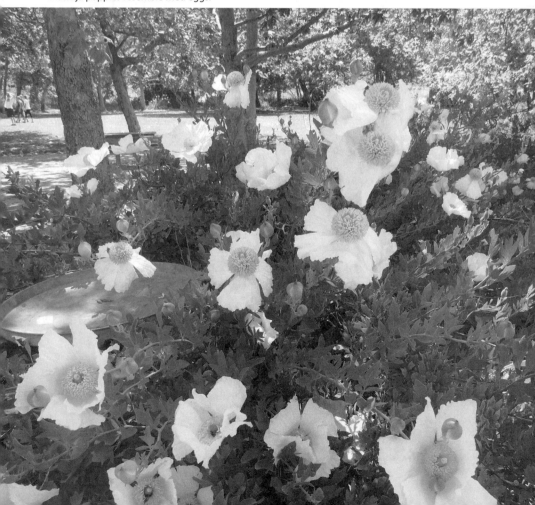

chapter 2

Upper Newport Bay

The marshes surrounding Upper Newport Bay represent tiny remnants of a much more extensive wetland that once stretched inland to the present city of Tustin. The Portolà expedition of 1769 (led by Gaspar de Portolà) and subsequent travelers passing up or down the coast avoided this soggy region and stuck to the base of the foothills, where the firm ground more than made up for the inconvenience of traversing ridges and ravines.

During the past 100,000 years or more, the Santa Ana River has wandered across the surface of the Los Angeles Basin, changing course many times in response to flooding and silt deposition. Around 30,000 years ago, the river (which at that time carried more runoff because of a wetter climate) carved out the basic form of the troughlike structure now occupied by Upper Newport Bay. Sediment carried by the river and dropped at the mouth of the trough formed a barrier island, today's Balboa Peninsula, enclosing (lower) Newport Bay.

The most recent natural shift in the Santa Ana River's course occurred in 1825, when a large flood redirected the flow west from Upper Newport Bay to essentially the place where it now reaches the ocean via artificial channel. Today the bay is fed by San Diego Creek, a small former tributary of the river.

For many millennia, decayed marsh vegetation (peat) accumulated along the upper bay shores. This material, mixed with fine silt washed down from the surrounding slopes and bluffs, has created soil conditions conducive to self-sustaining wetlands.

Hemmed in by bustling traffic arteries, high-rise office buildings, residential areas, and the Irvine campus of the University of

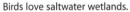
Birds love saltwater wetlands.

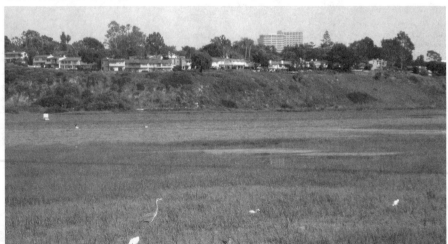

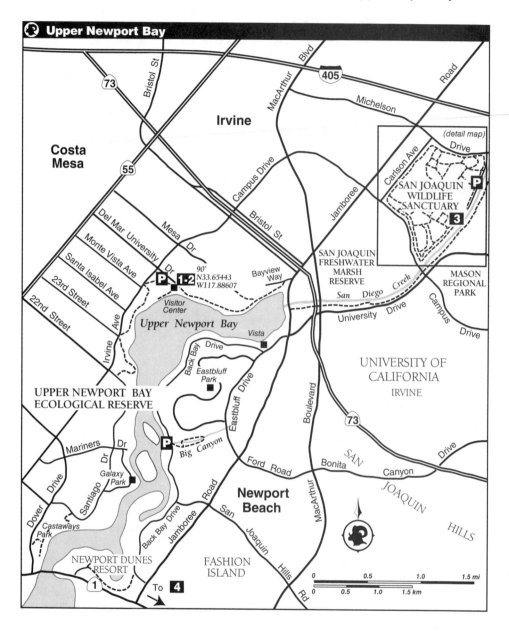

Upper Newport Bay

California, Upper Newport Bay exists in a kind of time warp. Coyotes and mule deer still roam the periphery, while myriads of migratory birds use the productive marshes as a stopover or winter home.

The future of the wetlands around Upper Newport Bay has been assured by the establishment of three protected areas. One of them, the Upper Newport Bay Ecological Reserve, encompasses most of the bay's saltwater marshes. Just upstream along the channelized San Diego Creek are two more areas, protecting only a fraction of the freshwater marsh that once extended inland for several miles. Some 200 acres of the marsh became UC Irvine's San Joaquin

Freshwater Marsh Reserve in 1970, now managed as a research reserve accessible only to qualified researchers. The adjacent and newer San Joaquin Wildlife Sanctuary, on the other hand, has been designed for extensive use by recreationalists and amateur naturalists. An amazing 10 miles of wide, smoothly graded trails crisscross the wildlife sanctuary, which covers 300 acres of diked ponds, natural riparian habitat, and artificially created native habitats.

Buck Gully is part of the Newport Beach trail system. Although it doesn't really fit in with the other waterfront trails, the lovely trail is included in this chapter for lack of a more suitable home.

---

trip 2.1   Upper Newport Bay Nature Preserve

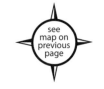

see map on previous page

Distance	2.7 miles (loop)
Hiking Time	1½ hours
Elevation Gain	200'
Difficulty	Easy
Trail Use	Cyclists, dogs, good for kids
Best Times	All year
Agency	OC Parks: UNBNP

DIRECTIONS To reach Upper Newport Bay's Muth Interpretive Center, exit the Costa Mesa Freeway (Highway 55) at Del Mar Avenue in Costa Mesa, and go east toward the bay. In 0.5 mile, Del Mar becomes University Drive. Continue 0.4 mile to reach the interpretive center parking lot just past Irvine Avenue.

Were it not for public protest in the 1960s and '70s, Upper Newport Bay would surely have become yet another of Orange County's residential harbor communities. Instead, the State of California purchased 752 acres of Irvine Company land in 1975, thus establishing the Upper Newport Bay Ecological Reserve. An astounding 100 species of coastal and mudflat fish, as well as some 200 species of birds, frequent the shallow waters of the bay.

The well-designed Muth Interpretive Center offers exhibits explaining the significance of the estuary. Naturalists organize a variety of activities, including Tideland Tykes, birding, kayak tours, and service projects. Register for free in advance at **lets gooutside.org.**

The west side of the preserve is laced with a spiderweb of trails squeezed between the wetlands and Irvine Avenue. The longest, most interesting walk in the preserve involves making a loop of up to 3 miles along these trails. Follow the trail from the east end of the parking area down through a native butterfly garden to the Muth Interpretive Center. Below the interpretive center, you can follow a trail west along the wetlands. It soon climbs onto the bluff to circle the head of a ravine and reach a vista point. There's a good view of the broad sweep of the bay's channels and marshy islands, the steep bluffs rising from the far (east) shore, and the rolling San Joaquin Hills beyond.

Incised into the roughly 10-million-year-old marine sedimentary cliffs on the far side is a canyon that contained the largest assemblage of invertebrate fossils ever found in western North America. From sea level to their highest summits, the San Joaquin Hills exhibit eight distinct marine-terrace levels. You may recognize some of these, though massive grading for construction has greatly altered the land's natural contours. During excavation for the Fashion Island shopping center at Newport Center (a cluster of high-rises), a great deal of petrified wood was uncovered.

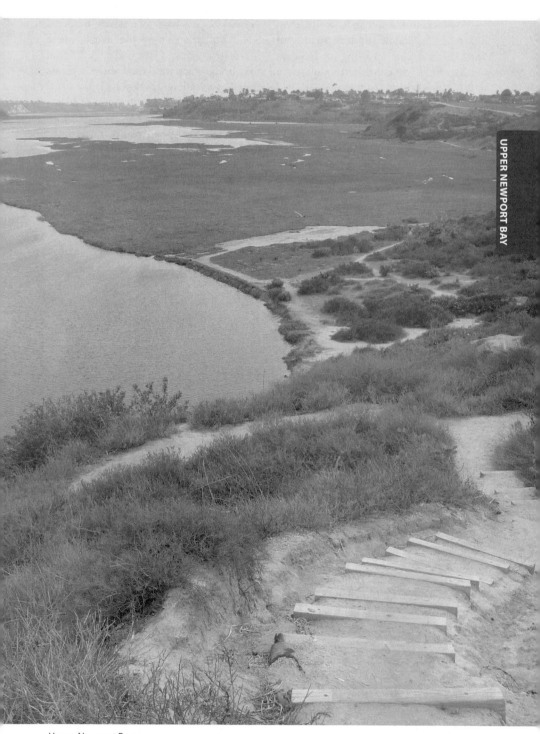

Upper Newport Bay

At an easily missed fork just beyond, descend back to the wetlands, which teem with bird life. Follow the trail southward along the shoreline, crossing an inlet on a bridge, until you are forced away near a bluff-top subdivision. At the far south end of the trail, you can reach an alternative trailhead on Santiago Drive.

Loop back north along the paved Bayview Trail that parallels Irvine Avenue. This route is popular with cyclists and joggers, but hikers may prefer to veer onto the broad dirt bluff-top path between Bayview and the wetlands. Whatever route you take, you'll eventually find yourself back at the parking area.

The north shore features a bayshore bikeway connecting Bayview Way with the west segment of University Drive. At one point, you pass over a massively timbered wood bridge spanning the marsh where it pinches against a steep, dry bluff. From that bridge, you can view three separate tiers of vegetation. The lowest is the usual low-growing, salt-tolerant group of plants like pickleweed and cordgrass. Just above the reach of the tide are plants typical of the coastal uplands, such as wild buckwheat, mulefat, and cattails. Above the level of the bridge, the bluff slope supports a dense growth of native coastal sage scrub vegetation: California sagebrush, lemonade berry, elderberry, prickly pear cactus, and cholla cactus (a coastal variant of the same cactus that grows abundantly throughout the California and Southwest deserts).

---

trip 2.2 Newport Back Bay Loop

Distance	10 miles (loop)
Hiking Time	4 hours
Elevation Gain	300′
Difficulty	Easy
Trail Use	Cyclists, dogs
Best Times	All year
Agency	OC Parks: UNBNP

see map on p. 21

DIRECTIONS To reach Upper Newport Bay's Muth Interpretive Center, exit the Costa Mesa Freeway (Highway 55) at Del Mar Avenue in Costa Mesa, and go east toward the bay. In 0.5 mile, Del Mar becomes University Drive. Continue 0.4 mile to reach the interpretive center parking lot just past Irvine Avenue.

A great way to get to know Upper Newport Bay is to take the Back Bay Loop that circles the wetlands. This paved route, heavily used by cyclists and joggers, features panoramic bluff-top views, intimate marshside experiences, and diverse bird-watching opportunities. There are many places to start, but this description assumes you're following a counterclockwise loop beginning at the interpretive center.

Like Trip 2.1, this trip begins at the parking area for the Muth Interpretive Center. It's worth a short detour down to the center, where you can find spotting telescopes, interpretive exhibits, activities for children, and knowledgeable volunteers. When you're ready to begin, your first goal is to reach the corner of Irvine Avenue and Santiago Drive, 1.1 miles from the start. Hikers will favor the narrow footpaths that hug the edge of the marsh (see Trip 2.1), but cyclists must take the wide paved path paralleling Irvine Avenue.

The trail ends at the intersection with Santiago Drive. Hikers can avoid busy Irvine Avenue by veering onto Santiago

Drive and following it through a residential neighborhood. Where Santiago abruptly veers left and becomes Polaris Drive, continue onto a paved walking and biking path, and immediately reach a T-junction where you turn left (1.6 miles). Cyclists may prefer to follow Irvine Avenue, then turn left onto Dover Drive at Mariners Park. Near Westcliff Drive, turn left onto the paved path to rejoin the route described above.

The next 0.8-mile stretch to the Pacific Coast Highway (Highway 1) begins with a spectacular bluff-top pathway leading to Castaways Park. Pay your respects at the Marine Corps memorial, then navigate the maze of trails through the park to find the one leading southwest steeply down to Dover Drive. The Back Bay Loop leads south on the paved sidewalk to meet the PCH.

Turn left and follow the sidewalk path over the bay bridge, then make your first left onto North Bayside Drive. Just before the west entry gate at Newport Dunes Resort Marina, veer right onto another paved walking and riding path that leads behind the RV resort. When it emerges at the east entry gate, continue to Back Bay Drive, and turn left onto the road, 1.2 miles from Dover Drive.

You now follow Back Bay Drive along the east side of the bay. After passing the Back Bay Science Center in 0.3 mile, the road narrows to become one-way northbound for cars, with a wide lane on the side for self-powered travelers. This is also the terminus of the Mountains to Sea Trail (Trip 18.2). In 1 mile, reach the Big Canyon parking area with a small boardwalk. If you have time for a detour, a 0.5-mile loop on a gravel road visits a small freshwater marsh on the east side. In the early morning, bird calls almost drown out the sound of traffic, and cottontail rabbits frequent the trail.

In another 1.9 miles, make a steep ascent to a vista point on Eastbluff Drive. Turn left and follow the Back Bay Loop along Eastbluff Drive. Make your first left onto Jamboree Road, where a paved trail resumes on the west side of the road. As you approach a bridge, the San Diego Creek and Mountains

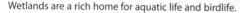
Wetlands are a rich home for aquatic life and birdlife.

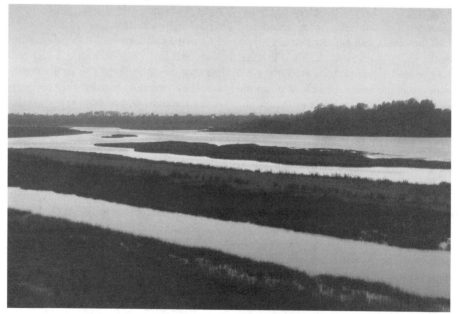

to Sea Trail veer left and then crosses under the bridge, but you stay on the Bayview Trail atop the bridge. Sometimes you will see remarkable numbers of mullets jumping high out of the water at this confluence of freshwater and saltwater. Mullets do not eat flying insects, so scientists are unsure why they like to jump.

Soon turn left onto Bayview Way, and find the trail again. A short spur on the right leads to streetside parking. The trail briefly splits with a paved bike path on the left and a dirt equestrian route on the right, which then rejoin before a long bridge and boardwalk. Cross the Santa Ana Delhi Channel, and reach the parking area where you began.

trip 2.3 San Joaquin Wildlife Sanctuary

Distance	2–4 miles (loop)
Hiking Time	1–2 hours
Elevation Gain	Negligible
Difficulty	Easy
Trail Use	Good for kids
Best Times	All year, open dawn–dusk
Agency	IRWD

DIRECTIONS Exit the 405 Freeway at Jamboree Road. Go south for 1 mile and turn left on Campus Drive. In 1 mile, make a U-turn at University Drive and an immediate right onto Riparian View, and follow it to the parking area for the wildlife sanctuary. Note that construction projects may change the preferred access at some point in the future.

As one of the richest wetland areas along the Southern California coast, the San Joaquin Wildlife Sanctuary offers an uncommon opportunity to come into contact with a natural ecosystem in the midst of Orange County's high-rise urban core. Amid willows, bulrushes, and mulefat, you can spy on ducks, geese, and shorebirds, listen to songbird serenades, and perhaps even observe a bobcat and her kitten. You can thrill to the graceful antics of herons and egrets and the soaring flights of hawks and falcons.

Make no mistake, though, the entire 300-acre wetland, in its present incarnation, is an urban park, planted densely with native trees and shrubs and irrigated with recycled water from the state-of-the-art wastewater treatment plant. Starting in the early 1990s, the Irvine Ranch Water District, with the support of the Irvine Company and the Sea and Sage chapter of the Audubon Society, began an ambitious project to transform the former duck-hunting-club property into a naturalistic landscape typical of Orange

County's original lowland and upland habitats. That effort resulted in a dense system of more than 11 miles of wide, smooth, wheelchair-accessible trails, restrooms, resting benches galore, and, most importantly, first-class habitat for birds.

A nesting platform high on a pole in Pond 4 has attracted a pair of ospreys, which you may see diving for large fish in the ponds. Audubon volunteers have installed 100 nestboxes throughout the sanctuary to attract tree swallows, and they conduct a monthly bird census that has documented nearly 300 species of resident and migratory birds.

Start at the Audubon House nature center (open daily) by the parking lot, and pick up a free map. Naturalists offer regularly scheduled interpretive walks, and kids of all ages love the summer bat walks.

The most direct way to the heart of the sanctuary is to begin on Fledgling Loop, a broad dirt road starting by the parking area that leads between Ponds A–E. These ponds are used to hold treated water from the

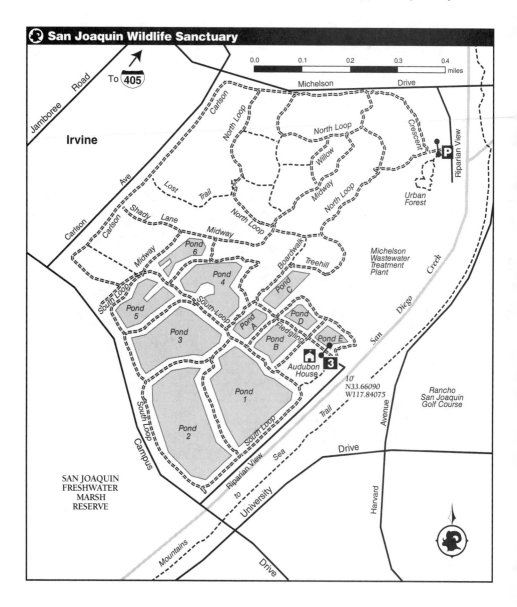

San Joaquin Wildlife Sanctuary

Michelson Wastewater Treatment Plant and act as emergency storage areas, but Ponds E and D are usually kept shallow to provide rare freshwater habitat for birds. These are favorite spots for bird photographers, especially in spring when shorebirds nest on the mudflat. (Note that visitors are required to stay on the established trails; don't cut your own path down to the water.)

Watch for signs identifying the most common native plants along the trail, especially mulefat, California sagebrush, and coyote bush. Bladderpod and California wild rose are also plentiful. The three dominant trees in the sanctuary are willows (with long, skinny leaves), cottonwoods (with heart-shaped leaves), and sycamores (with white bark and hand-shaped leaves).

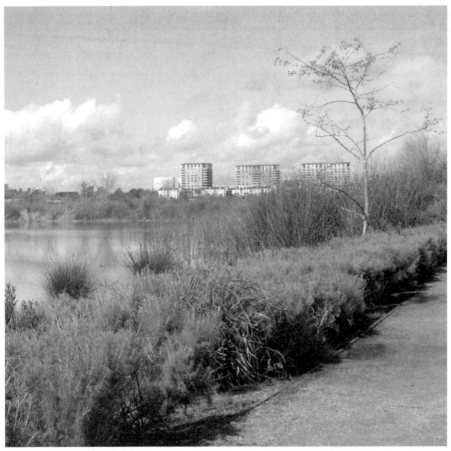

Pond 1, San Joaquin Wildlife Sanctuary

Photo: Trude Hurd

At a T-junction in 0.2 mile, turn right along Pond C, then veer left to follow a boardwalk through the wetlands. This is one of the more likely places to spot a resident bobcat. Lizards, butterflies, and dragonflies have the right-of-way here! Watch for splendid reflections of the willows in the placid waters.

A web of trails continues from the end of the boardwalk. Following specific directions would be difficult, and there's no need to take a particular route because all of the sanctuary is interesting. Plan your loop to include some of the large ponds (1–4) on the southwest side of the sanctuary, which attract white pelicans, great blue herons, and other large fish-eating birds. These ponds contain water pumped in from San Diego Creek and help filter excess nitrates before the water is pumped back into the creek, which empties at Newport Back Bay. The thousands of American crows you may see roosting in trees at dusk represent an explosion in population, thanks to the plentiful food that they forage in neighboring communities.

A typical loop will cover 2–4 miles. Although most junctions are signed, it's very easy to get lost in the dense web of trails through tall native vegetation. Monitor your progress on your map, and be sure to carry some water if the day is warm.

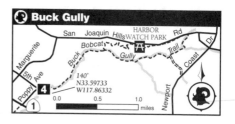

trip 2.4 **Buck Gully**	
Distance	5 miles (semiloop)
Hiking Time	2½ hours
Elevation Gain	600′
Difficulty	Moderate
Trail Use	Cyclists
Best Times	All year
Agency	City of Newport Beach

DIRECTIONS From the Pacific Coast Highway (Highway 1) in Newport Beach, turn northeast onto Poppy Avenue. Proceed 0.3 mile, and park on the street before 5th Avenue.

Lined by multimillion-dollar mansions on the adjacent ridges, Buck Gully Reserve was acquired in 2005 to protect a slice of open space in the San Joaquin foothills. Most verdant in winter and spring, the canyon is pleasant any time of year. The trail system was improved in 2013 to protect the rich coastal sage scrub ecosystem. Beware of the extensive stands of poison oak found near the trail.

The gated and signed Buck Gully Trail begins on the east side of Poppy Avenue just north of 5th Avenue. Descend the paved road to a sign marking the start of the dirt trail along the canyon. In 1.2 miles, pass the Bobcat Trail on the left, by which you will return. In another 0.8 mile, stay left at a fork where another dirt road climbs to Newport Coast Drive. The Buck Gully Trail soon veers north to meet San Joaquin Hills Road in 0.5 mile at a signed trailhead with no street parking.

To make a loop, turn left and follow the sidewalk west along the road. In 0.7 mile, join a paved trail leading to a gazebo with a compass rose. Transmission lines partially obscure the views of the mansions across the canyon. Don't be lured down the gated road toward one of the transmission line towers. Instead, continue west and rejoin the sidewalk before reaching the signed Bobcat Trail in 0.2 mile near Harbor Watch Park. Benches at the trailhead provide a good place to rest and take in views of the canyon, Newport Bay, and the ocean.

Descend the Bobcat Trail, initially a powerline service road. At a fork, stay right on a narrower trail. In 0.6 mile, cross a footbridge to the signed junction with the Buck Gully Trail. Turn right and retrace your steps to the trailhead.

Lemonade berry

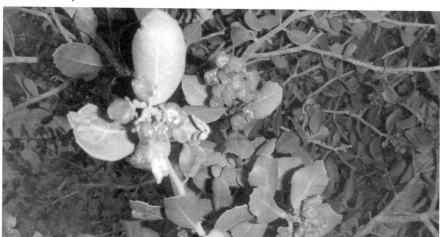

chapter 3

Crystal Cove State Park

outh of Newport Bay, the shoreline topography, so flat and uninspiring back along the north county coast, becomes bold and dramatic. Cliffs provide a backdrop for restless surf breaking upon smooth, sandy beaches and rocky reefs or surging into secluded coves. In the hills behind the wave-cut cliffs, you can see, imprinted on the slopes, a muted stairstep pattern of earlier cliffs that used to border the ocean long before this area was uplifted to its present height.

From Corona del Mar through the posh communities of Laguna Beach and Laguna Niguel to Dana Point, rustic cottages, opulent ocean-view homes, gated housing complexes, and swank hotels blanket most of the coastline. Interspersed within these thickly populated areas lie conspicuously blank areas on the street maps—sensuously curved hills and lush valleys that represent what nearly all of southern Orange County was like a century ago. Fortunately, some large pieces of the undeveloped land

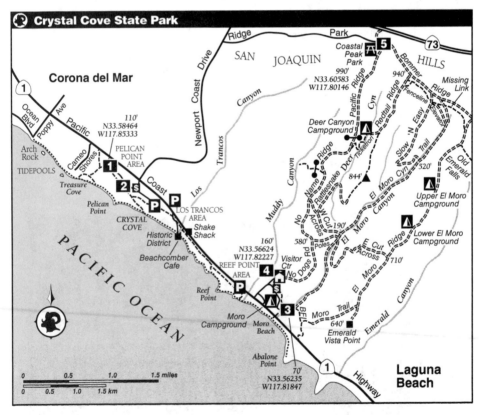

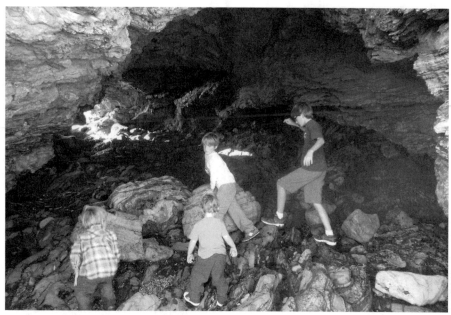

Searching for pirate treasure in Crystal Cove

will never succumb to the ever-rising tide of suburbia. Over the past three decades, several large parcels of undeveloped land near Laguna Beach have passed into public ownership.

Crystal Cove State Park was the first large parcel to be set aside. Besides a 3-mile stretch of bluffs and ocean front, the park reaches back into the San Joaquin Hills to encompass the entire watershed of El Moro Canyon—2,200 acres of natural ravines, ridges, and terrace formations. In the back-country (El Moro Canyon) section of the park alone, visitors can explore 18 miles of dirt roads and paths open to hikers, equestrians, and mountain bikers. Several more miles of paved bike path and trail lace the coastal bluff tops and descend to the beach.

Surrounding Crystal Cove State Park, several large parcels of undeveloped land in the San Joaquin Hills, owned for many decades by the Irvine Company, have passed into public ownership. These parcels, now incorporated into units called Laguna Coast Wilderness Park, Aliso and Wood Canyons Wilderness Park, and Irvine

Open Space Preserve, are covered in Chapters 4, 5, and 11. This 20,000-acre area, collectively known as the South Coast Wilderness, is one of the treasures of Orange County.

Crystal Cove State Park is open for day use from dawn to dusk. You can park along the beach and enjoy some tidepooling or beach-walking. Or you can drive up to the parking area adjoining the visitor center just east of the Pacific Coast Highway (Highway 1), and start your exploration of the backcountry sector of the park from there. Mountain biking is both permitted and popular in Crystal Cove's backcountry section, not only on fire roads and former fire roads, but also on the narrow, single-track trails. This situation is unusual for state parks, which often reserve the narrow trails for hiking use only.

Visitors can camp at Moro Campground or rent a cottage at the seaside Historic District in the park. Hike-in camping in the park is available at the Lower El Moro, Upper El Moro, and Deer Canyon primitive-camping sites.

The park's interpretive program includes occasional lectures and weekly outdoor activities, such as bird-watching sessions, tidepool walks, and canyon hikes. As at any California state park, expect to pay a substantial parking fee for attending events or just exploring on your own. These fees go toward maintaining the park's facilities and infrastructure, which are designed to accommodate heavy use.

An alternative access point for those who just want to hike, run, or bike the trails is to start from Coastal Peak Park atop the San Joaquin Hills. From Highway 1 northwest of Crystal Cove State Park, head north on Newport Coast Drive for 2.4 miles, then turn right onto Ridge Park Road and continue 1.6 miles to the end, where you can find free street parking. From here, the Bommer Ridge fire road through Laguna Coast Wilderness Park offers access to the top of the Crystal Cove trail network. Remember that any loop from here will be uphill on the return.

---

trip 3.1   **Corona Rock-Hop**

see map on p. 30

Distance	2.4 miles (out-and-back)
Hiking Time	2-plus hours
Elevation Gain	100'
Difficulty	Moderate
Trail Use	Good for kids
Best Times	Low tide; October–March
Agency	CCSP
Permit	CCSP parking fee required

DIRECTIONS At the intersection of the Pacific Coast Highway (Highway 1) and Newport Coast Drive, south of Corona del Mar, turn west into Crystal Cove State Park (at the Pelican Point entrance). Bear right beyond the entrance station to reach Lot 1, the northernmost parking lot on the coastal bluff.

Some of the finest tidepools in Orange County—indeed in all of Southern California—await you on this short, absorbing, and probably time-consuming, rock-hopping trek between the Pelican Point area of Crystal Cove State Park and Little Corona City Beach in Corona del Mar. Wear an old pair of rubber-soled shoes or boots (boots are better for ankle support), and expect to get wet below the ankles. Don't turn your back to the incoming waves; otherwise, you may get even wetter.

Successful tidepool gazing requires both good light (midafternoon is best) and negative tides. These conditions occur during either new or full moons from October through March. On about 20 afternoons each year, the tide drops to less than minus 1 foot (zero is defined as the average of the tides across the United States), which is low enough for you to examine marine life in the intertidal zone. Plan to start your walk about an hour before a predicted low tide.

These tidepools are remarkably pristine, and your good manners will help keep them healthy. Tidepool explorers should take care not to step on living creatures and should be especially watchful for delicate sea anemones that can be hard to recognize. Remember not to pick up, touch, or poke the tidepool life. Don't turn over rocks because the creatures living under them need to stay there, and those on top of the rocks won't fare well if they find themselves under them. Please don't collect shells.

Rocky reefs are exposed frequently along Crystal Cove State Park's beachfront, but not to the degree found along a 0.5-mile stretch of coast just north of the park. As you pay your parking fee, you may be able to pick up a brochure with pictures to help you identify tidepool life. Docents also sometimes lead walks on weekends coinciding with low tide, and you might consider joining one of these walks at Pelican Point before continuing up to Little Corona Beach.

From the northernmost Pelican Point parking area (lot 1), a paved bike path—lined with native planted shrubs and spring wildflowers—swings toward the edge of the bluff. Soon there's a split: left toward the beach, right toward a viewpoint overlooking the ocean. For the rock-hopping trip, descend to the beach and head up the coast over boulders and finlike rock formations beside a sea cave into the tidepool area, 0.6 mile from the parking area. The rock formations in the tidepools and the nearby cliffs are thinly bedded shales, gently tilted and sometimes fantastically contorted, dating back about 12 million years. In most but not all places in the intertidal zone, this rock affords good traction even when wet.

In the intertidal strip itself, a few dozen steps from high-tide to low-tide level encompass a complete spectrum of marine plants and animals adapted to the various degrees of inundation and exposure. In the high intertidal zone, hardy species like periwinkle snails, limpets, mussels, barnacles, and green sea anemones are found. Some of these creatures are adapted to survival in habitats moistened only by the splash of breaking waves. Shore crabs patrol these bouldered spaces, but they'll likely be hiding.

Closer to the surf, the middle intertidal zone features rock depressions called tidepools, and luxuriant growths of surfgrass, which look like bright, shiny green mats of long-bladed grass. The tidepools serve as refuges for mobile animals like fish, shrimp, and the sluglike sea hare, as well as some of the relatively immobile animals like urchins and various shellfish. Here, the effects of biological erosion (or weathering) are apparent in the many pits and cubbyholes in the rocks occupied by various creatures.

In the low intertidal zone, many kinds of seaweeds thrive, including the intriguing sea palm. Animal life, however, is usually concealed beneath the rocks. Look for sea stars, sea urchins, sponges, worms, chitons, snails, abalones, and hermit crabs. If you're very lucky, an octopus may come your way. Remember that all marine life, shells, and rocks are protected.

CRYSTAL COVE STATE PARK

Giant keyhole limpet

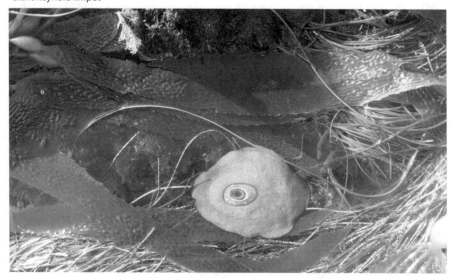

On your way up toward Little Corona Beach, you pass two picturesque sea stacks just offshore, both pierced by wave action. The first is known as Ladder Rock and the second Arch Rock, but either could just as well have been called Bird Rock for the ever-present pelicans and other avian life. Ladder Rock is 0.3 mile up the coast, and Arch Rock is another 0.3 mile beyond.

If you are traveling with small children or are becoming weary of navigating slippery rocks, the sea cave in the cliffs near Ladder Rock is a good turnaround point because you have seen the best of the tidepools and rock formations. If you still have energy, continue up the coast to the small Cameo Shores Beach, which, except during low tides, is only accessible via a locked gate from the private community. Continue past more tidepools to Shorecliff Beach, then past even more to Little Corona Beach by Arch Rock.

You can retrace your steps from Little Corona Beach, or use roads to complete a loop by walking up the beach access trail and veering right onto Poppy Avenue to reach the Pacific Coast Highway (Highway 1) in 0.4 mile. From here, Pelican Point is 1 mile southeast on the highway. If you didn't arrange a bicycle shuttle, you could take OC Transit Bus #1 to avoid walking along the busy road; the bus stops at Poppy Avenue and at Pelican Point Drive, where a trail shortcuts back into the state park.

trip 3.2 Crystal Cove Beaches

Distance	2–5.5 miles (loop)
Hiking Time	1–3 hours
Elevation Gain	100'
Difficulty	Easy–moderate
Trail Use	Good for kids
Best Times	All year
Agency	CCSP
Permit	CCSP parking fee required

see map on p. 30

DIRECTIONS There are three separate entrances to the bluff-and-beach section of Crystal Cove State Park: Pelican Point, Los Trancos, and Reef Point. All three are clearly marked with large brown signs posted on the Pacific Coast Highway (Highway 1) between Corona del Mar and Laguna Beach. For the longest loop, enter via Pelican Point on the west side of the PCH opposite Newport Coast Drive, turn right beyond the entrance station, and park in lot 2.

Hemmed in by 80-foot cliffs on one side and the restless surf on the other, Crystal Cove State Park's 3 miles of sandy beachfront seem strangely detached from the busy world above. Aside from the quaint beachfront-cottage community at Crystal Cove, recognized on the National Register of Historic Places, the midportion of the beach is largely free of encroachment by man-made structures. Come early in the morning, or anytime on a cold or rainy day, and you may have the beach all to yourself. The bluff tops represent the first (other than the one being cut now at beach level) of several successively higher and older marine terraces extending back into the interior San Joaquin Hills. Stay on the designated paths so as not to trample the sage scrub plant and wildlife community that has been reestablished here. Much of this vegetation looks brown and drab in summer and fall, when

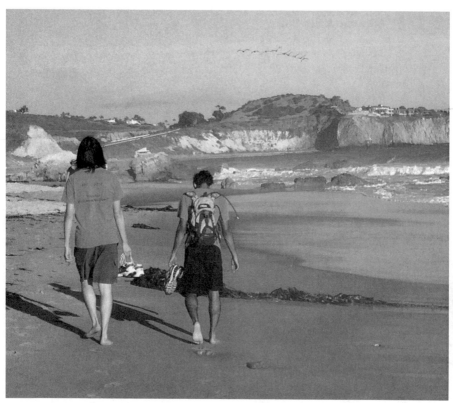

Crystal Cove State Beach

it is dormant, but it turns green and color-ful during the rainy season.

The tops of the bluffs are excellent for watching gray whales migrate along the shore from December through February, although it is not unusual to see whales spouting just off the coast at other times of year. Using binoculars, scan the ocean sur-face out to a distance of 1 or 2 miles. Early- to mid-morning light (sidelight) is best for this.

Below the cliffs on the gently shelv-ing beach, you can scuff through warm, squeaky sand above the high-tide line, tip-toe through beached kelp along with flocks of nervous shorebirds, or cool off in the undulating wash of the surf. Swimmers and surfers should beware of the rocky reefs submerged at higher tides. During low tides, the rocky reefs are exposed, promis-ing tidepool discoveries.

To explore the entire length of the beach, park at one of the lots at Pelican Point, pick a trail down to the sand, and follow the beach southeast. Pass the historic district, where you can find upscale refreshments at the Beachcomber Café near the mouth of Los Trancos Creek. Pass between the rocks and cliffs at Reef Point, and continue east over Moro Beach to the lifeguard headquar-ters near Abalone Point, nearly 3 miles from the start. On your way back, take the trail up to Reef Point and walk along the bluffs, enjoying the overlooks. Pass the bustling Shake Shack in the historic district, and continue back to your vehicle. For a shorter loop, you can trim off either end.

see map on p. 30

trip 3.3   Emerald Vista Point

Distance	4.6 miles (loop)
Hiking Time	2½ hours
Elevation Gain	800'
Difficulty	Moderate
Trail Use	Backpacking, cyclists, equestrians, good for kids
Best Times	October–May
Agency	CCSP
Permit	CCSP parking fee required

DIRECTIONS Crystal Cove State Park's visitor center and backcountry trailhead is located just east of the Pacific Coast Highway (Highway 1), 2 miles north of Laguna Beach and 3 miles south of Corona del Mar. The entrance driveway is well marked, and a traffic light has been installed here for safety. Follow the road as it veers right and passes the entrance station. Continue past Moro Campground and down the hill, then turn left (east) and drive to the trailhead parking near a picnic area at the end of the road.

On the most transparent winter days, the view from Emerald Vista Point spans more than 200 miles of Southern California coast and extends out to sea for a distance of 100 miles or more. Beyond Dana Point to the southeast, the low profile of San Diego's Point Loma can be traced along the curving shoreline, while offshore the diminutive Coronado Islands (just south of the international border) barely rise above the ocean haze. Southwest and west stand two big islands, San Clemente and Santa Catalina, the former a gently rising blister on the ocean surface,

the latter a bold headland sprawling across 25 degrees of ocean horizon. Over the top of the upthrust Palos Verdes peninsula and through the often murky Los Angeles Basin to the northwest, you can sometimes spy the Santa Monica Mountains and the faint blue coastline reaching west toward Santa Barbara.

If you plan to make this a backpacking trip, make a reservation at **reserveamerica .com** for Crystal Cove State Park Primitive Tent Camping (Lower or Upper Moro trail camps), or get a permit in person at the visitor center. The camping fees are

Prickly pear cactus at Emerald Vista

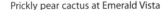

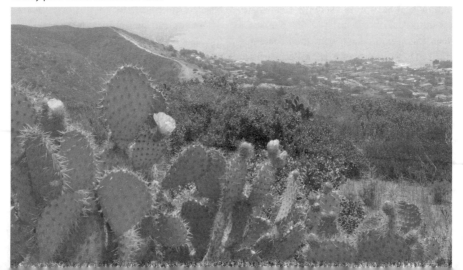

hefty considering the scrubby, waterless campground with a strenuous approach to a ridge miles from the beach.

From the top of the trailhead parking area, take the wide path up El Moro Canyon, then very quickly turn right on the narrow BFI Trail ("Big F. Inline"), and go up a grassy slope to the south. After sharply gaining about 200 feet of elevation, you connect with a service road winding up the west spur of El Moro Ridge. Continue climbing up the service road for 0.7 mile, then make a sharp right on a spur leading south to a small antenna facility on the shoulder of the ridge. Your views of Emerald Bay, the city of Laguna Beach, and out over the ocean are most panoramic here.

For a longer, more leisurely descent, follow the service road 0.7 mile farther north along El Moro Ridge (signed MORO RIDGE ROAD), then veer left down the East Cut-Across road to El Moro Canyon in 1.2 miles. Turn left there, and go down-canyon 1 mile to reach the wide trail leading out of the canyon and back toward the visitor center.

If you are backpacking, you'll travel farther north up El Moro Ridge. Add another mile for the round-trip to the Lower El Moro trail camp, or 2.8 miles round-trip if you're heading to the Upper El Moro trail camp.

---

trip 3.4 **El Moro Canyon Loop**

Distance	8 miles (loop)
Hiking Time	4½ hours
Elevation Gain	1,400′
Difficulty	Moderately strenuous
Trail Use	Cyclists, equestrians
Best Times	October–May
Agency	CCSP
Permit	CCSP parking fee required

see map on p. 30

DIRECTIONS Crystal Cove State Park's visitor center and backcountry trailhead is located just east of the Pacific Coast Highway (Highway 1), 2 miles north of Laguna Beach and 3 miles south of Corona del Mar. The entrance driveway is well marked, and a traffic light has been installed here for safety. After passing El Moro School, don't take the main road that veers right toward the entrance station. Instead, continue straight to the parking area by the ranger station, where you pay your day-use fee.

On this grand, looping tour of the Crystal Cove backcountry, you'll enjoy wide-ranging views from the spine of a prominent ridge along the way up, and you'll admire upper El Moro Canyon's fine oak woodlands on the way back down.

From the ranger station parking lot, take the dirt road leading east (No Dogs Road) toward a dry, scrub-covered ridge. After you climb a little, and if the morning marine-layer clouds have evaporated, fine views will open up of lower El Moro Canyon, the surrounding hills, and the blue ocean. Hawks and ravens soar on the updrafts generated on the sun-warmed slopes.

After 0.9 mile, the Poles Trail (a power-line road) on the right drops straight down into El Moro Canyon. Stay left and proceed generally north along the ridgeline. At the next intersection (1.5 miles), turn right on the West Cut-Across road. Descend only 0.2 mile, and then turn left on Rattlesnake Trail. It contours around a steep ravine (Deer Canyon), then climbs to the nose of the ridge between El Moro and Deer Canyons and ascends the steep rocky slope. All but the most gnarly cyclists hike-a-bike on this stretch.

As you approach an 844-foot high point on the ridge, the hike takes on a wilder

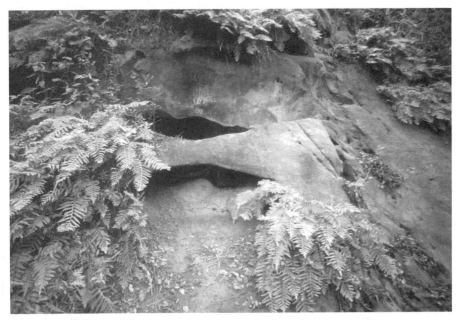

Fern grotto in El Moro Canyon

character. The narrow trail passes delicately sculpted outcrops of sandstone. The native coastal sage scrub vegetation crowding the trailside exudes a warm, spicy odor. In spring, the colorful blooms of sticky monkeyflower, goldenbush, and paintbrush play counterpoint to the muted greens of the sages, buckwheat, laurel sumac, and lemonade berry. Two kinds of cacti appear: common coastal prickly pear cactus and the somewhat uncommon coastal cholla cactus, whose easily detached bristling joints may snag the skin, clothing, or shoes of careless passersby.

At one point along the ridge, most of the near and far suburban landscapes are temporarily veiled from sight by intervening ridges; for a moment, you can picture southern Orange County as it was about a century ago. On clear days, Mount San Antonio (Old Baldy) pokes up behind a nearby ridge to the north, and Santa Catalina Island seems to float out at sea like a mountain range cast adrift from the mainland.

Up a little farther, join the Redtail Ridge fire road, and you can look down upon Deer Canyon trail camp nestled in a grove of sycamores in the shallow canyon to your left. Still farther up the ridgeline, a gate across the road marks the boundary between the state park and the Laguna Coast Wilderness Park. Shy of this gate, however, you pick up the narrow Fenceline Trail on the right leading southeast toward El Moro Canyon, parallel to the boundary fence. After 0.4 mile on this trail, you join a road coming in from the left. Keep straight momentarily, and turn left at the next junction to take the more scenic "Elevator Trail" east-side descent into upper El Moro Canyon, rather than the less scenic west-side descent called Slow 'n Easy Trail.

A steep (average 20% for 0.3 mile) grade follows, the bane of mountain bikers and hikers traveling either up or down. But afterward, you can let gravity repay you in a gentle way as you make a much more gradual descent along the bottom of El Moro Canyon.

Upper El Moro Canyon is far and away the most beautiful attraction in the park's backcountry. You stroll past thickets of willow, toyon, elderberry, and sycamore, all brightly illuminated by the sun; then suddenly plunge into cool, dark, cathedral-like recesses overhung by the massive limbs of live oaks. In one such recess, several shallow caves, adorned with ferns at their entrances, pock a sandstone outcrop next to the road. Prior to the establishment of the California missions, coast-dwelling Indians gathered acorns, seeds, and wild berries in this canyon. These foods, coupled with the abundant marine life nearby, provided a balanced and healthy diet.

Continue down El Moro Canyon to the trailhead at its mouth, then veer right onto the trail ascending the bluff back to the visitor center.

---

trip 3.5 **Deer Canyon Loop**

Distance	3.6 miles (loop)
Hiking Time	2 hours
Elevation Gain	600'
Difficulty	Moderate
Trail Use	Backpacking, cyclists, equestrians
Best Times	October–May
Agency	CCSP

see map on p. 30

DIRECTIONS This trip begins at the Pacific Ridge Trailhead near Coastal Peak Park atop the San Joaquin Hills. From Highway 1, follow Newport Coast Drive northeast for 2.4 miles. Turn right onto Ridge Park Road, and proceed 1.4 miles to park on the street by the park and trailhead.

Crystal Cove State Park's parking fee is comparable to other beach parking, but it's mighty high compared with entry fees for nearby wilderness parks. The Pacific Ridge Trailhead is increasingly popular because it is outside the park and avoids the hefty parking fee. This trip describes the shortest loop you might make into the park from the Pacific Ridge Trailhead. A brief study of the map will suggest many other options, including challenging treks to the sea of 10 miles or more.

The Deer Canyon loop route along the west edge of Crystal Cove's backcountry sector explores the park's higher ridges and valleys. Since there's little shade and views are the primary attraction, the hike is by far most rewarding on clear, cool winter or early spring days. Backpackers have the option of staying overnight at Deer Canyon's trail camp, near the halfway point of the loop. Make a reservation in advance at reserveamerica.com for Crystal Cove State Park Primitive Tent Camping, or get a permit in person at the visitor center.

From the three-way junction at the trailhead, pick up the Pacific Ridge Trail that leads south along a ridge. The vast area of luxury homes comes into view on your right, a stark contrast with the open, protected lands of the South Coast Wilderness on your left. Soon enter land belonging to Laguna Coast Wilderness Park. At 1.4 miles, pass a gate where the path enters Crystal Cove State Park and changes to No Name Ridge Road.

Just beyond, look for the narrow, rutty "Ticketron" trail branching left. Ticketron makes a radical drop (at least for mountain bike riders) toward the floor of shallow Deer Canyon, then settles into an easy grade as it approaches the trail camp, which features a picnic bench, a composting toilet, and sites to pitch a tent down near a scraggly line of live oaks and sycamores.

CRYSTAL COVE STATE PARK

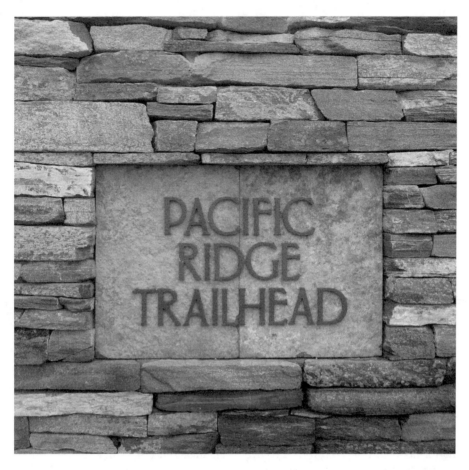

Beyond the campground, a short, steep climb leads to Redtail Ridge Trail, which is a fire road to the left (north). Follow this path north to a T-junction with Bommer Ridge Road, where you turn left and loop back to the trailhead.

chapter 4

Laguna Coast Wilderness Park

The quintessentially coastal town of Laguna Beach blankets pillowy hills that rise abruptly from the sea to an elevation of nearly 1,000 feet. Many of its finest houses cling precipitously to ledges cut into the steep slopes. Other houses seemingly defy gravity by resting upon cantilevered platforms or spidery networks of steel poles. There is an almost universal striving to capture a piece of the view, which without a doubt encompasses one of California's most dramatic stretches of coastline.

Laguna Beach residents have faced disasters periodically. The Laguna Beach Fire destroyed hundreds of homes in 1993. A landslide on a waterlogged slope destroyed or destabilized dozens of hillside homes in early 2005.

Laguna residents have also been fiercely protective of the natural environment around their coastal town. In the 1980s and '90s, they spearheaded a campaign to protect thousands of acres of land in and around Laguna Canyon slated for development. Those efforts reached a dramatic crescendo in 1989 when more than 8,000 people marched down the road through Laguna Canyon protesting the Irvine Company's plan to build a huge housing development there. In what many regard as a win–win outcome, the company was allowed to proceed with massive urban development elsewhere, and large parcels of land, such as the Laguna Coast Wilderness Park, were created with the help of grants, donations, and park bond funds. The park now forms the heart of the South Coast Wilderness.

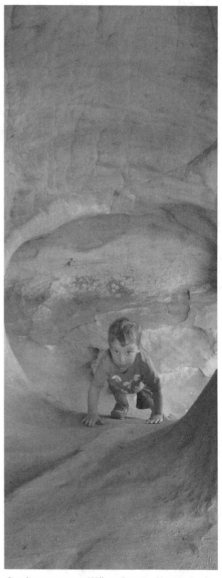

Sandstone cave at Willow Canyon Staging Area

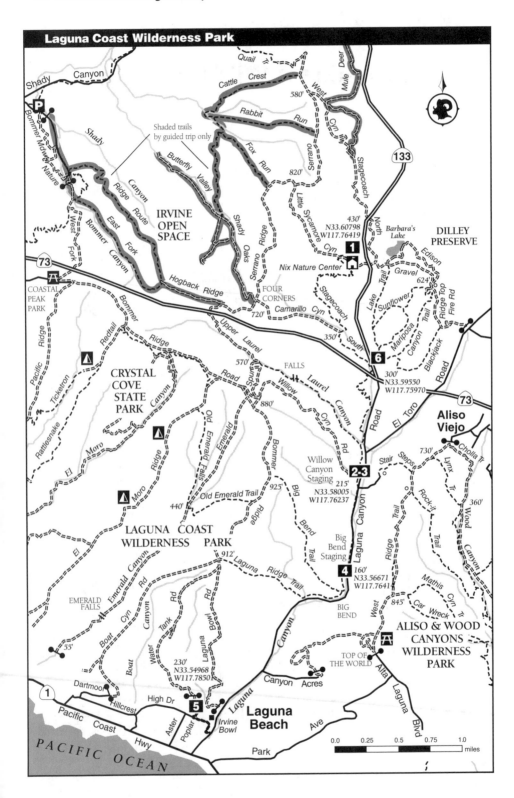

Laguna Coast Wilderness Park

Shady
Canyon

Quail

Cattle Crest

Rabbit Run

580'

West

Mule

Deer

Cyn Trl

Stagecoach

133

Serrano

Fox Run

Butterfly Valley

820'

Shady
Oaks

Serrano Ridge

Little Sycamore

Cyn

430'
N33.60798
W117.76419

1

Nix Nature Center

Barbara's
Lake

DILLEY
PRESERVE

Edison

Gravel

624'

Shaded trails
by guided trip only

IRVINE
OPEN
SPACE

Shady

Canyon
Route

Ridge

East

Fork

Bommer Canyon

West
Fork

Bommer Ridge Nature

P

73

COASTAL
PEAK
PARK

Hogback Ridge

FOUR
CORNERS
720'

Camarillo Cyn

Stagecoach

Lake Trail

Sunflower

Mariposa

Canyon Trail

Blackjack

Ridge Top
Fire Rd

South

350'

6

300'
N33.59550
W117.75970

73

Aliso
Viejo

Pacific Ridge

Redtail

Bommer

Ridge

Upper Laurel

570'

FALLS

Laurel

Willow

Cyn

Canyon Rd

880'

CRYSTAL
COVE
STATE
PARK

Ticketron

El Moro

Moro Ridge

Old Emerald Falls

Emerald

Bommer Ridge

Willow
Canyon
Staging
215'
N33.58005
W117.76237

730'

Stair Steps

Cholla Tr

Lynx Tr

Rock-it Trail

360'

Wood Canyon

Rattlesnake

El

Moro

Old Emerald Trail

440'

925'

Big

Bend Trail

2-3

Ridge Trail

Mathis Cyn Tr

LAGUNA COAST
WILDERNESS PARK

912' Laguna Ridge Trail

Big
Bend
Staging

4

160'
N33.56671
W117.7641

845'

Car Wreck

West Trail

EMERALD
FALLS

Emerald Canyon Rd

Boat Cyn

Water Canyon Rd

Tank Rd

Laguna Bowl Rd

BIG
BEND

ALISO & WOOD
CANYONS
WILDERNESS
PARK

55'

230'
N33.54968
W117.7850

Canyon

Canyon Acres

TOP OF
THE WORLD

Alta Laguna Blvd

1

Dartmoor

Hillcrest

High Dr

Aster

Poplar

5

Irvine
Bowl

Laguna
Beach

Canyon

Ave

Park

Pacific Coast Hwy

PACIFIC OCEAN

0.0   0.25   0.5   0.75   1.0
miles

Nix Loop

Distance	4.4 miles (loop)
Hiking Time	2½ hours
Elevation Gain	800′
Difficulty	Moderate
Trail Use	Hiking only
Best Times	October–May
Agency	OC Parks: LCWP
Permit	OC Parks parking fee required

DIRECTIONS Park at the Nix Nature Center on the west side of Laguna Canyon Road (Highway 133), 1.1 miles north of the 73 Toll Road.

Starting at the James and Rosemary Nix Nature Center, this loop tours sage scrub slopes and a ridgeline offering far-reaching views. The center is the headquarters for the Laguna Coast Wilderness Park; visit **ocparks .com** for a schedule of interpretive events.

Many trails radiate from the parking area. Be sure to start up Little Sycamore Canyon from the trailhead to the right of the center. Promptly cross Marys Trail (an interpretive nature trail), then cross it again before making a steep ascent into the canyon. The sycamores on the canyon floor are stunted, perhaps by the sandstone bedrock that lays just beneath the soil. Your path leads through tall laurel sumac shrubs and through other coastal sage scrub, including

black and white sage, California sagebrush, bush sunflower, and California everlasting. The hill to the north is pockmarked with small caves once used by the Tongva tribe of Native Americans.

In 1 mile, reach the top of the canyon, and turn right onto the Serrano Ridge Trail at post #29. The ridge offers expansive views from Santiago Peak to the San Gabriels and the Palos Verdes Hills, including the high-rises and countless subdivisions of Irvine. Turkey vultures favor this ridge, riding the thermals in search of carrion. You'll also likely encounter mountain bikers making a loop from Quail Hill. Pass the Rabbit Run Trail leading west into the Irvine Open Space Preserve; this trail is closed to the

Serrano Ridge

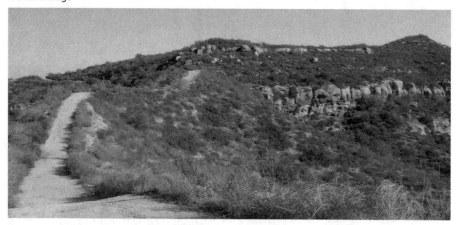

public except by guided tour and on special access days.

In 1.1 miles, drop to a saddle where you can turn right onto the West Canyon Trail. The road descends to a junction with the Mule Deer Trail (access to which is also restricted) and some utility roads, then undulates southward through the sage scrub. In another 1.5 mile, pass under two highway bridges. Parallel the busy Highway 133 for 0.5 mile to a junction at the edge of Dilley Preserve, where you turn right and pass under another set of highway bridges to return to the nature center.

| trip 4.2 | Laurel Canyon Loop |

see map on p. 42

Distance	3.5 miles (loop)
Hiking Time	2 hours
Elevation Gain	700'
Difficulty	Moderate
Trail Use	Good for kids
Best Times	All year
Agency	OC Parks: LCWP
Permit	OC Parks parking fee required

DIRECTIONS Park at Laguna Coast Wilderness Park's Willow Canyon staging area on the west side of Laguna Canyon Road, 3 miles north of Laguna Beach. This point is 5 miles south of the 405 Freeway, 0.7 mile south of the 73 Toll Road, and 0.2 mile south of the intersection of El Toro and Laguna Canyon Roads.

The best single hike within the Laguna Coast Wilderness Park is surely the secluded Laurel Canyon loop. Though it lies close to the San Joaquin Hills Transportation Corridor tollway, that roadway and much of its associated urban development is hidden from both sight and sound along most of the route.

Volunteers frequently staff a booth at the Willow Canyon staging area, offering tips

Banshee Rock, in Laurel Canyon, was formed by sandstone weathering.

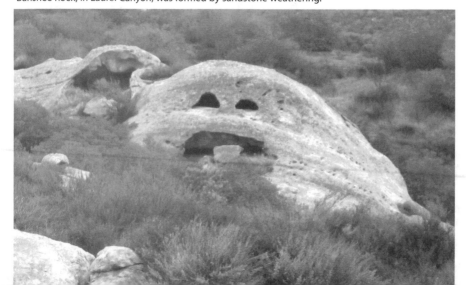

about the logistics of hiking in the park as well as the area's natural history. Follow the fire road beyond—Willow Canyon Road, which gains nearly 600 feet of elevation in the next 1.5 miles. Springtime wildflowers bloom in profusion along this stretch, which cuts along east- and north-facing slopes smothered in thick chaparral.

At 1.5 miles, turn right on the first intersecting pathway. Traverse a grassy meadow, and then follow the trail as it plunges down through more dense growths of chaparral toward the narrow bottom of Laurel Canyon. The deeper you go, the more you gain a sense of seclusion. Once you arrive in the canyon bottom (2 miles), don't miss the turn onto the narrow trail that branches right and goes down (not up) the canyon.

Graced with gorgeous oaks and sycamores (and copious amounts of poison oak), Laurel Canyon has recovered from the extremely hot, fast-moving Laguna Beach Fire of October 1993. Nearly all of the vegetation you see here is no stranger to periodic fires. Centuries ago, coastal Southern California landscapes, such as this one, were visited by fire every decade or so.

At 2.4 miles, you pass near the lip of a dramatic dropoff—a seasonal waterfall nearly 100 feet high. During the extraordinarily wet winter of 2005, hikers beheld a spectacular sight of plunging water, but most years, this declivity sports only a modest trickle.

Past the lip of the falls, you swing to the left side of the canyon bottom and descend along a dry, south-facing slope. By 3 miles, you emerge in a grassy meadow that is either green, golden, or transitional in color, depending on the season. Cavernous sandstone outcrops dot the meadow on the left and the slope on the right. The shapes of some suggest grotesque skulls and other figures. The path through the meadow soon flanks busy Laguna Canyon Road, climbs south to an exposed earthquake fault, and returns you to your starting point.

---

trip 4.3   ## Emerald Canyon

Distance	8 miles (out-and-back)
Hiking Time	4 hours
Elevation Gain	1,400'
Difficulty	Moderately strenuous
Trail Use	Cyclists, equestrians
Best Times	November–May
Agency	OC Parks: LCWP
Permit	OC Parks parking fee required

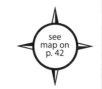

see map on p. 42

DIRECTIONS Park at Laguna Coast Wilderness Park's Willow Canyon staging area on the west side of Laguna Canyon Road, 3 miles north of Laguna Beach. This point is 5 miles south of the 405 Freeway, 0.7 mile south of the 73 Toll Road, and 0.2 mile south of the intersection of El Toro and Laguna Canyon Roads.

Equally as beautiful as El Moro Canyon in neighboring Crystal Cove State Park, Emerald Canyon receives much less visitation. Entry to the lower end of the canyon by way of Laguna Beach's city streets is blocked by a formidable fence, so it's only accessible from above.

Both hikers and mountain bikers can follow the route as described here. Hikers and gonzo mountain bikers, either on the way out or the way back if they choose, can also follow a somewhat longer variant of the route by utilizing the singletrack Old Emerald Trail.

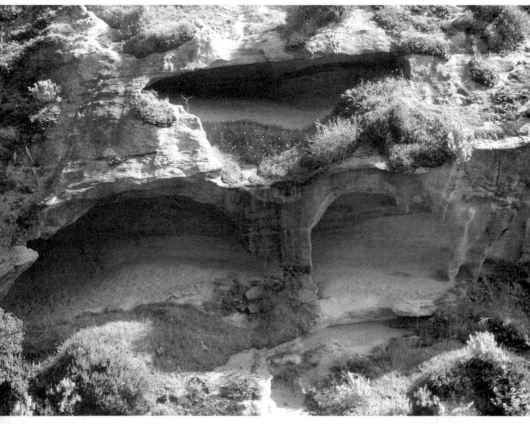

Sandstone caves, Emerald Canyon

Follow Willow Canyon Road 1.5 miles to the Laurel Canyon turnoff, but stay straight (south) and climb 0.1 mile to an intersection with Bommer Ridge Road. Turn right, proceed 0.1 mile to a dip in the road, and turn left onto Emerald Canyon Road. That "road"—essentially a wide trail—descends along the top of the ridge for a mile, through growths of sage, encelia, and monkeyflower blooming in shades from orange to yellow.

After a mile on the descending ridge, you arrive on the canyon bottom, at a signed junction where the narrow Old Emerald Trail branches left. The next 1.5 miles of travel down-canyon is along a more moderate grade, and the scenery is simply gorgeous. Gnarled oaks and sycamores (survivors of repeated firestorms) line the trail, and dense willows flank the canyon's seasonal stream. Take care not to brush against the luxuriant poison oak lining the trail. About halfway down this easy stretch, note the spacious cave pocking a large sandstone outcrop on the left, across the canyon bottom.

At 4.2 miles from the start, you arrive at a place where the trail curls sharply downward and a 20-foot-tall waterfall lies to the right. More like a "dry" fall in most years, it comes alive only with sustained heavy rains. This is a good spot to take a break, and afterward return the way you came. The remaining half-mile down to and back from the secure fence at the edge of Laguna Beach is worth exploring only if you have energy to spare.

trip 4.4 **Big Bend Loop**

Distance	3.9 miles (loop)
Hiking Time	2½ hours
Elevation Gain	1,100′
Difficulty	Moderate
Trail Use	Hiking only
Best Times	November–May
Agency	OC Parks: LCWP
Permit	OC Parks parking fee required

see map on p. 42

DIRECTIONS Park at Laguna Coast Wilderness Park's Big Bend parking lot on the west side of Laguna Canyon Road, 2 miles north of Laguna Beach and 2 miles south of the 73 Toll Road.

Both the beginning section on Big Bend Trail and the ending section on Laguna Ridge Trail will test the mettle of any hiker due to their combination of steepness and roughness. Although mountain bikes are technically allowed on the route, much of your effort would go into slinging your bike over your shoulder and slip-sliding down the steepest grades. You might as well walk!

The low-growing coastal sage scrub and grassland vegetation on the slopes and ridges hereabouts does little to block views of the ocean, hills, and distant mountains. This is a hike best taken, then, whenever the air is beautifully transparent.

From the Big Bend staging area, head south and start climbing immediately on the Big Bend Trail, a wide fire road. At 0.2 mile, just as you cross under some power lines, note the obscure path to the left. You will arrive at this spot again near the end of the hike. Turn right and head straight

Laguna Ridge Trail

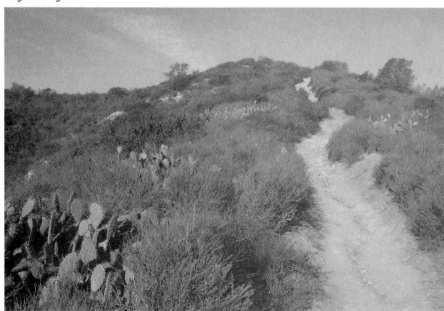

up the hill. Stay right at an immediate fork where a powerline road veers left.

The Big Bend Trail takes you ever upward along a ridgeline on a course absolutely committed to gaining elevation as quickly as possible. A couple of flat stretches along the way allow you to catch your breath and look around. Before long, cars and buildings in Laguna Canyon below begin to look toylike. You may spot scallop fossils near your feet if your eyes are glued to the ground.

At 1.6 miles, you come to an intersection with the wide Bommer Ridge Road. Turn left and proceed south on a gently falling, then gently rising course to the intersection of Boat Canyon Road on the right (2.5 miles from the start). On the left, just past Boat Canyon Road but before the next intersecting road on the right, take the narrow Laguna Ridge Trail, which goes briefly up a 912-foot knoll, then suddenly and precipitously plunges down to Laguna Canyon.

Rough and worn deeply into the sandstone bedrock, it approaches a 40% grade in a couple of spots. It, too, sticks to a plunging ridgeline. Near the bottom of that plunge, the trail veers left (east), almost reaching the pavement of Laguna Canyon Road (3.3 miles). The final leg goes up and down a couple of times, staying parallel to but decently clear of the busy roadway. At 3.7 miles, you meet Big Bend Trail, which leads 0.2 mile down to the starting point.

---

trip 4.5 **Laguna Bowl Loop**

Distance	4.1 miles (loop)
Hiking Time	2 hours
Elevation Gain	950'
Difficulty	Moderate
Trail Use	Cyclists, equestrians
Best Times	All year
Agency	OC Parks: LCWP

see map on p. 42

DIRECTIONS Follow Aster Street north from the Pacific Coast Highway (Highway 1) in Laguna Beach. Continue 0.3 mile to High Drive; go right one block, and turn left on Poplar Street. Follow Poplar to its end, and park on the street.

On many a fall or winter morning, a damp, opaque layer of air a few hundred feet deep lies over the low-lying Southern California coast. By 9 or 10 in the morning, the sun usually burns through this marine-layer fog, ushering in a fine day of mild sunshine. Sleepy-eyed hikers never know what they're missing unless they get an early start on a coastal hiking route, such as this one, that pokes above the cloud layer.

Squeeze through a gate at the east end of Poplar Street, and start up a very steep paved road. After 0.1 mile, the paved road enters a fenced water-tank and antenna facility, but a steep bypass trail skirts the fenced area on the right and keeps climbing. Soon that bypass joins the dirt Water Tank Road. You continue climbing, but more moderately. At about 0.4 mile and 550 feet of elevation, you enter Laguna Coast Wilderness Park property. The early morning boundary between fog and clear air often lies at about this level. If that is the case when you're there, then the next couple of miles will be an absolute delight.

Right at the boundary between clear air and cloud, look westward (opposite the rising sun), and you may see the upper arc of a colorless rainbow (the so-called white rainbow) that results from sunlight refracting through water droplets much smaller than those of falling rain. Another remarkable spectacle, called the "glory" or "Specter of the Brocken," is visible whenever you can

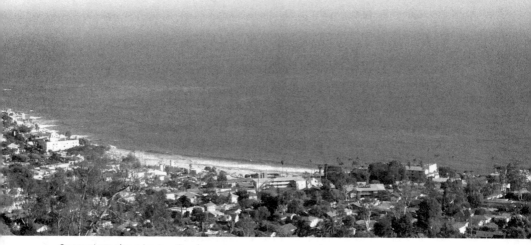

Ocean views above Laguna Beach

manage to cast the shadow of your own body onto a bank of fog. The ghostly specter is that of concentric rings of colored light at the spot exactly 180° away from the sun. The right conditions and optical geometry exist during the first hour or so after sunrise.

At 1.5 miles, you arrive at the junction of Bommer Ridge Road (to the left) and Laguna Bowl Road (to the right). Turn right, head south along the top of the ridgeline, and enjoy vistas of the blue ocean ahead or of tendrils of fog below, depending on the atmospheric conditions. At 2.2 miles, the road forks; take the right branch, staying on Laguna Bowl Road. Soon afterward, you commence a quick, steep descent that takes you past the fenced Irvine Bowl outdoor amphitheater and down to Laguna Canyon Road.

To complete the loop, you must follow city streets. Turn right, follow the sidewalk of Laguna Canyon Road for 0.25 mile, turn right on Acacia Drive, and immediately go right on High Drive. Follow High Drive for 0.25 mile, and turn right on Poplar Street to return to your car.

trip 4.6   **Dilley Preserve**

Distance	2.9 miles (loop)
Hiking Time	1½ hours
Elevation Gain	350′
Difficulty	Moderate
Trail Use	Good for kids
Best Times	All year
Agency	OC Parks: LCWP
Permit	OC Parks parking fee required

see map on p. 42

DIRECTIONS The Dilley Preserve parking area is on the east side of Laguna Canyon Road just north of the 73 Toll Road off-ramp. It can also be reached from Highway 1 by taking Laguna Canyon Road 4.4 miles north, or from the 405 Freeway by taking Laguna Canyon Road (also called Highway 133) 4 miles south.

The James Dilley Greenbelt Preserve, a unit within the Laguna Coast Wilderness Park, dates back to a landmark purchase by the City of Laguna Beach in 1978. Environmentalist James Dilley helped champion the concept of greenbelts, or parcels of open space between cityscapes.

The preserve's trail system is pieced together out of former bulldozed roads and current utility roads. The 2.9-mile loop described here covers the most interesting trails and touches upon the best sights the preserve has to offer. The first stretch (Canyon Trail) doubles as a portion of the 1.8-mile Bea Whittlesly Loop, a self-guided nature trail that features posts keyed to a brochure available at the Nix Nature Center or via your cell phone.

From the Dilley staging area, head east across a field of sage and buckwheat on the Canyon Trail, which at first gains elevation gradually and stays near the bottom of a small canyon dotted with gorgeous specimens of coast live oak and California sycamore. At about 0.7 mile, the trail begins a steeper ascent, curling upward through a patch of prickly pear cactus (look or listen for cactus wrens). At 1 mile, you arrive on top of a buried water reservoir on a 624-foot knoll. Take a look around. Leisure World lies to the east, the open spaces of the South Coast Wilderness sprawl to the south and west, and the winter-snow-capped summit of Mount San Antonio floats above the often hazy urban landscape to the north.

Next, slip down the slope northeast of the reservoir to reach a maintained gravel fire road following the ridgetop. Jog left, then immediately veer right onto the Edison road that stays more or less underneath the high-voltage power lines. That route takes you down to and then right along the shoreline of beautiful Barbara's Lake, the larger of two small lakes that constitute Orange County's only naturally formed inland bodies of water. They are geologically described as small sag ponds, located where the ground has subsided due to movements along a fault. Because Barbara's Lake is shallow and its drainage area

Watching for wildlife at Barbara's Lake

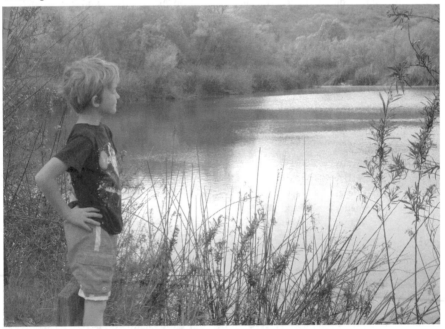

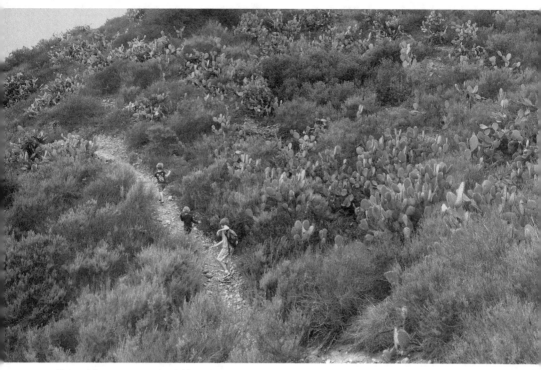

Young hikers tromp past prickly pear cactus.

small, it is believed that artesian springs on the its bottom help keep it full no matter what the season. It expanded in 2005 following the realignment and widening of Laguna Canyon Road. The old roadbed, which formerly divided the lake from Bubbles Pond, has been obliterated, and the two bodies of water have merged. Another lake, a seasonal body of water called Lake 1, lies about 0.5 mile north along Laguna Canyon Road.

At Barbara's Lake and elsewhere in the Laguna Coast Wilderness Park, large plaques feature original plein-air paintings by local artists. Ultraviolet-resistant coatings on the paintings have kept them from fading much over the years.

From the gravel road at the south end of Barbara's Lake (2 miles), you can make a side trip under Laguna Canyon Road's arched overpasses to reach the James and Rosemary Nix Nature Center on the far side. The strange cavities on the undersides of those overpasses are entrances into the hollow interiors of the concrete structures where bats and swallows live.

Our route, however, jogs left on the gravel road, then right onto the Lake Trail, which leads south back toward the trailhead. Pass a junction with the Sunflower Trail. Reach another junction with the Mariposa Trail within view of the parking lot. Veer left onto the Mariposa Trail and then right, down to the trailhead.

chapter 5

Aliso and Wood Canyons
Wilderness Park

Aliso Creek starts at the foot of the Santa Ana Mountains and flows down to the Pacific. Over the past 1.2 million years, the San Joaquin Hills have been pushed up along the coast by a blind thrust fault. The creek, which predated this uplift, continued to flow in its course, cutting the steep Aliso Canyon through the hills.

Orange County dedicated Aliso and Wood Canyons Wilderness Park in 1979 to protect Aliso Canyon, the surrounding ridges, and its most attractive major tributary. The park covers public-utility lands and other formerly private properties. It became an instant hit with all sorts of self-propelled travelers when it opened.

These trips will take you to some of the finest overlooks along the California coast and guide you into many a quiet canyon recess. You can also start at the headwaters and follow Aliso Creek all the way to the canyon (see Trip 18.3). Unfortunately, the lower end of the canyon is closed to public access because it is blocked by a private resort. Please observe park closure at sunset.

Pacific views from the Seaview Trail

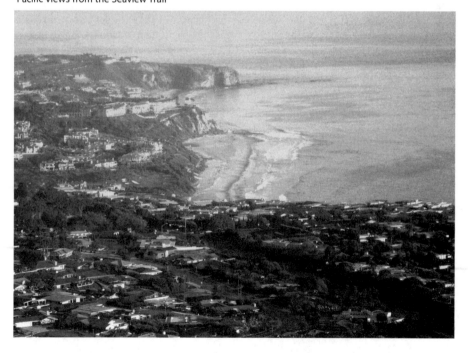

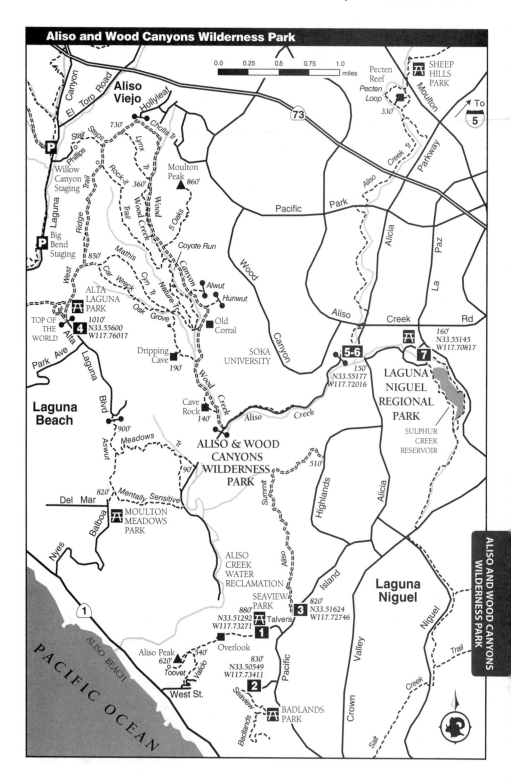

see
map on
previous
page

trip 5.1   **Seaview Park Overlook and Aliso Summit**

Distance	0.6 mile or 1.6 miles (out-and-back)
Hiking Time	½ hour or longer
Elevation Gain	50' or 500'
Difficulty	Easy or moderate
Trail Use	Dogs, good for kids
Best Times	All year
Agency	OC Parks: AWCWP

DIRECTIONS From Interstate 5, exit south on Alicia Parkway. In 5.9 miles, turn right on Pacific Island Drive, then in 1.2 miles, turn right again on Talvera Drive. Continue 0.3 mile west to its end at Seaview Park. If you are coming from the south via Crown Valley Parkway, turn north on Pacific Island Drive, and go 1.6 miles to Talvera Drive.

Starting from Seaview Park in the city of Laguna Niguel, this brief walk takes you past several interpretive panels annotating the common species of vegetation found throughout coastal Southern California. The path leads to a concrete platform offering a jaw-dropping view of the hills of Laguna Beach spilling down to the ocean. If you live in Orange County, this somewhat obscure overlook is a good spot to keep in mind when entertaining out-of-town relatives or friends.

Start walking at the west end of the grassy strip running along the brink of Aliso Canyon in Seaview Park. Follow a wide, ridge-running path going west. Notice the differences between the types of vegetation growing on the two sides of the path. Dense chaparral clings to the steep, north-facing slope to the right, which drops a sheer 800 feet to Aliso Creek. A sparser assemblage of mostly coastal sage scrub plants lies exposed to the sun's harshest rays on the left, south-facing, side of the path. Only a few minutes' walk takes you to the viewing platform, which is a good turnaround point if you want an easy hike.

Beyond the platform, a narrower trail continues: It pitches sharply downward, skirts a residential street, and drops to a four-way junction in a saddle. The unmarked path dropping to the left is the Valido Trail, which drops to a residential neighborhood on Valido Road. This pleasant walk would be recommended except that the Valido Trailhead lacks adequate parking. The signed Toovet Trail veers slightly left and contours around the hill. *Toovet* is an Acajchemem tribe word for "bush rabbit." The path would more aptly be named "Sewer Line Trail" because it leads to a foul-smelling dead end near a water tank and is not recommended.

Stay straight and make the short climb to Aliso Summit. From there, the ocean shore lies just 0.4 mile away and 600 feet below.

Aliso Peak

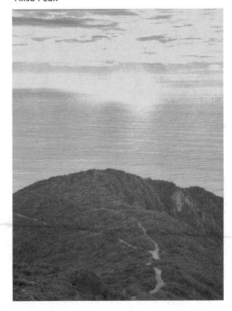

| **trip 5.2** | **Seaview and Badlands Trails** |

Distance	2.0 miles (out-and-back)
Hiking Time	1 hour
Elevation Gain	150′
Difficulty	Easy
Trail Use	Cyclists, equestrians, dogs, good for kids
Best Times	All year
Agency	OC Parks: AWCWP

see map on p. 53

DIRECTIONS From Interstate 5, exit south on Alicia Parkway. In 5.9 miles, turn right on Pacific Island Drive, then in 1.7 miles, turn right again on Ocean Way. Continue 0.3 mile west to its end, and park on the street nearby, taking care to observe parking restrictions. If you are coming from the south via Crown Valley Parkway, turn north on Pacific Island Drive and go 1.1 miles to Ocean Way.

The short but scenic Seaview and Badlands Trails provide million-dollar views from an ancient seashore now thrust far above the Pacific.

From the west end of Ocean Way, walk south past bollards on the signed Seaview Trail. After a short, steep descent, come to a junction. A spur on the right leads to a fire road, but this trip turns left and continues south on the Seaview Trail through coastal sage scrub overlooking the Pacific. You soon pass a cluster of picnic tables called Badlands Park, then, at 0.3 mile, reach a boardwalk with steps on the right signed for Badlands Trail.

The Seaview Trail continues briefly to an unceremonious end above Monarch Crest, but this trip turns onto the Badlands Trail beneath eroded cliffs. At the end of the boardwalk, the path turns to sand. In the Miocene era, 10 million years ago, this area was once a beach, but now it has been heaved 800 feet upward. At a unmarked fork, a path on the right leads to a Pacific Ocean overlook beside a sandstone outcrop.

After you have enjoyed the view, take the left path, which may initially appear unpromising but soon broadens into a well-maintained trail leading south atop the bluffs just west of a row of mansions. At the south end of the ridge, come to another vista point with terrific views of Dana Point. Salt Creek Beach is the prominent beach between you and the point. Catalina and San Clemente Islands may rise out of the mist.

You can continue as the trail loops north toward Monarch Crest and then east past more mansions before abruptly ending on a ridge with more fine views. Enjoy the sights and then return the way you came.

Watching the sun set at Badlands Park

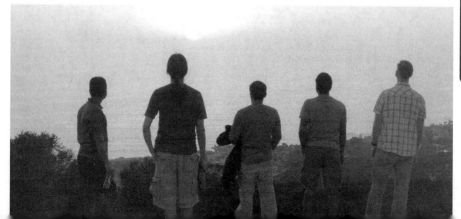

ALISO AND WOOD CANYONS WILDERNESS PARK

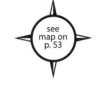

trip 5.3 **Aliso Summit Trail**

Distance	4.4 miles (out-and-back)
Hiking Time	2 hours
Elevation Gain	350'
Difficulty	Moderate
Trail Use	Cyclists, equestrians, dogs, good for kids
Best Times	All year
Agency	OC Parks: AWCWP

see map on p. 53

DIRECTIONS From Interstate 5, exit south on Alicia Parkway. In 5.9 miles, turn right on Pacific Island Drive, then in 1 mile, park on the shoulder opposite La Brise at the sign for the Aliso Summit Trail.

This neighborhood trail on the ridge overlooking Aliso Canyon doubles as a firebreak that separates the huge hilltop mansions from the fire-prone sage scrub in the canyon. The mellow hike is popular with locals because of its sweeping views. Cyclists connect with city streets for a hilly loop.

The broad trail makes one short switchback and then runs mostly level northward with views over lower Aliso Canyon and out to Catalina Island. As you pass a knoll on the left, step off the trail to the summit for good canyon views. As the trail bends eastward, views of the Santa Ana Mountains and the suburbs of Orange County replace ocean views. After 1.5 miles, the trail begins a steeper descent, passing a water tank and ending at the corner of Highlands Avenue and Ridgeview Drive. Those looking for an easy hike may wish to turn around before the descent.

Aliso Summit Trail

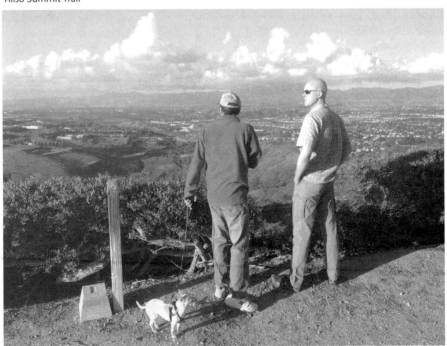

see map on p. 53

trip 5.4   **Top of the World Loop**

Distance	6 miles (semiloop)
Hiking Time	3 hours
Elevation Gain	1,000'
Difficulty	Moderate
Trail Use	Cyclists, equestrians
Best Times	All year
Agency	OC Parks: AWCWP

DIRECTIONS From the Pacific Coast Highway (Highway 1) in Laguna Beach 0.3 mile south of Laguna Canyon Road, turn east onto Legion Street. In 0.3 mile, stay right to merge onto Park Avenue. Follow Park Avenue as it curves up the hill for 1.6 miles, then turn left on Alta Laguna Boulevard, and follow it 0.2 mile to its end at Alta Laguna Park.

As you can see from the map, Aliso and Wood Canyons have several other access points besides the main Amwa Road staging area, and you can make enjoyable loops from any of them. This trip starts at the aptly named Top of the World trailhead and visits the west side of the wilderness park, providing the most direct access to its verdant heart. Expect panoramic views from the ridges, lovely oak-shaded paths on the canyon floors, and hordes of hikers and bikers nearly everywhere. If you have more time, you can lengthen this trip with pleasant excursions up the Wood Creek Trail, the Five Oaks Trail to Moulton Peak, or the Dripping Cave Trail to the cave where stagecoach robbers hid out during the days of the Wild West.

From the trailhead, head north on the West Ridge Trail, a broad fire road. In 0.6 mile, pass the Mathis Canyon Trail, by which you will return. In another mile, reach a water tank and microwave antenna site where you can turn right onto the Rock-it Trail. Initially a service road, it soon narrows and steepens as it descends. The exposed sandstone bedrock offers a stimulating ride for mountain bikers.

In 1.3 miles, reach a T-junction with the Coyote Trail on the bottom near a grove of

Car Wreck Trail

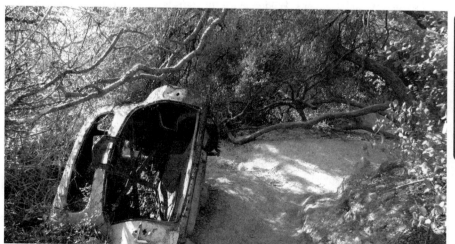

mistletoe-laden sycamores. Turn right and take the Coyote Run Trail for 0.3 mile to a junction with the Nature Trail. Cyclists must stay on the Coyote Run Trail, but hikers can veer left onto the Nature Trail, which climbs to follow the crest of a narrow ridge with excellent views over the sage scrub.

In either case, your path reaches the wide Mathis Canyon fire road in 0.6 mile near a bridge over Wood Creek. Turn right and head up the road for 0.3 mile, then stay left onto the Oak Grove Trail. A bench under some live oaks offers a relaxing place to rest before you climb out of the canyon. Just beyond, the trail changes names to Car Wreck Trail. This trail was constructed by volunteer mountain bikers in collaboration with park rangers and opened in 2010.

As you begin to climb, stay right at an unmarked junction to reach the wreck, turned on its side and half-buried. Make a 500-foot ascent directly up a steep and rocky ridge, a sweaty grunt that gonzo cyclists prefer to attempt downhill. When you rejoin the Mathis Canyon Trail in 0.9 mile, turn left, continue 0.1 mile to the West Ridge Trail, and return 0.6 mile to your starting point at Top of the World.

trip 5.5   Aliso and Wood Canyons Loop

see map on p. 53

Distance	10 miles (semiloop)
Hiking Time	5 hours
Elevation Gain	1,000'
Difficulty	Moderately strenuous
Trail Use	Cyclists, equestrians
Best Times	November–June
Agency	OC Parks: AWCWP
Permit	OC Parks parking fee required

DIRECTIONS The main Aliso and Wood Canyon Wilderness Park trailhead is located opposite Laguna Niguel Regional Park. From Interstate 5 in Laguna Hills, take Exit 90 and follow Alicia Parkway southwest for 4 miles, then turn right onto Amwa Road. Turn left into the wilderness park parking area (fee required).

Aliso and Wood Canyons Wilderness Park consists of more than 4,200 acres of shallow canyons, sandstone rock formations, narrow strips of oak and riparian woodland, and hillsides draped with aromatic sage scrub vegetation. Subdivisions and subdivisions-in-the-making press in along the park's long, narrow boundary, which is perforated by many neighborhood access points.

This trip takes you on a grand, looping tour of the Wood Canyon section of the park. The park's multiuse trails accommodate all sorts of self-propelled travelers. You will unavoidably encounter passing mountain bikes, though this route mostly avoids the trails favored by cyclists. Try to explore the park during the gorgeous green months of February through April. During summer, the midday hours are uncomfortably warm, though the early-morning and pre-sunset periods are often fairly cool.

The sole trail departing the parking lot takes you subtly downhill along the wide floodplain of Aliso Canyon. This first part is, frankly, unexciting. You follow the shoulder of the service road for about 0.7 mile, then diverge on a trail that stays within a short distance of the road. The glimpses you get of sandstone outcrops on hillsides to the north are intriguing. This sandstone was derived from layers of sand deposited in an offshore environment some 15 million years ago. Soon you will see a lot more of it at close range.

At 1.4 miles, you arrive at a major junction, with restrooms and benches, where the two canyons—Aliso and Wood—join. Head north on Wood Canyon Trail (the dirt road up Wood Canyon), and you soon spy, on the left, Cave Rock, a series of wind caves pocking a sandstone ledge. The 0.2-mile Cave Rock Trail on the left is worth taking for a close-up view. When weak sedimentary rock is exposed to air and dripping water, the effects of chemical weathering loosen the mineral grains that are cemented together in the rock. Winds then scour out hollows like those you see here.

Continue north on the Wood Canyon Trail until, at 2.2 miles, you find and follow the side trail on the left leading to Dripping Cave. This impressive overhang, tucked into a narrow ravine lined with poison oak, was the supposed hideout of 19th-century stagecoach and livestock thieves. Holes bored into the cave's walls once held pegs used to hang supplies, and the black color of its ceiling is evidence of past campfires.

Retrace your steps for a few paces, and veer left on the narrow trail going northwest. You contour across a steep hillside, pass some elaborately sculpted sandstone formations on the far side of a ravine, and drop precariously onto the flat floor of shallow Mathis Canyon. Turn left on the Mathis Canyon Trail, and stay right at the next split. A 500-foot, no-nonsense climb atop a narrow ridge ensues. But it may be eased by the pauses you take to admire the ever-widening views of Wood Canyon, an island of green or gold amid an endless suburban tapestry spreading inland. Hawks, ravens, and vultures patrol the air space around you, gliding by at close range or spiraling upward on thermals.

At 4 miles, the sweaty ascent ends as you reach the West Ridge Trail, a wide, graded fire road coming down from the Top of the World neighborhood in the city of Laguna

Beach. Turn right (north), and enjoy fine views of the sharp gash of Laguna Canyon to the left and the gentler watershed of Wood Canyon on the right. At 5.4 miles, find and follow the narrow Lynx Trail on the right (which is very steep in a couple of spots) down a ridge and into upper Wood Canyon. On this trail, the viewshed is pristine—there's no sign of anything other than precipitous hillsides clothed in dense chaparral and live oaks. The breeze blowing up the canyon often bears the scent of marine air tinged with sage.

At the bottom of the Lynx Trail, turn right on the Wood Canyon Trail. Close ahead, veer right 0.1 mile to a canyon overlook. At the overlook, you can join a parallel trail down the canyon open only to hikers (if you are on a mountain bike, stay on Wood Canyon Trail). Following a narrow strip of oak woodland and later the Coyote Run Trail, you reach—after nearly 2 miles of travel in shady Wood Canyon—Mathis Canyon Trail. Veer left to cross Wood Canyon's tiny creek and rejoin the Wood Canyon Trail. Continue south to the Aliso and Wood Canyons confluence, and from there return to the Alicia Parkway trailhead the way you came.

Mountain-biking Wood Canyon

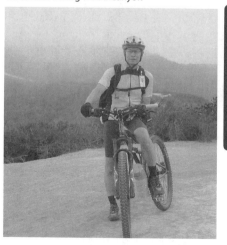

trip 5.6 Pecten Reef via Aliso Creek

see map on p. 53

Distance	7 miles (semiloop)
Hiking Time	3 hours
Elevation Gain	150'
Difficulty	Moderate
Trail Use	Cyclists, equestrians, dogs
Best Times	All year
Agency	OC Parks: AWCWP
Permit	OC Parks parking fee required

DIRECTIONS Park at the Aliso and Wood Canyon Wilderness Park trailhead. From Interstate 5 in Laguna Hills, take Exit 90 and follow Alicia Parkway southwest for 4 miles, then turn right onto Amwa Road. Turn left into the wilderness park parking area (fee required).

Pecten Reef is a limestone outcrop riddled with huge fossilized pecten shells (scallops) dating back to when this part of Orange County lay beneath a shallow tropical sea. The shortest hike to the reef is a 1.5-mile loop from Sheep Hills Park, but this longer trip offers a pleasant chance to explore Aliso Creek along the way.

During the Miocene period 6–16 million years ago, the eastern edge of the Pacific Plate was submerged beneath a shallow sea. Over time, sediments accumulated that are now known as the Monterey Formation. This formation is rich in fossils and oil. As the Pacific Plate has slipped northwest relative to the North American Plate, the Monterey Formation has been pushed up to form the western edge of California. Pecten Reef is an especially interesting part of this formation where Aliso Creek has exposed a fossil-rich limestone outcrop for your inspection. Please look at but do not take the fossils, so that others may enjoy them for generations to come.

From your vehicle, walk back on Amwa Road to the gated, signed start of the Aliso Creek Bikeway leading north along the west bank of the creek. You will follow this paved multiuse trail 3 miles to the reef. Aliso Creek teems with life, including snowy egrets and other waterfowl. The trail curves past various schools and parks, beneath Pacific Park's major overpass, and under the two bridges of Highway 73. Cross the creek on a wooden bridge, and stay left to soon reach the signed Pecten Loop Trail on the left. Continue 0.2 mile on the bikeway to a second signed junction for Pecten Loop on the left, on which you will make a counterclockwise loop.

Sharp-eyed hikers may find occasional fossils in the chunks of limestone along the trail. Unfortunately, thoughtless visitors have removed many of the specimens. As you curve around to the south side of the

Studying fossils at Pecten Reef

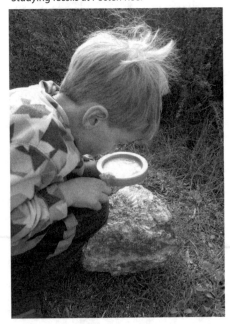

reef, watch for larger chunks of limestone studded with 4- to 6-inch diameter pecten fossils. Pass several unsigned trails leading onto the hill; the most defined makes a gradual climb past coyote gourds and limestone blocks to the top of the hill. Either finish the loop or descend the east side of the hill to rejoin the Aliso Creek Trail. It continues all the way to the foot of the Santa Ana Mountains (see Trip 18.3).

You can retrace your steps, or turn east before the bridge and pick up a trail that parallels Alicia Parkway back to the trailhead.

trip 5.7 Sulphur Creek Reservoir

Distance	1.7 miles (loop)
Hiking Time	1 hour
Elevation Gain	100'
Difficulty	Easy
Trail Use	Cyclists, equestrians, dogs, good for kids
Best Times	All year
Agency	OC Parks: LNRP
Permit	OC Parks parking fee required

see map on p. 53

DIRECTIONS Park at Laguna Niguel Regional Park. From Interstate 5 in Laguna Hills, take Exit 90 and follow Alicia Parkway southwest for 4 miles, then turn left onto Aliso Creek Road. Make the first right onto La Paz Road, then turn right again in 0.2 mile into the park (which charges a fee). After the entry station, turn left and park in the first major parking area across from a playground and picnic areas.

Birders and families will enjoy this mellow loop around the 44-acre Sulphur Creek Reservoir. The dam was completed in 1966 for water storage and fishing, and Laguna Niguel Regional Park opened around the lake in 1973. The lake is surrounded by oaks, sycamores, and eucalyptus, and is lined with bulrushes. The island in the center serves as a bird sanctuary.

From the picnic area, join a paved trail leading southeast along Sulphur Creek. The trail climbs past the dam's spillway and then turns to dirt as it follows the east side of the reservoir. At the far end of the lake, cross the creek on a bridge and reach a T-junction. Turn right and walk back along the west side of the lake. At times you can follow a path along the shore, while at other times, you'll have to join the paved road. Pass a dock with boat rentals. After the dam, drop down to a road junction, and turn right to return to your starting point.

Sulphur Creek Reservoir

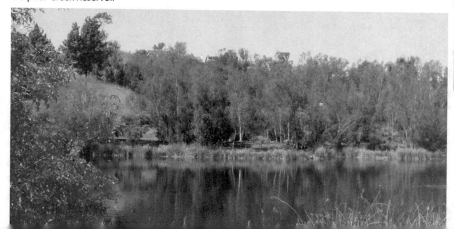

chapter 6

South Coast

Life seems to pass a little more slowly along Orange County's southernmost stretch of coastline. Somewhat removed from the snarling traffic and the crush of people farther up the coast, the narrow beaches and eroded cliffs are quite in tune with the rhythm of the surf and the tides. While Dana Point, Capistrano Beach, and San Clemente continue to fill up with elegant houses and condominium complexes spilling over the coastal bluffs and foothills, these communities still boast many miles of tranquil beach. Away from the focal points of activity, you can still enjoy a warm evening's stroll on the sand with nothing but shorebirds as companions.

This section describes four fine coastal walks in south Orange County, plus a fourth (San Onofre State Beach) just over the line in San Diego County, which is included because it is readily accessible to Orange Countians.

Dana Point tidepools

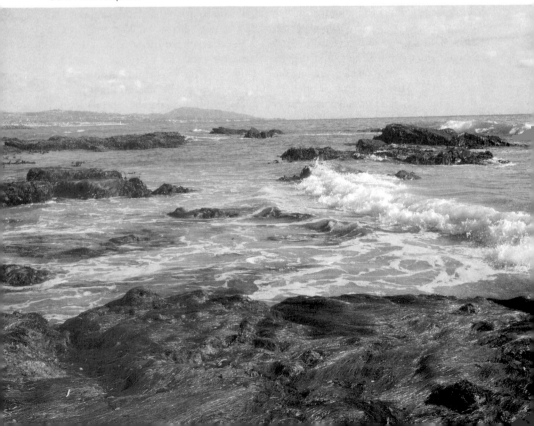

South Coast

| trip 6.1 | **Salt Creek Trail** |

Distance	7 miles (out-and-back)
Hiking Time	3 hours
Elevation Gain	500'
Difficulty	Moderate
Trail Use	Cyclists, dogs, good for kids
Best Times	All year
Agency	OC Parks: SCBP

DIRECTIONS This trip begins at Chapparosa Park in Laguna Niguel. From Interstate 5, exit west on Crown Valley Parkway. In 0.4 mile, turn left on Cabot Road, then in 0.6 mile turn right on Paseo de la Colinas. In 0.9 mile, turn left onto Golden Lantern Street. In 1.4 miles, turn right onto Chapparosa Park Road. Follow it all the way to where it ends and the trail begins at the far western end of the park.

Salt Creek Beach in Dana Point is a tremendously popular beach that draws surfers, swimmers, sunbathers, and families. At low tide, the tidepools are also worth exploring. Most visitors pay to park at the large lot between the Pacific Coast Highway (Highway 1) and Ritz-Carlton Drive, but those with a sense of adventure can combine exercise and relaxation via the Salt Creek Trail.

Although it is paved and weaves through a narrow canyon between housing developments, the Salt Creek Trail is beautifully landscaped with native sage scrub. It receives a great deal of use from walkers, joggers, cyclists, and even parents pushing jogging strollers.

From the end of Chapparosa Park Road, pick up the paved path leading down San Juan Canyon. In 0.8 mile, turn left at a junction, and then soon pass through a tunnel under Niguel Road. Stay right at a confusing junction beyond the tunnel, and climb onto the hillside overlooking Salt Creek. The native vegetation has been restored and now supports a population of native birds and animals. Rattlesnakes have been known to sun themselves on the pavement; they are an important part of the animal community, keeping rodent populations under control, and will leave you alone if you let them be. The trail undulates steeply at times before dropping and veering left to an underpass beneath Camino del Avion at 2.1 miles.

The next segment is squeezed between Monarch Beach Golf Links (famous for presidential visitors) and a housing development. At 3.1 miles, go through another tunnel under the Pacific Coast Highway (Highway 1), and follow signs for the public path through the golf course to stay on the Salt Creek Trail. You'll soon see a trail descending to the northern end of the beach. At 3.5 miles, arrive at the grassy Salt Creek Beach park where stairs and a path lead down to the beach.

Surfers at Salt Creek Beach

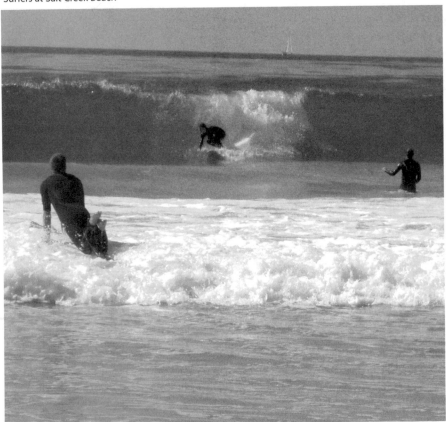

trip 6.2   San Juan Creek Trail

Distance	5 miles (one-way)
Hiking Time	2½ hours
Elevation Gain	150′ loss
Difficulty	Easy
Trail Use	Cyclists, equestrians, dogs
Best Times	All year
Agency	City of San Juan Capistrano

see map on p. 63

DIRECTIONS From Interstate 5, drive 1.8 miles east on Highway 74. Turn right on Avenida Siega, then in 0.2 mile right again on Calle Arroyo. Proceed 0.2 mile to a parking area between Cook Park and Mission Trails Stable.

The San Juan Creek Trail is a paved multiuse path following San Juan Creek from San Juan Capistrano to its mouth at Doheny State Beach. This trail is popular with joggers, cyclists, and families. Equestrians use the upper portion of the trail as far as Trabuco Creek. Many parks along the way offer alternate start or end points, and you may wish to set up a car or bicycle shuttle. You may also wish to use part or all of the trail for a trip to the beach, avoiding the hefty parking fee at Doheny.

San Juan Creek is noted for its steelhead trout. Once believed to be extinct in Southern California, this form of rainbow trout is born in fresh water, swims out to sea to live its adult life, and repeatedly returns to fresh water to spawn. Steelhead populations

Creekside trail

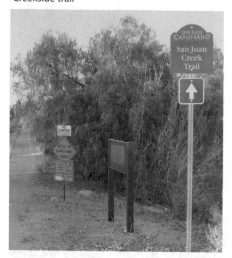

have been severely impacted by pollution and stream degradation, and they are now a protected endangered species. Fishing is prohibited, and efforts are in progress to restore their creek habitat.

The first portion of the trail has two options. A paved path parallels Calle Arroyo on the north side of a greenbelt. A dirt path runs along the bank of San Juan Creek on the south side of the greenbelt. Pick your path and head southwest. In 1 mile, cross La Novia Avenue and, soon after, pass Ortega Equestrian Center. Beyond the equestrian center, the dirt path drops into the San Juan Creek wash and becomes poorly defined, so rejoin the paved path before the stables and follow it along Calle Arroyo, then continue as it turns left into the Paseo Tirador cul-de-sac and then resumes as a trail at the end of the street.

The San Juan Creek Trail soon dips to pass under I-5. Reach Descanso Veterans Park at the confluence with Trabuco Creek, which you cross on a wooden bridge. The Trabuco Creek Trail leads north from here, but this trip continues southwest atop the levee along San Juan Creek.

Pass beside Mission Bell, Creekside, and Del Obispo Parks, all of which could be alternate trailheads. Finally, the trail dips beneath the Pacific Coast Highway (the underpass may occasionally be flooded at high tide) and ends between the mouth of San Juan Creek and the lifeguard station at Doheny State Beach.

SOUTH COAST

see map on p. 63

trip 6.3	**Dana Point Headlands**

Distance	1.4 miles (out-and-back)
Hiking Time	1 hour
Elevation Gain	Negligible
Difficulty	Moderate
Trail Use	Good for kids
Best Times	Low tide; October–March
Agency	OIDP

DIRECTIONS From the Pacific Coast Highway (Highway 1), just west of Dana Point's "downtown," turn south on Street of the Green Lantern. Drive two blocks south to Cove Road and turn left. Cove Road descends to Dana Point Harbor Drive and Dana Cove Park, where the beach walk begins.

The sea cliffs at Dana Point are revered by historians as the site where Spanish vaqueros threw hides over the cliffs and down to waiting ships as described in Richard Henry Dana's *Two Years Before the Mast.* The sheer cliffs remain, but the 2,500-slip Dana Point Marina occupies much of the coastline below. Just west of that marina, though, you'll find a fine wild stretch of rocky beach and dramatic headland, a little piece of old California that you can fully explore during low tides.

Just beyond the starting point, the Dana Cove Park parking lot, you'll find a replica of the *Pilgrim,* the sailing ship that author Dana sailed on during the early 1800s, and the Ocean Institute museum. Beyond the museum, descend a stairway to the beach and, tide permitting, pick your way westward over storm-tossed boulders and under the looming cliffs toward the rocky headland of Dana Point itself. The mostly metamorphic rocks underfoot, a variety of colors and textures, have eroded out of the conglomerate cliffs.

There's a sea cave at the end of the walkable section (0.7 mile from the start of the beach) and plenty of small sea stacks just

Sea cave at Dana Point

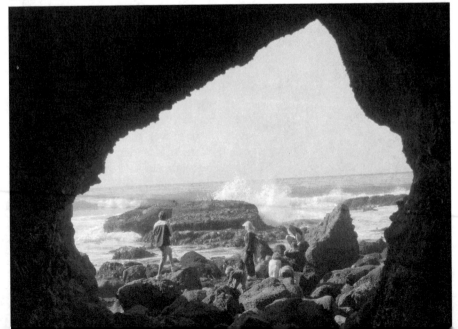

offshore that catch the incoming waves and breakers. The tidepools here are of fair quality. Travel beyond the sea cave is more difficult, but with a low enough tide, you may be able to reach the smooth sand of Strand Beach beyond.

The **Ocean Institute** (see Appendix 4) offers interpretive hikes to the tidepools and sea cave. Call for their current schedule.

trip 6.4 San Clemente State Beach

Distance	3.1 miles (loop)
Hiking Time	1½ hours
Elevation Gain	150'
Difficulty	Easy
Trail Use	Good for kids
Best Times	All year
Agency	SCSB
Permit	State-beach parking fee required

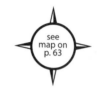

see map on p. 63

DIRECTIONS From southbound Interstate 5, exit at Avenida Calafia in San Clemente, and drive west 0.25 mile. Then turn left into the San Clemente State Beach entrance. Pay your day-use or camping fee, and follow signs to the day-use parking at the west end of the road.

From Dana Point to San Mateo Point, a long, gently curving stretch of sand and surf beckons surfers, swimmers, sunbathers, and strollers. In the north half, both the old coast highway and the tracks of the Santa Fe Railroad follow the beach. South into San Clemente, the highway turns inland, while the tracks, chiseled along the base of tan cliffs, continue near the high tide line.

South of San Clemente State Beach, the coastline is scenic and isolated, and it receives few visitors—good reasons why ex-President Richard Nixon located his "Western White House" here. Only the sudden thunder of a passing train, every half-hour or so, disturbs the beachgoer's reverie of curling breakers, shifting sands, and salt-laden breezes.

On the loop route described here, you begin by walking on the sand but return via an inland route that skirts the mouth of San Mateo Creek.

From the day-use area of San Clemente State Beach, descend to the sand on either of the two trails that drop 120 feet through gaps in the cliff wall. The cliffs, consisting of marine deposits about 15 million years old,

form the blunt edge of the marine terrace on which much of the city of San Clemente rests. The forces of erosion, including the not-insignificant pitter-patter of countless bare feet down the paths and the chiseling of inscriptions in the rock, help to loosen sand grains and hasten their return to the sea.

Cross the tracks through an underpass, and head south along the beach onto a posted stretch overlooked by a row of modern homes. Although the upper beach is private here, California law protects public use and passage below the mean-high-tide line.

Tall palms and cypress trees on the left conceal most of the former Western White House, but a round structure—the "Card Room," where Nixon and Dwight Eisenhower used to enjoy card games—is prominently perched on the cliff edge.

The cliffs peter out at San Mateo Point, where Orange County ends and San Diego County begins. At high tide, you may have to squeeze between the waves and the rocks supporting the train track. In the water gap just ahead lies the marshy mouth of San Mateo Creek. On the right is Trestles Beach

Sunset at San Clemente State Beach

(part of San Onofre State Beach), a favorite of surfers. Ahead a little and back of the white sand lies a shallow, cattail-fringed pond where San Mateo Creek comes to an inglorious end after winding more than 20 miles from the southern Santa Ana and Santa Margarita Mountains. Only during wet periods does the flow of water breach the sand to reach the ocean. This a good place to watch migratory birds, especially in winter.

Head inland now by crossing under the low railroad trestle that gave the beach its name. Pick up a paved service road and bike path, often clogged with surfers portaging their boards. After 0.3 mile, you reach the main bicycle path paralleling Interstate 5 through Camp Pendleton. Turn left (north) here, and after 0.2 mile you'll come up to Avenida del Presidente, the west frontage road of I-5. Stay left to follow the road another 0.8 mile north to Avenida San Luis Rey, where a pedestrian pass-through on the left leads to the fenced San Clemente State Beach campground. Pass the short nature trail looping through a butterfly garden, and continue straight onto the Access Trail for the final 0.2 mile back to the day-use parking.

trip 6.5   San Onofre State Beach

Distance	1–6 miles (loop)
Hiking Time	1–3 hours
Elevation Gain	150'
Difficulty	Easy to moderate
Trail Use	Good for kids; dogs allowed north from Trail 1 and south from Trail 6
Best Times	All year
Agency	SOSB
Permit	State-beach parking fee required

see map on p. 63

DIRECTIONS From Interstate 5 south of San Clemente, exit west on Basilone Road. Follow the west-side frontage road (Old Highway 101) south for 3 miles to the main state beach entrance.

San Onofre State Beach is perhaps best known as a busy camping spot midway between the Los Angeles and San Diego metropolitan areas. More than 300 campsites serve the needs of traveling motorists, touring bicyclists, and (rarely) backpackers headed up or down the coast.

The state beach includes three parcels of land leased from the US Marine Corps, whose Camp Pendleton base sprawls for 17 miles down the coast from San Clemente. A north coastal section extends from the Orange County line (Trestles Beach) to the San Onofre Nuclear Generating Station. The second, most heavily used section lies south of the power station and consists of 3 miles of beach and ocean bluffs just west of Interstate 5. The 300 or so campsites here occupy the roadbed of the former US Highway 101, and all are impacted by noise from Interstate 5 and Amtrak trains. A third parcel of state park territory lies inland along Cristianitos Road. It includes quiet and serene San Mateo Campground.

The San Onofre Nuclear Generating Station produced 2 gigawatts of electricity for Southern California, as much power as a massive coal-fired plant. The steam generators were upgraded in 2009, but within three years they were shut down because of premature wear. The power plant, situated close to millions of people, was considered risky due to nearby faults, potential tsunamis, operational safety issues, and stored radioactive waste. Southern California Edison eventually chose to decommission the generators rather than bring them back online, but the spherical containment buildings will remain a prominent landmark for years to come.

It's worth taking at least a brief look at the sage scrub vegetation on top of the bluffs. These are fairly dense and undisturbed stands, accented with taller shrubs, such as laurel sumac, lemonade berry, toyon, and tree tobacco. Red and sticky monkeyflower plants here produce a variety of colors—red, orange, salmon pink, and yellow—during the spring bloom. The red variety is a great attractor of hummingbirds. Bladderpod, a familiar plant of California's deserts, also makes a home among the sage scrub here.

Several dirt roads or pathways, designated Trails 1–6, travel through ravines or breaks in the bluff wall to reach the white-sand beach below. There, the sounds and sights of civilization are gone, and you're left to explore a primeval stretch of coastline. Strolling along the water's edge, you may spot dolphins, sea lions, and harbor seals. Schad and his companions once watched a pair of dolphins cavort in the surf less than 50 feet from the shore here. (Trail 5 has repeatedly washed out and is closed indefinitely at the time of this writing.)

A secluded stretch of beach south of the southernmost trail, Trail 6, extending into Camp Pendleton historically was used as a clothing-optional beach in honor of Saint Onuphrius Magnus, the naked hermit

SOUTH COAST

who roamed the Egyptian desert. California Parks rangers began issuing citations in 2008, and the status of this section remains contentious.

Watch for sea anemones in the shallow tidepools near the bottom of Trail 1. In the northern reaches of the beach, north of Trail 1 and extending as far as the nuclear power plant, the eroded cliff faces rising over the beach are especially interesting and photogenic. In color and form, some are reminiscent of the formations in Utah's Bryce Canyon National Park.

At a point 0.6 mile south of the power plant, note how the line of bold cliffs ends suddenly. Look upward through the vegetation to discover the Cristianitos Fault, a crack in the Earth that extends some 25 miles inland. To the right (south) side of the fault's inclined surface, you'll see brownish Monterey shale, a fine-grained sedimentary rock deposited some 15–20 million years ago. To the left of the fault is the off-white San Mateo sandstone, laid down an estimated 5 million years ago. Above both of these formations lies a flat, continuous layer of boulders deposited in a marine environment about 120,000 years ago, along with other land-laid deposits on top of the bouldery layer. The undisturbed nature of these upper layers has assured geologists that the Cristianitos Fault has been inactive for at least 120,000 years and is almost certainly not a threat to the power plant's stability and safety. Other faults, however, are known to exist several miles to the southwest. These offshore faults are thought to be extensions of ones exposed on land known to have been active in historic times.

You can spend as little as a half-hour or as much as half a day exploring the 3-plus miles of beachfront that lies below the bluffs. Remember that it is easier to walk this sandy stretch during low tide, taking advantage of the wet, hard-packed sand just above the reach of the surging waves.

San Onofre State Beach

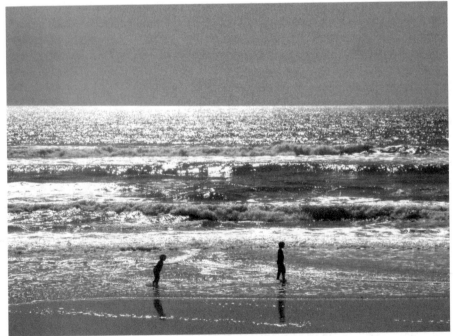

chapter 7

Chino Hills State Park

Seen from the air, the Chino Hills look like a rumpled bedsheet tossed near the northern brow of the higher Santa Ana Mountains. If they weren't cleanly separated from the Santa Anas by the broad trench of Santa Ana Canyon, these hills and their extensions to the north, the Puente Hills, would certainly be considered the northernmost expressions of the Peninsular Ranges.

Rapidly eroding, yet exhibiting a rather graceful, rounded topography, the Chino Hills consist of 5- to 15-million-year-old marine sedimentary rocks uplifted fairly recently by movements along the Whittier Fault zone to the west and along lesser faults to the east. These sediments—called the Puente Formation—extend as far as 13,000 feet beneath the surface of the Chino Hills.

For the past two centuries, the rolling, grassy swells and wooded ravines of the Chino Hills have been used for cattle and sheep grazing. They were originally part of lands assigned to Mission San Gabriel; they were later incorporated into various Spanish land grants or reserved as lands in the public domain. Private ranching interests acquired most of the land by the mid-20th century. By the 1970s, however, ranching was in decline everywhere around Southern California, and tract houses began popping up like mushrooms around the base of the hills. The setting aside of open space and parkland suddenly became an urgent priority.

In 1975, Orange County established the 124-acre Carbon Canyon Regional Park on the west edge of the Chino Hills. Following suit, the State of California in 1977 began a feasibility study for a large park in the Chino Hills. In 1981, the state acquired its first parcel, and by 1984 Chino Hills State Park was opened to the public. After the expenditure of more than $100 million,

Coyote in Chino Hills State Park

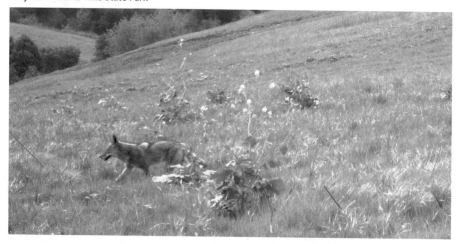

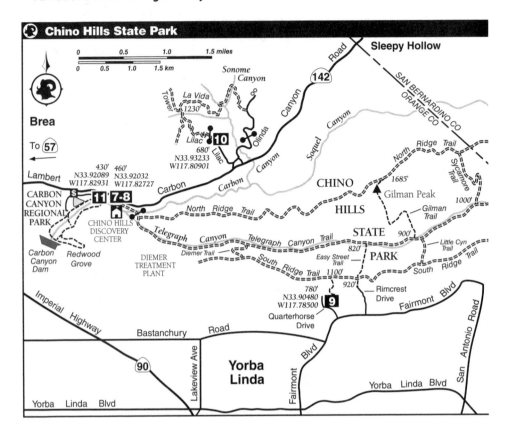

nearly 14,000 acres of state parkland stretch from Carbon Canyon Regional Park to the eastern edge of the Chino Hills in San Bernardino and Riverside Counties. The park remains almost entirely undeveloped, containing just one small drive-in campground, an equestrian staging area, and scattered picnic tables and outhouses.

Aside from its recreational potential, Chino Hills State Park contains important plant and wildlife habitats. About 10% of the park is classified as southern oak woodland, a plant community that has been greatly affected by California's population explosion. Some of the best remaining stands of the California walnut, a tree whose native range is confined to the Los Angeles Basin and surrounding foothills, are found in the larger canyons of the park.

Wildlife includes mule deer, foxes, rabbits, coyotes, bobcats, badgers, mountain lions, and rattlesnakes. Several rare or endangered species of birds may visit the park, including the southern bald eagle, peregrine falcon, least Bell's vireo, California gnatcatcher, and the coastal cactus wren. From a biological perspective, the Chino Hills are regarded as a key link in a natural wildlife corridor stretching between the Whittier and Puente Hills in the Los Angeles Basin to the Santa Ana Mountains in Orange and Riverside Counties.

The 2008 Freeway Complex Fire burned across 95% of Chino Hills State Park. Started almost concurrently at both ends of the park by automobile exhaust on dry brush and an unmaintained power line, it was fanned by hot Santa Ana winds into an inferno that consumed 187 homes. The grassland and sage scrub in the park has evolved to periodically burn, and it is now going through the natural stages of regeneration. However,

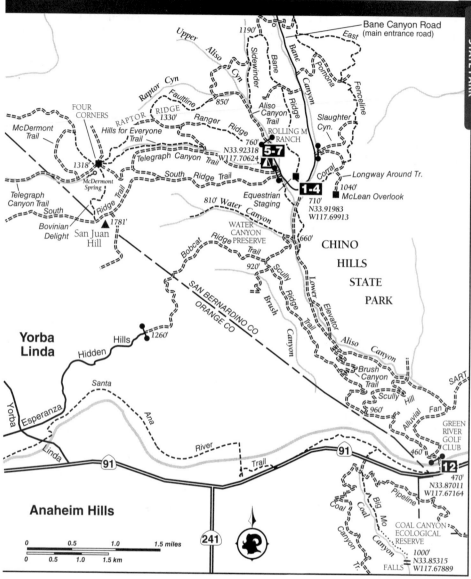

the interval of fires in the area has shortened due to human causes over the past century. Planners are studying how to mitigate the fire risk to protect both the ecosystem and the surrounding communities.

Chino Hills State Park is popular with hikers, equestrians, and especially mountain bikers, all of whom enjoy the park's primitive character. Dirt roads and old cowpaths lace the open ridgelines and thread through the shady canyons. Some 90 miles of dirt roads and trails are open to mountain bikers as well as hikers and horse riders. Certain singletrack (narrower) trails may be closed to cyclists or equestrians. Trail signs and the allowed trail uses are now posted throughout the park, and an improved trail map (available when you enter the park) makes navigation relatively easy. The major trails and roads feature mileposts stating the distance (by way of the most direct route) from Rolling M Ranch.

The Chino Hills State Park Discovery Center forms the western gateway to the park and is the best place to find a ranger or ask questions. On the northeast side, in San Bernardino County, the gravel road that long served as the main entrance is finally being paved and is scheduled to reopen in April 2015. A third designated entrance to Chino Hills State Park can be found at Quarterhorse Drive in a suburban neighborhood of Yorba Linda. Other entrances to the state park are more obscure.

trip 7.1 Bane Rim Loop

see map on pages 72–73

Distance	7 miles (loop)
Hiking Time	3½ hours
Elevation Gain	1,300'
Difficulty	Moderately strenuous
Trail Use	Cyclists, equestrians
Best Times	November–May
Agency	CHSP
Permit	State-park day-use fee required

DIRECTIONS Exit Highway 71 at Soquel Canyon Parkway in Chino. Drive west on Soquel Canyon Parkway 1 mile to Elinvar Drive. Turn left and then left again onto Sapphire Road after 0.2 mile, and then immediately turn right onto Bane Canyon Road entering Chino Hills State Park. Proceed 2.6 miles to the Lower Aliso Day Use Area, the first trailhead parking area on the left with picnic gazebos. If you reach the equestrian staging area, you've gone 0.2 mile too far. *Note that the Bane Canyon entrance is scheduled to be closed for paving until April 2015.*

Bane Canyon cuts through the northeast portion of the park. The ridges on either side of the canyon offer terrific views, especially in the spring when the park is green and wildflowers are blooming. This loop hike, the long way to McLean Overlook, features walks on both ridges.

From the parking area, find a trail on the north side of the road that leads 0.1 mile west to the equestrian staging area. Pick up the Bane Ridge Trail, and follow the undulating ridge, which is steep in places, as it leads north for 2.3 miles. The panoramic views of the largely undeveloped hills are a

Chino Hills

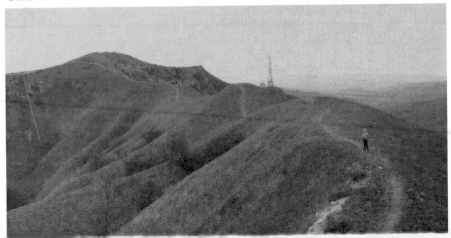

striking contrast to the heavily built lands outside the park. Pass a utility road near the three high-voltage transmission lines, then the unsigned Sidewinder Trail on the left. Your path broadens into a service road and descends to Bane Canyon Road.

Cross the paved road, and continue east up a dirt road that curves up to the ridge. At a ridgetop junction in 0.4 mile, turn sharply right and follow the ridge south for 0.2 mile. At a signed junction, the East Fenceline Trail descends to the east, but this trip continues south on the dramatic narrow ridge. In 0.5 mile, reach a vista point atop a hill where the trail ends at a powerline road called the Pomona Trail.

Turn left onto the Pomona Trail, and follow it southeast for 0.6 mile, descending to an old windmill where you again meet the East Fenceline Trail. Turn right and follow the trail south as it weaves along the fence separating the state park from private ranchland. In 0.8 mile, cross dirt Slaughter Canyon Road; in another 0.6 mile, the trail ends at a T-junction with a dirt road known as the Longway Around Trail. Turn left and head up the road, passing the Corral Trail in 0.1 mile and reaching McLean Overlook in another 0.2 mile. Enjoy a snack at the picnic bench, and survey the eastern end of the park from the knoll.

Return to the Corral Trail, and follow it down 0.5 mile to Lower Aliso Canyon, where you turn right and reach your starting point in 0.1 mile.

trip 7.2	**McLean Overlook**

Distance	1.8 miles (out-and-back)
Hiking Time	1 hour
Elevation Gain	350'
Difficulty	Easy
Trail Use	Cyclists, equestrians, good for kids
Best Times	All year
Agency	CHSP
Permit	State-park day-use fee required

see map on pages 72–73

DIRECTIONS Exit Highway 71 at Soquel Canyon Parkway in Chino. Drive west on Soquel Canyon Parkway 1 mile to Elinvar Drive. Turn left and then left again onto Sapphire Road after 0.2 mile, and then immediately turn right onto Bane Canyon Road entering Chino Hills State Park. Proceed 2.6 miles to the Lower Aliso Day Use Area, the first trailhead parking area on the left with picnic gazebos. If you reach the equestrian staging area, you've gone 0.2 mile too far. Note that the Bane Canyon entrance is scheduled to be closed for paving until April 2015.

Worthwhile as an introductory hike, this short stroll takes you to McLean Overlook, a knoll featuring a commanding view of about half of Chino Hills State Park's more than 14,000 acres.

From the trailhead parking area, walk south on the broad Lower Aliso Canyon Trail. In 0.1 mile, veer left onto the signed Corral Trail, which climbs a ridge to meet an old dirt road called Longway Around Trail in 0.5 mile. This steep stretch may tax young hikers. Turn right on the road, and continue more gently 0.3 mile to the overlook.

The view encompasses most of the Aliso Canyon drainage. You see rolling, grass-covered hills flanking a shallow valley lined with tall sycamores. In spring, the green hills are tinted by the blue-purple flowers of lupine and accented by yellow bands of blooming invasive wild mustard. The grass abruptly turns tawny gold in April or May. By early fall, after months of fierce sunshine and desiccating winds, it's difficult to believe these same sere hills could ever be green again.

Their clay soils are derived from bedrock consisting mainly of weak siltstone. These soils expand when wet and are especially prone to creeping and sliding when water-logged. You'll notice many examples of recent slumping and gullying on the slopes. Look also for evidence of much older and larger landslides. These big ones probably developed during the last Pleistocene glacial stage (20,000–10,000 years ago) when Southern California's climate was much wetter.

trip 7.3   Water Canyon

see map on pages 72–73

Distance	3.6 miles (out-and-back)
Hiking Time	2 hours
Elevation Gain	300'
Difficulty	Moderate
Trail Use	Good for kids
Best Times	November–May
Agency	CHSP
Permit	State-park day-use fee required

DIRECTIONS Exit Highway 71 at Soquel Canyon Parkway in Chino. Drive west on Soquel Canyon Parkway 1 mile to Elinvar Drive. Turn left and then left again onto Sapphire Road after 0.2 mile, and then immediately turn right onto Bane Canyon Road entering Chino Hills State Park. Proceed 2.6 miles to the Lower Aliso Day Use Area, the first trailhead parking area on the left with picnic gazebos. If you reach the equestrian staging area, you've gone 0.2 mile too far. *Note that the Bane Canyon entrance is scheduled to be closed for paving until April 2015.*

If you're searching for the single most intriguing spot in the Chino Hills, you may find it in the upper reaches of Water Canyon. Concealed in the inky depths of this steep-walled ravine, massive sycamores and oaks reach skyward, casting a perennial chill. Except for the occasional buzz of a small aircraft and the rustle of leaves in the breeze overhead, the silence and stillness are absolute. The 2008 Freeway Complex Fire incinerated many of the mature trees in the canyon, but new trunks have been

Water Canyon

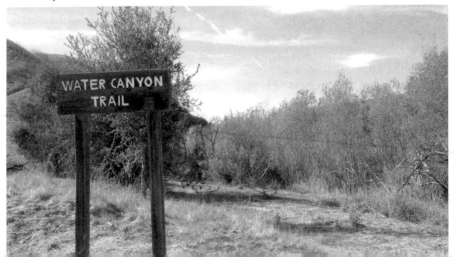

rising rapidly and the canyon is beginning to return to its former beauty.

From the trailhead, start heading south on the wide trail (dirt road) along the shallow valley known as Lower Aliso Canyon. In 0.7 mile from the campground, you dip to cross Aliso Canyon's seasonal stream. On the other side, you join another road at a T-intersection. Turn right, go about 100 yards to a hairpin turn, and turn right again on the narrow trail up Water Canyon. This is one of the few trails in the park reserved for hikers; equestrian and bike traffic is prohibited.

The trail starts on the south side of the creekbed but soon crosses a bridge to the north side and remains there for the rest of the walk. Lining Water Canyon is a narrow finger of riparian willow and sycamore growth, flanked by grizzled oaks and well-proportioned walnut trees. After a short mile, you pass a thicket of prickly pear cacti so dense it forms a trailside wall. This is a good turnaround point for a casual hike.

The trail, which may or not have benefited from recent maintenance, may be partially hidden beyond this point by seasonal grasses, especially after a wet winter season. Intrepid hikers can continue another half-mile up along the shady canyon bottom and reach the darkest heart of the canyon, flanked by steep slopes on both sides. Watch out for poison oak, stinging nettles, and rattlesnakes. The pristine little patch of wilderness in upper Water Canyon is as close—and as far—from modern civilization as you will find anywhere around the LA metropolitan area.

---

trip 7.4   **Lower Aliso Canyon Loop**

Distance	10 miles (loop)
Hiking Time	5 hours
Elevation Gain	1,500'
Difficulty	Moderately strenuous
Trail Use	Cyclists, equestrians
Best Times	November–May
Agency	CHSP
Permit	State-park day-use fee required

see map on pages 72–73

DIRECTIONS Exit Highway 71 at Soquel Canyon Parkway in Chino. Drive west on Soquel Canyon Parkway 1 mile to Elinvar Drive. Turn left and then left again onto Sapphire Road after 0.2 mile, and then immediately turn right onto Bane Canyon Road entering Chino Hills State Park. Proceed 2.6 miles to the Lower Aliso Day Use Area, the first trailhead parking area on the left with picnic gazebos. If you reach the equestrian staging area, you've gone 0.2 mile too far. *Note that the Bane Canyon entrance is scheduled to be closed for paving until April 2015.*

Lower Aliso Canyon extends from the heart of Chino Hills State Park southeast to the Santa Ana River. The canyon and overlooking ridge take you back to California's ranching days when civilization seemed remote. This trip describes a long loop on fire roads out along the rolling ridge and back via the gentle canyon. Like most hikes in Chino Hills, this trip is especially attractive in the spring when the hills are green and the wildflowers are in bloom. Signage in this remote corner of the park may be poor or missing, so pay attention to your map. Those desiring a shorter trip can shave off some distance by closing the loop on the Scully Hill or Brush Canyon Trails. The Lower Aliso Canyon Trail is also very popular with mountain bikers.

From the trailhead, pass through a gate onto the Lower Aliso Canyon Trail, a broad fire road. Head south 0.7 mile, and cross a bridge over the Water Canyon creek to reach a T-junction. Turn right onto the Scully Ridge Trail, which passes the Water Canyon Trail at a hairpin turn and climbs onto the ridge. The next 4.7 miles follow the delightfully undulating ridge, steep in places. The higher parts offer expansive views over Chino Hills State Park and out to the four major mountain ranges of Southern California: the San Gabriels, San Bernardinos, San Jacintos, and Santa Anas. This is a great place to appreciate the significance of Chino Hills State Park. Were it not for the advocacy of many volunteers and the state's investment, the canyons and ridges would be covered with yet more housing subdivisions. Stay right at three junctions; the first two short-cut down to Lower Aliso Canyon, while the third is just a powerline access road.

At the end of the ridge, drop steeply to the floor of the Santa Ana River Canyon. Stay left on a partially paved road leading toward a gate out of the park onto train tracks and the Green River Golf Course. Just before the gate, veer left onto the possibly unsigned Alluvial Fan Trail, a narrow path along the fenced park border. Follow this trail 1.1 miles to its end at the Lower Aliso Canyon fire road.

Turn left and walk back up the gently sloping canyon. The canyon gets its name from the Spanish word for alder, which is found along the seasonal creek. Native sycamores and live oaks also grow in the canyon. The nonnative grasses and attractive but invasive and fire-prone mustard plants are reminders of the canyon's ranching history. Lower Aliso Canyon is a vital link in the wildlife corridor between the Santa Ana Mountains and the Chino and Puente Hills, and you may see scat testifying to the trail's nocturnal users. The many service hatches and roads along the canyon are part of the Metropolitan Water District pipeline that carries water from the Colorado River to Southern California. Part of the pipeline construction near San Juan Hill during the 1950s involved boring a tunnel 6,800 feet in length and 15 feet in diameter.

Pass the Scully Hill and Brush Canyon Roads on the left, and in 1.7 miles reach a Y-junction on the canyon floor. The Lower Aliso Canyon Trail stays left on the canyon floor, while the Elevator Trail, a pipeline service road, parallels it through hilly terrain before rejoining. In another 1 mile, watch for a narrow path on the right leading to Bane Canyon. Take this more scenic and slightly shorter path for 0.6 mile until it rejoins the Lower Aliso Canyon Trail, and continue 0.3 mile to the trailhead where you began.

VARIATION

Using the Brush Canyon or Scully Hill cut-off reduces this loop to 6.5 or 8.5 miles, respectively.

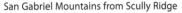

San Gabriel Mountains from Scully Ridge

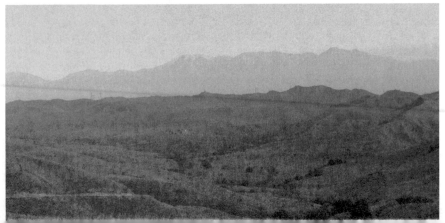

trip 7.5 Upper Aliso Canyon

Distance	3.8 miles (loop)
Hiking Time	2 hours
Elevation Gain	700'
Difficulty	Moderate
Trail Use	Cyclists, equestrians, good for kids
Best Times	November–May
Agency	CHSP
Permit	State-park day-use fee required

see
map on
pages
72–73

DIRECTIONS Exit Highway 71 at Soquel Canyon Parkway in Chino. Drive west on Soquel Canyon Parkway 1 mile to Elinvar Drive. Turn left and then left again after 0.2 mile, and then immediately right on Bane Canyon Road entering Chino Hills State Park. Continue 3 miles to the Rolling M Ranch (former park office) at the end of the road, where parking is available. *Note that the Bane Canyon entrance is scheduled to be closed for paving until April 2015.*

On this pleasant loop through the upper reaches of Aliso Canyon, you'll appreciate the fine vistas (on clear days at least) of miles of empty hill country presided over by the snowdusted summits of the San Gabriel Mountains.

From Rolling M Ranch, hike north past a gate, and continue on an old dirt road up the west bank of sycamore-lined Aliso Canyon. At 0.7 mile, the Sidewinder Trail forks right, but you stay on the old road as it soon bends

Golden star, Aliso Canyon

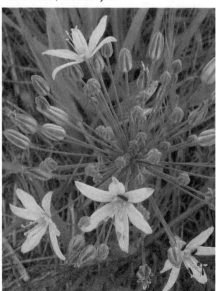

decidedly west up along the bottom of a shallow tributary called Raptor Canyon. A few willows and an occasional walnut tree are all that the canyon musters for display here.

At 1.1 miles, the road veers right and zigzags up the slope to the north. Stay left on the Faultline Trail that strikes west up a grassy ridge just south of Raptor Canyon. After passing a windmill, you begin a stiff climb of about 500 vertical feet, up through tall-growing grasses, topping out on Raptor Ridge. On the way up, you can look out over the upper reaches of Raptor Canyon, smothered in a rich, dark growth of live oak and walnut trees. True to its namesake, you'll probably notice a hawk or two cruising on updrafts in the canyon.

At 2 miles, atop Raptor Ridge, the trail descends a little, and you meet a powerline access road. Turn left (east), walk 0.3 mile, and then go right on a road that drops into the wooded drainage to the south. At the bottom (2.8 miles), turn east and return toward your starting point by way of the gently descending Telegraph Canyon Trail (a graded dirt road). When you reach the paved entrance road, turn left and complete the remaining 200 yards back to Rolling M Ranch.

trip 7.6   Hills for Everyone Trail

Distance	4.6 miles (loop)
Hiking Time	2½ hours
Elevation Gain	700'
Difficulty	Moderate
Trail Use	Good for kids
Best Times	October–June
Agency	CHSP
Permit	State-park day-use fee required

see map on pages 72–73

DIRECTIONS Exit Highway 71 at Soquel Canyon Parkway in Chino. Drive west on Soquel Canyon Parkway 1 mile to Elinvar Drive. Turn left and then left again after 0.2 mile, and then immediately right on Bane Canyon Road entering Chino Hills State Park. Continue 3 miles to the Rolling M Ranch at the end of the road, where parking is available. *Note that the Bane Canyon entrance is scheduled to be closed for paving until April 2015.*

The Hills for Everyone Trail (reserved for hikers—mountain bikes and equestrians are prohibited), commemorates a conservation group with the same name that was instrumental in the establishment of Chino Hills State Park. The trail runs up an unnamed tributary of Aliso Canyon, beautifully shaded by live oak, walnut, sycamore, elderberry, and toyon. **Note:** *This trail was severely damaged after*

Tired hikers

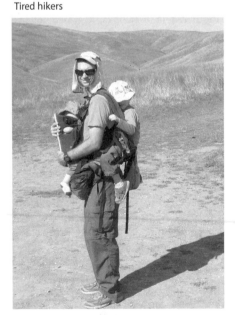

the 2008 wildfire and is closed until further notice. Check with a ranger before considering this trail.

From the parking lot next to Rolling M Ranch, walk south on the paved entrance road for 200 yards, then turn right (west) on the Telegraph Canyon Trail, a maintained dirt road closed to motor traffic. After a nearly flat 0.9 mile of travel, veer right onto a dirt road crossing the creek on a bridge, then make an immediate left onto the Hills for Everyone Trail. For the next 1.3 miles, you stick close to the ravine bottom, first on its right, then on its left. During the wet season, water trickles down the bottom, nourishing a moist, dark understory of wild berry vines, ferns, nettles, watercress, and other water-loving plants. Near the top of the trail at 1,318 feet, filtered sunlight illuminates wild grapevines draped among the oak trees.

At the top you come to a saddle, part of a major watershed divide. Several trails converge in this area. Raindrops falling to the west are routed down Telegraph Canyon to Carbon Canyon, while rain falling to the east goes into Aliso Canyon. Although these hills quickly absorb most of the precipitation they receive, all of the excess eventually makes its way to the Santa Ana River.

Just west of the saddle is McDermont Spring, a small stock pond filled with cattails.

An old windmill groans nearby as it pumps water into a metal tank. Most of the old stock ponds in the park have been allowed to silt up, but this one is maintained for passing horses and the local wildlife. Look for frogs, pond turtles, and a host of birds in the area before you return. To make a loop, take Telegraph Canyon Road back east, then stay on it or South Ridge, both of which terminate yards south of where you began.

trip 7.7   Telegraph Canyon Traverse

Distance	8 miles (one-way)
Hiking Time	4 hours
Elevation Gain/Loss	650'/900'
Difficulty	Moderately strenuous
Trail Use	Cyclists, equestrians
Best Times	November–May
Agency	CHSP
Permit	State-park day-use fee required

see map on pages 72–73

DIRECTIONS This trip requires a car shuttle. Leave a vehicle at the Chino Hills Discovery Center at the west end of the trip. Exit the 57 Freeway at Lambert Road in Brea, and drive east. After 2 miles, Lambert Road becomes Carbon Canyon Road. Continue straight ahead an additional 1 mile to the Chino Hills Discovery Center on the right. Then shuttle around to the trailhead at the east end. Continue on Carbon Canyon Road for 7.2 miles to its end, then turn right onto Chino Hills Parkway. In 1.5 miles, turn right on Pipeline Avenue. In 1.7 miles, turn left on Soquel Canyon Parkway. In 0.7 mile, turn right on Elinvar Drive. In 0.2 mile, just after Elinvar turns left, turn right onto Bane Canyon Road into Chino Hills Sate Park, and follow it 3.2 miles to the Rolling M Ranch parking area at the end of the road. *Note that the Bane Canyon entrance is scheduled to be closed for paving until April 2015.*

Whether you are a hiker, equestrian, or mountain biker, more than 8 miles of superb scenery are yours to enjoy on this one-way trek over the Chino Hills. Telegraph Canyon is long enough, wild enough, and beautiful enough (especially in its upper reaches) to provide a close approximation to a true wilderness experience. Try this trip sometime on a late autumn afternoon, after the first rains of the season, when the sun's warm rays illuminate the gold and green sycamores, and the cool breeze has a tangy, woodsy aroma.

Walk south on Bane Canyon Road past the campground entrance to the gated Telegraph Canyon Trail. Make your way up Telegraph Canyon to Four Corners and McDermont Spring, the headwaters of Telegraph Canyon.

Navigational matters are very simple thereafter: Just stroll down the bottom of the canyon 5.4 miles until you reach the canyon's mouth, then continue out to the Discovery Center.

Telegraph Canyon

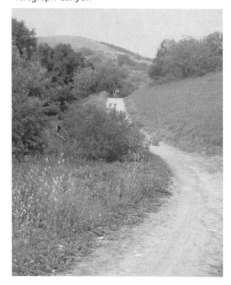

trip 7.8 **Gilman Peak**

Distance	8 miles (out-and-back)
Hiking Time	4 hours
Elevation Gain	1,400'
Difficulty	Moderately strenuous
Trail Use	Cyclists, equestrians
Best Times	October–June
Agency	CHSP
Permit	State-park day-use fee required

see map on pages 72–73

DIRECTIONS Exit Highway 57 at Lambert Road in Brea, and drive east. After 2 miles (where it intersects Valencia Avenue), Lambert Road becomes Carbon Canyon Road. Continue straight ahead 1 more mile to the Chino Hills State Park Discovery Center and staging area on the right.

Gilman Peak's bald summit, barely poking over lesser ridges, affords a breathtakingly spacious view of Southern California on a clear day. To the southwest lies the wide mouth of Santa Ana Canyon, scored by a broad flood channel carrying runoff that originates far inland amid the San Bernardino Mountains. Beyond, the vast urban plain of Orange County, resting on a large sheet of alluvium, slopes gently toward the ocean. Northward, the gaunt San Gabriel Mountains, snowcapped in winter, rise boldly over foreground hills and valleys. In the southeast, the Santa Ana Mountains form a broad, dusky blister on the horizon. *Note that at the time of this writing, the North Ridge Trail is temporarily closed due to severe erosion.*

From the Discovery Center, start hiking or riding on a dirt road slanting southeast, just below the grade of the highway. Following this route, you skirt a former citrus orchard. Orange County was named for its once vibrant citrus industry, but as the cost of water and the value of land rose, orchards became less profitable for fruit and more valuable as real estate.

In 0.2 mile, reach a fork beyond a gate. Telegraph Canyon lies straight ahead, but you veer left and start climbing on the North Ridge Trail, a dirt road. There are many California walnut trees in the next couple of miles, their wispy branches swaying and their compound leaves shimmering in the

breeze. These trees, which cling to north-facing slopes, offer welcome shade during the warmer months. They are deciduous, dropping their leaves by late fall and regaining them in early spring. Be aware of poison oak thickets growing alongside the trail.

By 2 miles into the hike, the trail stays higher on the ridgeline, which is bald save for grass and low-growing sage scrub vegetation. After you pass over a couple of smaller bumps on the ridge, Gilman Peak appears ahead, its summit accessible by way of a wide side trail from the northeast.

Lupine

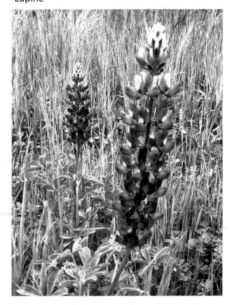

Hikers can turn this hike into a loop. Follow the narrow Gilman Trail (bikes prohibited) southwest from Gilman Peak, and soon plunge down the steep ridge to Telegraph Canyon. Turn right and return by way of the Telegraph Canyon Trail. This option adds 0.5 mile.

trip 7.9   San Juan Hill

see map on pages 72–73

Distance	7 miles (out-and-back)
Hiking Time	3½ hours
Elevation Gain	1,600'
Difficulty	Moderately strenuous
Trail Use	Cyclists, equestrians
Best Times	November–May
Agency	CHSP
Permit	State-park day-use fee required

DIRECTIONS From the 57 Freeway, take Yorba Linda Boulevard east for 5.1 miles, then turn left on Fairmont Boulevard, and go 1.2 miles. Turn left onto Quarter Horse Road; in 0.2 mile, watch for the Quarter Horse Staging Area on the right.

This is a straightforward hike to the high point of Chino Hills State Park, 1,781-foot San Juan Hill, from the Quarter Horse Staging Area in Yorba Linda. It is a bit longer than a route from the Rolling M Ranch, but it requires less driving.

This hike formerly began on Rim Crest Drive, but the park has relocated the trailhead to Quarter Horse to reduce the parking burden in the residential neighborhood. Unfortunately, the Quarter Horse trailhead adds a stiff hill climb and increases the distance by 0.6 mile each way.

Start up an unsigned dirt track alongside the gated paved water district road. In 0.25 mile, reach the signed Chino Hills State Park boundary next to the covered reservoir. Look back for a view of Catalina Island over the broad Orange County coastal plain. In another 0.2 mile, turn right at a V-junction and immediately reach South Ridge Road. From here, you can see San Juan Hill as the high point to the east near some transmission line towers. Telegraph Canyon is to the north, and Gilman Peak is the undistinguished high point on the ridge beyond.

Turn right, heading east along the South Ridge toward San Juan Hill. For 3 miles, the trail's gently curling course takes you through a nearly treeless landscape. Tall grasses and wild mustard on both sides of the trail sway in the stiff afternoon breezes typically blowing up Santa Ana Canyon from the west. This fact is not lost on kite flyers, who sometimes practice their art here. Keep an eye out for small herds of deer that roam this section of the park. Your road also doubles as a utility access for a buried Southern California Gas pipeline.

Drop for 0.2 mile to a saddle where the Easy Street Trail departs to the north, and Rim Crest Drive is beyond a gate to the south. In another 0.9 mile, pass the Little Canyon Trail on the north. Watch for a variety of utility spurs on either side.

Eventually, you crest a hill and views of San Gorgonio open to the east. Pass the Bovinian Delight Trail on the left. Where the South Ridge Road curves around the left (north) side of San Juan Hill, take the narrow side trail on the right leading 0.1 mile to the San Juan Hill summit. If not for the presence of the transmission line towers to the east, this would be one of the best panoramic viewpoints in Southern California. You can pick out the high points of the four surrounding counties: Santiago Peak in Orange County to the south, San Jacinto in Riverside County to the east, San Gorgonio in San Bernardino County to the northeast, and San Antonio (Old Baldy) in Los Angeles County to the north. There are excellent views over Orange County's coastal plain to the southwest. To the north stands the crest of the San Gabriel Mountains, capped with snow in the winter. From left to right, mountain climbers will pick out a host of cherished peaks: Mt. Wilson, Twin Peaks, Mt. Williamson, Mt. Islip, Mt. Hawkins, Mt. Baden-Powell, Iron Mountain, Mt. Baldy, Ontario Peak, and Cucamonga Peak.

Return the way you came, or loop back through Telegraph Canyon via the Bovinian Delight and Easy Street Trails. This loop takes about the same amount of time and is a good way to enjoy the scenic canyon.

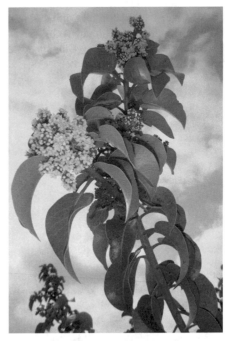

Sugarbush in bloom near San Juan Hill

see map on pages 72–73

trip 7.10 Sonome Canyon

Distance	3.9 miles (loop)
Hiking Time	2½ hours
Elevation Gain	1,100'
Difficulty	Moderate
Trail Use	Cyclists, equestrians
Best Times	November–May
Agency	CHSP

DIRECTIONS Exit the 57 Freeway at Lambert Road in Brea, and drive east. After 2 miles (where it intersects with Valencia Avenue), Lambert Road becomes Carbon Canyon Road (Highway 142). Continue straight ahead an additional 2.6 miles, then turn left onto Olinda Place. Make an immediate left onto Lilac Road, and follow it to the gated end where you park on the shoulder in a residential neighborhood.

The Sonome Canyon sector of Chino Hills State Park, annexed in 1996, is separated from the rest of the park by Carbon Canyon Road, but it still serves as an important wildlife linkage to Tonner Canyon to the northwest. The area was incinerated in the 2008 Freeway Complex Fire, but some of the oaks in the canyon survived and the grasslands are rich with spring wildflowers. This clockwise loop is a good workout with lots of ups and downs. The trip follows old service roads in Chino Hills State Park and loops back through the neighborhood.

Walk past the gate and continue up Lilac Road, which is now a dirt service road.

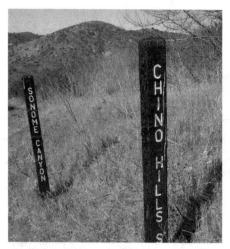

Sonome Canyon burn zone

Make a steep climb to meet a powerline service road on the ridge. Stay right, then veer right again at an easy-to-miss junction just beyond (if you find yourself on the powerline road, you've missed it). You now drop down into Sonome Canyon. After crossing the canyon, climb again to a T-junction with a paved water tank service road. Turn right and follow the steep road down to a gate at the top of Olinda Drive, 2.9 miles from where you started. Continue down through a neighborhood, then turn right on Olinda Place and right again on Lilac Lane to close the loop.

trip 7.11 Carbon Canyon Nature Trail

see
map on
pages
72–73

Distance	2.6 miles round-trip (loop)
Hiking Time	1½ hours
Elevation Gain	50'
Difficulty	Easy
Trail Use	Cyclists, equestrians, dogs, good for kids
Best Times	All year
Agency	OC Parks: CCRP
Permit	OC Parks parking fee required

DIRECTIONS Exit Highway 57 at Lambert Road in Brea, and drive east. After 2 miles (where it intersects Valencia Avenue), Lambert Road becomes Carbon Canyon Road. Continue straight ahead an additional 0.6 mile to Carbon Canyon Regional Park's entrance on the right (south) side of the road. After passing the fee kiosk, turn left and proceed 0.6 mile to the trailhead parking area past the nature center at the extreme east end of the park.

Carbon Canyon Regional Park, one of the many smaller units of Orange County's far-flung regional park system, has enough room for one significant hiking trail. An unlikely grove of coast redwood trees, nursed from seedlings and planted in 1975, lies at the end of this self-guiding nature trail. Indigenous to the California coast only as far south as Monterey County, their survival in this rather dry corner of Orange County is quite remarkable.

A typical suburban recreational facility, the park features various sports facilities, picnic grounds, and pedestrian and bike paths. The entire park lies within the flood zone of the Carbon Canyon flood-control dam, which may someday protect urbanized areas downstream. The park also happens to lie squarely within the Whittier Fault zone, a major splinter of the San Andreas Fault. Although not part of Chino Hills State Park, the park is described in this chapter due to its proximity.

The Nature Trail begins at a kiosk at the east end of the regional park. (Be careful not to take the other nearby trail paralleling the road to the state park.) Follow the designated path through a grove of planted pines, past

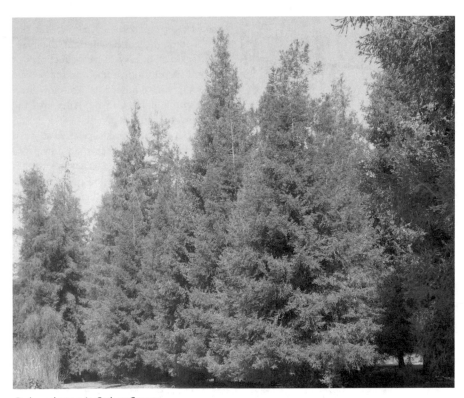

Redwood grove in Carbon Canyon

a second trailhead sign, and as it takes a hard right down into the bed of Carbon Canyon. The tiny stream is flanked by a variety of water-loving plants. Beware that stinging nettles and large poison oak bushes mingle with the more attractive vegetation.

After what could be a muddy creek crossing, the nature trail continues west, hugging a dry hillside on the left and dense riparian vegetation on the right. The hillside hosts graceful native walnut trees and nonnative pepper trees, along with nonnative fennel, mustard, and castor bean. Trailside benches make great places to hear and watch the lively bird activity. Occasional steep trails come down from the adjacent neighborhoods. The trail bends left into an arm of the

basin just above Carbon Canyon dam. Here, you find the curious stand of redwoods, a picnic bench, and a drinking fountain. Subsurface water in the basin may keep these redwoods alive, but without the rain and fog drip they are accustomed to in their native habitat, they look a bit thin and dusty.

If you stay on the trail all the way to its far end near the flood control dam, you can make a loop back on the Vista Trail along its base. When you reach the tall control tower, turn right onto another wide dirt path that leads back to the southwest end of the park near a dirt parking area, volleyball courts, and a picnic ground. Turn right on the sidewalk, and follow it back between the lagoon and creek to your vehicle.

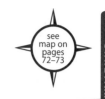

trip 7.12 Coal Canyon

Distance	6 miles (out-and-back)
Hiking Time	3 hours
Elevation Gain	600'
Difficulty	Moderate
Trail Use	Hiking only
Best Times	December–April
Agency	CHSP

see map on pages 72–73

DIRECTIONS From the 91 Freeway in Corona, take Exit 44 for Green River Road, and turn west. After 1 mile, park on the right side of Green River Road near the turnoff for the Green River Golf Club.

For at least three decades, the Coal Canyon diamond interchange on the Riverside Freeway through Santa Ana Canyon was a virtual joke, featuring ramps to and from nowhere. "Nowhere" might have been replaced by subdivisions spreading eastward from Yorba Linda and Anaheim Hills, but that hasn't happened, and likely will never. The Coal Canyon undercrossing, it was discovered, was the one and only practical wildlife corridor between 40,000 acres of undeveloped lands in the Chino and Puente Hills to the north and a half-million acres of wild land in the Santa Ana Mountains to the south. Mountain lions were using it to avoid being flattened by an endless river of cars, 10–12 lanes wide. Biologists increasingly insist that preserving habitat corridors (links like this one), even lowly ones, such as freeway crossings and tunnels, are essential to the regional survival of migratory wild animals.

Coal Canyon's freeway ramps were closed in 2003. The asphalt strip of the putative parkway underneath is gone, and a wide stretch of Coal Canyon south of the freeway is now friendlier to both migrating creatures and hikers curious enough to visit. Formerly under private ownership, the canyon was purchased by California State Parks for preservation. The upper portion is now designated an ecological reserve. This trip is most enjoyable during late winter and early spring when the sage scrub is green and flowering and a small waterfall may be running.

Mountain bikes are allowed on the dirt road but not in the ecological reserve. This trip can be done as a multisport adventure, pedaling along the Santa Ana River Trail and the lower portion of the canyon, then hoofing it up the wash through the reserve.

From the parking space on Green River Road, walk west for 0.2 mile to the end of the road, and continue on the paved Santa Ana River bike trail that closely parallels the freeway. Endure the roaring traffic on your left for the next few minutes. The wide Santa Ana River concrete flood channel lies on your right, and beyond that lie the green spaces of the golf course.

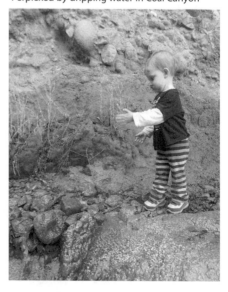
Perplexed by dripping water in Coal Canyon

When you reach the Coal Canyon crossing after 1.2 miles, walk underneath the overpasses, and continue south into Chino Hills State Park territory. Just beyond the entrance gate, veer left onto a dirt truck trail leading up Coal Canyon's wide floodplain, staying to the left of the canyon's sand- and gravel-coated stream bed. In another 0.2 mile, stay right onto the signed Big Mo Trail, an old jeep track, where the better Pipeline Road climbs east out of the canyon. (Big Mo was a 200-year-old Tecate cypress killed by wildfire in 2002.)

After a mile of uphill hiking, just short of where the canyon significantly narrows, reach the end of the road at the Coal Canyon Ecological Reserve boundary. From here, the trail virtually disappears, but you may be able to pick out a faint path behind the sign that briefly follows the rim of the rocky wash before dropping into it. Proceed 0.5 mile farther upstream, following a silvery strand of water (if there is any), to where the canyon walls soar and pinch in tightly. There—in the wettest time of the year—the sound of spattering water heralds your arrival at a sublime grotto graced with a 20-foot-high shower of crystal-clear water. It pours off a mineralized stalactite shaped like the spout of a teapot *(see photo)*. This is a rare sight in a location that seems unlikely for a waterfall.

Turn around and reverse your tracks to the entrance gate.

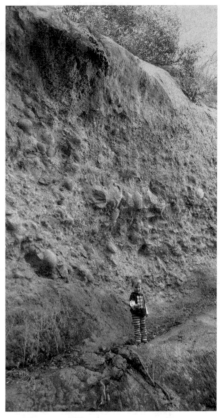

Teapot Spout Falls

chapter 8

Santiago Creek and Anaheim Hills

On the eastern fringes of Anaheim and the city of Orange lie several picturesque city and regional (county) parks—all within a half-hour drive of most parts of metropolitan Orange County. This is classic urban–wildland interface country: suburban housing developments spreading into the foothills of the Santa Ana Mountains, with little beyond but miles of profoundly empty land. This empty land has been pierced by the 241 Toll Road—but at the same time, most of it has received permanent protection and is now within the 20,000-acre Irvine Ranch Open Space (see Chapter 10) and the Cleveland National Forest (see Chapter 15).

Live oaks in Oak Canyon

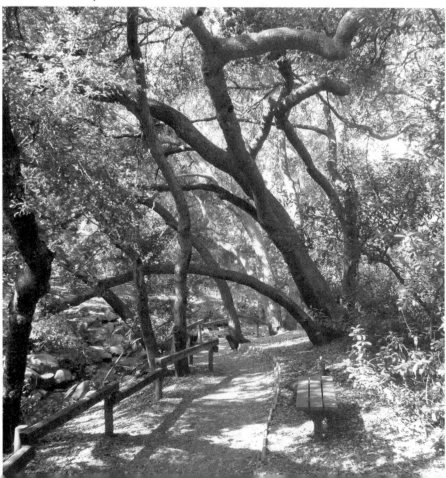

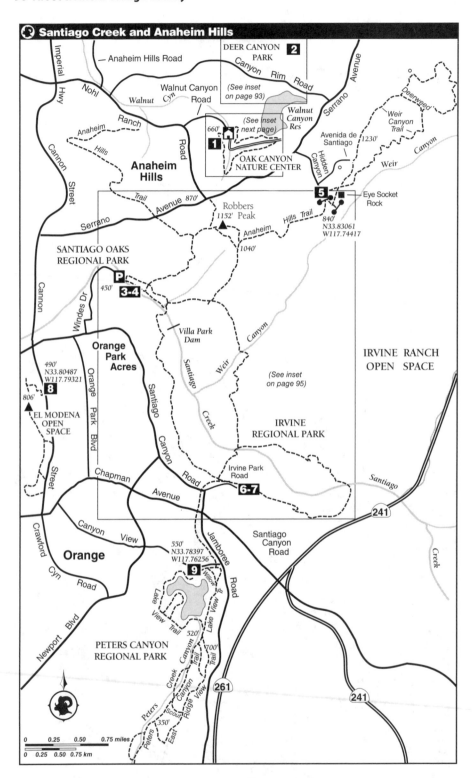

Santiago Creek and Anaheim Hills

Imperial Hwy

Anaheim Hills Road

Nohl

Walnut

Walnut Canyon Road

Walnut Cyn

DEER CANYON PARK **2**

Canyon Rim Road

Serrano Avenue

(See inset on page 93)

Anaheim Ranch

Anaheim Hills

Cannon Street

660'

(See inset next page)

1

Walnut Canyon Res

Deerweed

Weir Canyon Trail

1230'

Avenida de Santiago

OAK CANYON NATURE CENTER

Hidden Canyon

Weir Canyon

Anaheim Hills

Road

Trail

Avenue 870'

Robbers 1152' Peak

Anaheim

Hills Trail

5

840'
N33.83061
W117.74417

Eye Socket Rock

Serrano

SANTIAGO OAKS REGIONAL PARK

1040'

Cannon

Windes Dr

450'

P

3-4

Villa Park Dam

Weir

Canyon

IRVINE RANCH OPEN SPACE

Orange Park Acres

490'
N33.80487
W117.79321

8

806'

EL MODENA OPEN SPACE

Orange Park Blvd

Santiago

Canyon

Road

Santiago

Creek

(See inset on page 95)

IRVINE REGIONAL PARK

Santiago

Chapman

Irvine Park Road

6-7

Street

Avenue

Santiago

241

Crawford Cyn Road

Canyon View

Orange

550'
N33.78397
W117.76256

9

Jamboree Road

Santiago Canyon Road

Creek

Newport Blvd

Lake View Trail

Willow Tr

Lake View Trail

520'

700'

PETERS CANYON REGIONAL PARK

Peters Creek

Canyon Trail

Scout Ridge View Trail

East

350'

261

241

0   0.25   0.50   0.75 miles
0   0.25   0.50   0.75 km

trip 8.1   ## Oak Canyon Nature Center

Distance	1.5–2 miles (out-and-back or loop)
Hiking Time	1–1½ hours
Elevation Gain	200–300'
Difficulty	Easy
Trail Use	Good for kids
Best Times	All year
Agency	OCNC

DIRECTIONS Exit the Riverside Freeway (Highway 91) at Imperial Highway in Anaheim Hills. Drive south 0.7 mile to Nohl Ranch Road. Turn left there and go 1.7 miles east to Walnut Canyon Road. Turn left and continue 0.5 mile to the end of the road, where abundant free parking is available.

The tiny (58-acre) gem that is Oak Canyon Nature Center squeezes between a golf course and a reservoir on one side and a suburban housing tract on the other. Small children have plenty of room to roam on the tightly nested 4 miles worth of hiking trails here. Parking is free, but the nature center requests a small entrance donation. For adults, this is a park to savor slowly. Habitats include a trickling stream shaded by coast live oaks and hillsides coated with chaparral and sage scrub vegetation. Following a heavy rainfall season, the wildflowers, especially sticky monkeyflower, can be spectacular.

The primary mission of the Oak Canyon Nature Center is education. It offers a slew of workshops and hikes for families and individuals year-round. On certain summer evenings, the Center organizes "Nature Nights," twilight walks followed by presentations in the center's outdoor amphitheater.

A few steps from the parking lot will take you to a beautifully rustic interpretive center, nestled under spreading oaks. When it is open on Saturdays, you can view some exhibits and pick up a detailed trail map.

On the grounds of the nature center, numerous short trails diverge from the Main Road, a wide path paralleling a small stream in the bottom of Oak Canyon (a tributary of Walnut Canyon). You can go about 0.7 mile to the end of Main Road, then pick another route for your return trip. The Stream Trail meanders through

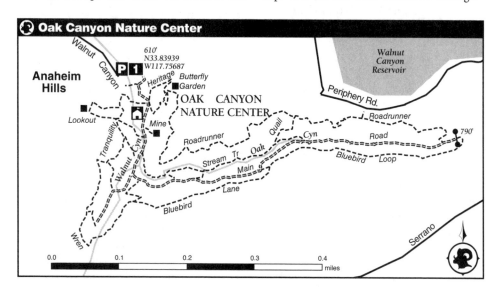

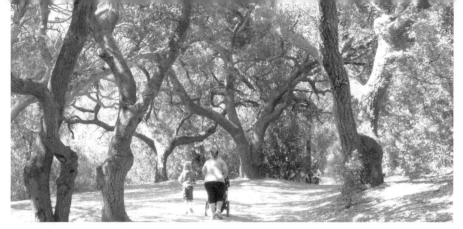

Oak Canyon

the thick of the riparian and oak woodland habitats, while the Roadrunner Ridge ascends onto the steep slopes overlooking the ravine bottom. The loop around the outermost perimeter of Oak Canyon Nature Center measures about 2 miles in length. (Note that the Bluebird Trail on the south side ends outside a gate at the east edge of the park. Walk back through the

gate to rejoin the main road or the Roadrunner Ridge Trail.)

In summer, you'll find little of interest high on the shadeless, scrub-covered slopes but a lot to enjoy down amid the oaks. In spring, you'll want to gravitate toward the slopes on the south side, where a variety of blooming native plants stands shoulder to shoulder.

trip 8.2 Deer Canyon Park Preserve

Distance	2.8 miles (loop)
Hiking Time	1½ hours
Elevation Gain	500'
Difficulty	Moderate
Trail Use	Cyclists, equestrians, dogs, good for kids
Best Times	All year
Agency	City of Anaheim

DIRECTIONS Exit Highway 91 south on Weir Canyon Road. In 0.9 mile, turn right on Serrano Avenue, then immediately right again onto Canyon Creek Road. In 0.5 mile, turn left on Sunset Ridge, then in 0.2 mile, turn right on East Hollow Oak Road. Proceed 0.4 mile and park on the street where the road ends at a gated community. Be sure to observe signed parking restrictions.

Deer Canyon Park is a little-known 103-acre wilderness tucked in the canyon between the heavily developed hills. This Anaheim city park receives little maintenance and has taken on a charmingly wild feel. The slopes are covered in native sage scrub, which blooms in the spring, and the stream is lined with sycamores, oaks, willows, mulefat, and cottonwoods. The canyon is a refuge for coyotes, rabbits, deer, and other animals

squeezed by urban development. The major trails are oddly all named Anaheim Hills, yet they do not connect to the better-known Anaheim Hills Trail near Robbers Peak. The long, skinny canyon is not conducive to loop hikes entirely within the park, so this trip connects two branches of the canyon via the sidewalk on streets overlooking it.

Unless you live in the area and you enter from one of many neighborhood access

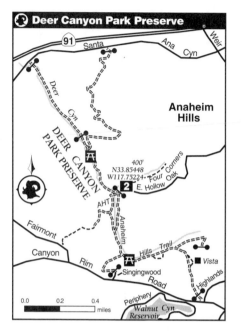

Deer Canyon Park Preserve

Anaheim
Hills

DEER CANYON
PARK PRESERVE

400'
N33.85448
W117.75224 · Four Corners
E. Hollow Oak

AHT

Anaheim

Fairmont

Canyon

Rim

Hills Trail

Singingwood

Road

■ Vista

Highlands

Periphery

0.0   0.2   0.4

miles

Walnut Cyn
Reservoir

Turn left and follow Fairmont, then veer left onto Canyon Rim Road and continue along it above the canyon. You'll eventually pass Walnut Canyon Reservoir on the opposite side of the road. In 1 mile, immediately before reaching a road called The Highlands, turn left onto another gated dirt road signed Anaheim Hills Trail to reenter Deer Canyon Park.

Follow the streamside road down the canyon. In 0.3 mile, come to a fork where the road crosses the stream. Veer right and make a short, steep climb to a knoll with a bench where you can take in the canyon views, then descend northeast on a trail that soon rejoins the road. Stay left at another road junction shortly beyond, and continue down the canyon. In 0.2 mile, watch for a half-overgrown picnic ground on the left with hitching posts and, remarkably, an operational drinking fountain.

After the picnic area, pass a trail on the left leading up to Singingwood Drive. Continue down the canyon floor, staying right at another junction, to reach the trailhead where you began.

points, the easiest parking is on Hollow Oak Road. Be sure to enter the park at the Deer Canyon sign on the south side of the road, not on the Four Corners Trail on the north. Pass through the gate, and come to an immediate T-junction with an old paved road. Don't take either fork; instead, join the signed Anaheim Hills Trail on the opposite side of the junction marked with a wooden fence.

Follow the Anaheim Hills Trail signs as you weave through a series of intersections. Stay left at a fork in 0.1 mile. Climb a hill to a T-junction with a dirt road. Both directions are signed Anaheim Hills, but this trip goes right to a powerline service road on the ridgeline. Turn left on this road, and follow it up to another tower near a housing development. Where the road ends, 0.4 mile from the start, merge onto a narrower footpath, which drops to follow a rutted gas pipeline road at the bottom of a slope between two housing developments. Beware of the large poison oak bushes growing beside the trail. In another 0.3 mile, the trail ends on Fairmont Boulevard.

Elderberry

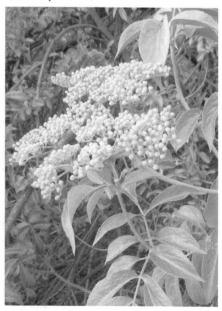

trip 8.3

Santiago Oaks Regional Park

Distance	0.8-plus miles (loop)
Hiking Time	1 hour
Elevation Gain	100'
Difficulty	Easy
Trail Use	Cyclists, equestrians, dogs, good for kids
Best Times	All year
Agency	OC Parks: SORP
Permit	OC Parks parking fee required

DIRECTIONS Exit Highway 55 at Katella Avenue in Orange. Go east on Katella (which quickly becomes Villa Park Road and finally Santiago Canyon Road) a total of 3 miles to Windes Drive on the left (north). Follow Windes Drive straight into the park. Pay your day-use fee at the entrance, drive past a traffic circle, and park in the lot beyond.

What Santiago Oaks Regional Park lacks in sheer size is more than adequately compensated for by its rare beauty. Its core is made up of two former ranch properties acquired in the mid-1970s. A small Valencia orange grove and many acres of ornamental trees planted around 1960 on these properties complement the natural riparian and oak woodland communities along Santiago Creek.

As you approach the park entrance on Windes Drive (just north of Santiago Canyon Road), the outlying subdivisions quickly fade from sight and a lush strip of riparian vegetation featuring willows and sycamores presided over by steep, scruffy slopes comes into view on the left.

The park is laced with several miles of trail, the best of which stay close to the wooded bottomlands of Santiago Creek. The multiuse trails (which allow hiking, biking, and horseback riding) stay generally north of Santiago Creek, while the hiking-only, self-guiding Windes Nature Trail and its Pacifica Loop extension are south of the creek, adjacent to the nature center. Because of the diversity of its habitats, Santiago Oaks is a delightful birding spot, with species ranging from the tree-dwelling western bluebird and acorn woodpecker to the water-loving

Windes Trail

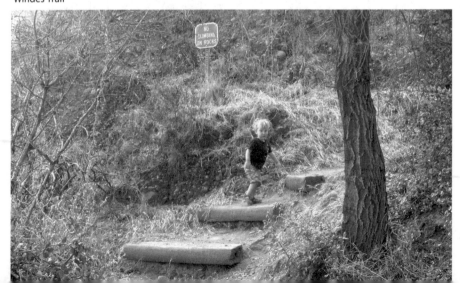

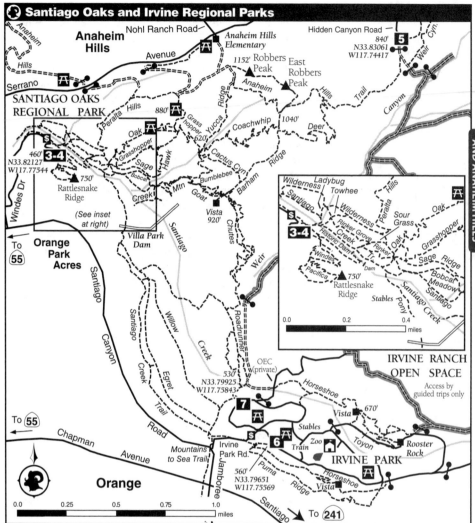

great blue heron. On occasion, vultures and ospreys, as well as some common hawks, may be seen soaring overhead.

For a short (0.8-mile) introduction to the park, return to the traffic circle, and pick up the Santiago Creek Trail, which has concrete stepping pads that help you cross the creek. Follow it southeast past several side trails to a major intersection with the Oak Trail on the left in 0.3 mile. The Heritage Oak, a 250-year-old coastal live oak, stood here until the 2007 Windy Ridge

Fire swept through the park and burned it. New sprouts are emerging from its trunk. Most of the park has recovered well, and new oaks have been planted. Follow the Oak Trail north, then take the first left onto the Rinker Grove Trail. Wander through the pleasant forest of eucalyptus, pepper, and other exotic trees, then jog right on the Sour Grass Trail and immediately left to continue on Rinker Grove until it ends at the Towhee Trail. Turn left and you soon emerge back on the Santiago Creek Trail and follow it back across the creek to the trailhead.

Another pleasant 0.7-mile loop starts at the nature center. From the end of the parking lot, you can stroll up past some oak-shaded picnic sites to the superb nature center, which is housed in a nicely refurbished 70-year-old ranch house. From here, the Windes Trail and Pacifica Loop Trail meander steeply up to the northern summit of Rattlesnake Ridge, an isolated, erosion-resistant block of mostly conglomerate rock. A slice of Pacific coastline can be glimpsed from the high point of the trail, and a fenced lookout point nearby offers a view almost straight down on Santiago Creek and the rest of the park.

Below the picnic area, you can walk upstream along the shaded creek bank on the Historic Dam Trail to reach a small rock-and-cement dam dating from 1892. This dam replaced an earlier one, built in 1879, that was part of one of Orange County's first irrigation systems. The surviving dam is a historical curiosity, dwarfed by the large Villa Park flood-control dam a short distance upstream, as well as Santiago Reservoir farther upstream.

Longer trails radiate outward from Santiago Oaks Regional Park toward Irvine Regional Park to the southeast, and up the slopes east and northeast into a county-owned tract formerly called Weir Canyon Wilderness Park that has been incorporated into Santiago Oaks. Massive suburban development is taking place on and beyond these slopes—yet thousands of acres in this same area have been preserved as part of the Irvine Ranch Open Space.

---

trip 8.4	**Robbers Peak**

Distance	5 miles (loop)
Hiking Time	2½ hours
Elevation Gain	1,000'
Difficulty	Moderate
Trail Use	Cyclists, equestrians, dogs
Best Times	November–May
Agency	OC Parks: SORP
Permit	OC Parks parking fee required

see maps on p. 90 and p. 95

DIRECTIONS Exit the 55 Freeway at Katella Avenue in Orange. Go east on Katella (which quickly become Villa Park Road and finally Santiago Canyon Road) a total of 3 miles to Windes Drive on the left (north). Follow Windes Drive straight into Santiago Oaks Regional Park, the starting point. Pay your day-use fee at the entrance, drive past a traffic circle, and park in the lot beyond.

The name "Robbers Peak" commemorates the notorious outlaws Joaquin Murrieta, Three Finger Jack, and others of the late 1800s. According to legend, these bandits swept down out of the hills, terrorized farmers below, and preyed upon passengers traveling the Butterfield Stage. From Robbers Peak, they could easily spot and evade sheriff's posses by slipping into the rugged ravines and canyons leading back toward the Santa Ana Mountains.

Robbers Peak is on private land. Despite a long and continuing tradition of visitation by hikers, the landowner now discourages access. Instead, this trip climbs to an almost equally high point on public land on the same ridge just to the southeast. From this height, you get a panoramic view of the lowlands to the south and west—a composite of disappearing pastoral landscapes and spreading suburban sprawl. On clear days, the panorama includes the blue arc of the Pacific Ocean and Santa Catalina Island.

There's a trivially easy way to reach Robbers Peak from a public-access gravel roadway starting at Nohl Ranch Road and Serrano Avenue on the east edge of Anaheim Hills Elementary School, but the looping route described here is much more scenic and exciting. Of the many existing options, this one offers superb views and diverse territory. Its many potentially confusing junctions were marked when the route was last scouted, but signs have been known to vanish. Don't worry if you lose the trail described here, but continue until you can identify a junction marked on the map.

Begin hiking at Santiago Oaks Regional Park's parking lot at the end of Windes Drive. From the traffic circle at the entrance to the parking lot, follow the broad path east and then north to cross Santiago Creek at the first opportunity, and continue along the Santiago Creek Trail, with Santiago Creek on your right for 0.6 mile. At that point, you reach a major trail junction where Pony and Santiago Creek Trail continues south, bound for Irvine Regional Park, and the Oak Trail veers left.

Go left and, shortly thereafter, reach another complex trail junction where you can continue up the Oak Trail on graded switchbacks. As you climb, the massive Villa Park flood-control dam comes into full view, along with its spillway on the far side. At full capacity (which it has not yet ever reached), the floodwaters backing up behind this dam would inundate about half of Irvine Regional Park. Pass a shaded picnic bench, and continue up to a signed junction with the Grasshopper Trail where the ridge turns north.

In the interest of a scenic tour, you now give up much of the elevation you just earned. Take the switchbacking Grasshopper Trail southeast into the canyon below. At a junction on the bottom, veer left, then make an immediate right onto the Coachwhip

Trail, which switchbacks vigorously up to reach Barham Ridge.

Turn left on the Barham Ridge Trail, and promptly pass junctions with the Anaheim Hills Trail on the left and then the right. Continue straight onto the hill ahead, and climb past a transmission line tower to the eastern summit of Robbers Peak. North of the summit, subdivisions press against the sage-dotted hills and canyons. Southward, a big swath of nearly untouched landscape has become a designated part of the Irvine Ranch Open Space.

To make a figure-eight loop, retrace your steps on the Barham Ridge Trail, and continue southwest down the scenic ridge. Pass the Cactus Canyon Trail on the right and the Chutes Trail to Irvine Regional Park on the left. Shortly beyond, reach the Mountain Goat Trail on the right. Continue a few more paces to the scenic overlook at the end of Barham Ridge before returning to descend the Mountain Goat Trail.

New Robbers Peak

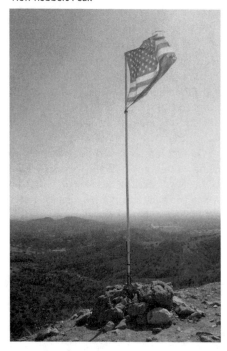

The Mountain Goat Trail has two intersecting options: a graded switchbacking path favored by equestrians and a rutted trail almost straight down the ridge favored by gonzo mountain bikers. Pick your preference. Both rejoin before a junction with the Bumblebee Trail, then fork again before rejoining on the floor of Santiago Canyon.

Turn right and follow the Bobcat Meadow Trail along the north side of the canyon, passing several trails on both sides. At the complex junction where you originally took the Oak Trail, continue along the canyon's edge on the Wilderness Trail. After more junctions on both sides, turn left onto the Ladybug Trail, and follow it down a short flight of stairs to the Santiago Creek crossing where you began near the parking lot.

---

see map on p. 90

trip 8.5 Weir Canyon Loop

Distance	4 miles (loop)
Hiking Time	2 hours
Elevation Gain	700'
Difficulty	Moderate
Trail Use	Cyclists, equestrians, dogs, good for kids
Best Times	November–May
Agency	OC Parks: SORP

DIRECTIONS From the 91 Freeway, exit south on Weir Canyon Road. In 0.9 mile, turn right on Serrano Avenue. In 2 miles, turn left on Hidden Canyon Road. After 0.5 mile, the road turns right and becomes Overlook Terrace. Find curbside parking at or near this spot, where there is access to the Weir Canyon Trail.

The Weir Canyon Trail skims an undeveloped ridge of the Anaheim Hills overlooking Weir Canyon, drawing significant numbers of hikers, equestrians, and mountain bikers. This trail is part of Santiago Oaks Regional Park and connects to the rest of the park through an extensive web of trails.

On foot, proceed on the gated dirt road going south from Overlook Terrace (not the Weir Canyon Trail at the kiosk to the left, by which you will return). Immediately, there's a split. The right fork is the Anaheim Hills Trail going to Santiago Canyon—take the left fork and, after only 100 yards, come to the Weir Gate blocking all traffic. Beyond lies Irvine Ranch Open Space property that is accessible only on guided tours. Just before this gate, find the narrow trail on the left and climb up a hill. Immediately to the left, look for a pair of closely spaced wind caves carved into a massive outcrop like the vacant eye sockets of a human skull. Shortly beyond, climb to an unsigned junction where you turn right onto the Weir Canyon Trail. You will return to this junction at the end of the loop.

For the next 2 miles, you follow the trail's crooked course as it undulates and contours in and out of ravines. The wide floor of Weir Canyon lies below. A rich assemblage of sage scrub vegetation, dotted here and there with coast live oaks, smothers the slopes hereabouts. Strangely weathered sedimentary strata crop out in many places along the trail, lending an otherworldly feel to the journey, especially in early morning mist. Throughout these hills and extending higher into the Santa Ana Mountains, such outcrops provide nesting sites for swifts, hawks, and other birds. This crooked stretch is fun for

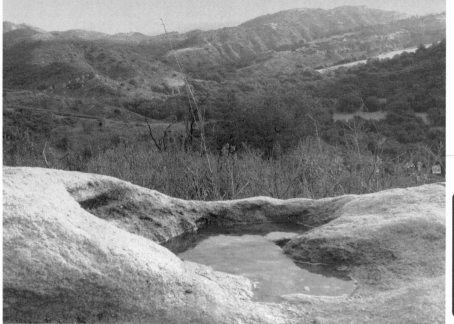

Weir Canyon

kids—though it's good to keep an eye out for mountain bikers. Watch for the Deerweed Cutoff Trail on the left, which allows you to shave a mile off the loop if you are short on time.

At 2.4 miles from the start, the trail climbs, swings sharply left, gains a viewful ridgeline, and follows that ridgeline southwest. Fingers of suburbia reach upward toward the trail on the north.

At 3.4 miles from the start, the trail pitches downward on the ridgeline. A spur on the right leads to a trailhead at the east end of a residential street called Avenida de Santiago, but your loop continues southwest. The steep old and switchbacking new Weir Canyon Trails split, cross, and rejoin in 0.25 mile. Pick either one, and then descend to the junction near the start, and turn right to reach the trailhead.

trip 8.6   Irvine Regional Park

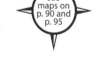

see maps on p. 90 and p. 95

Distance	3 miles (loop)
Hiking Time	1½ hours
Elevation Gain	200'
Difficulty	Easy
Trail Use	Cyclists, equestrians, dogs, good for kids
Best Times	All year
Agency	OC Parks: IRP
Permit	OC Parks parking fee required

DIRECTIONS From Interstate 5 in Irvine, exit north on Jamboree Road, and follow it 6 miles to the end. Stay right onto Irvine Park Road into the park. After passing the entrance gate (request a park map), veer right at the first junction, and then turn left into the first parking lot (Lot #7).

Alternatively, the park can be reached from the either of the eastern toll roads (241 or 261) by exiting at Santiago Canyon Road and taking it 1 mile northwest, then turning right on Jamboree Road and proceeding 0.25 mile. Or from the 55 Freeway in Orange, take Chapman Avenue east 4.2 miles, then turn left on Jamboree Road and proceed 0.25 mile.

For more than a century, Irvine Park has drawn Orange Countians up into the foothills of the Santa Ana Mountains. Once a meeting place for the early settlers (then known as the Picnic Grounds), it became Orange County Park in 1897 when early rancher James Irvine donated 160 acres of prime oak and sycamore groves fronting Santiago Creek. Now named Irvine Regional Park, it has grown to 477 acres and hosts thousands of visitors on busy weekends. The entrance road, on the eastern fringe of the city of Orange, is located at the north end of Jamboree Road.

Aside from picnic and playground areas, a lagoon with paddleboats, the small but

Kids of all ages love Rooster Rock.

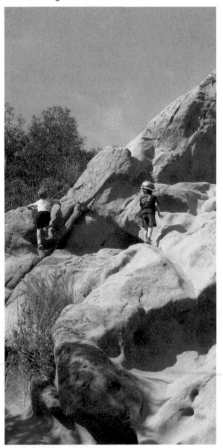

kid-friendly Orange County Zoo, a train ride, and wildlife and historical exhibits—it's possible to find some off-the-beaten-path hiking here. Several miles of paved and unpaved trails suitable for bicycling, hiking, and horseback riding follow Santiago Creek and wind around the perimeter of the park. For a pleasant introduction, try the following loop:

From Parking Lot #7, look southeast for a trail between wooden fence posts. Follow it, climbing steeply, to join the wide Horseshoe Loop Trail. Turn left, pass a junction with the Puma Ridge Trail, and make a switchbacking ascent to a lookout point beside an old water tank.

Descend, crossing a private road, and join a paved road leading east, north across Santiago Creek, and back west. Despite its nearly 100 square miles of drainage, the creek's broad, open bed is almost always dry, partly because much of the upstream surface flow has already seeped into porous soils, and partly because Irvine Lake (Santiago Reservoir) impounds water upstream. There's still enough water underground, however, to keep the oaks, sycamores, and other trees in the park looking healthy. The biggest oaks in the park are as old as 800 years.

Shortly before you reach an outcrop of sandstone called Rooster Rock, Horseshoe Loop veers right and resumes its dirt tread to climb a dry bluff. Kids and the young at heart will enjoy scrambling on the cliffs and exploring the small caves at Rooster Rock.

From here, the path has numerous poorly signed junctions, but any route north and east will suffice. Continue about 0.4 mile to reach a shaded viewpoint beside the Toyon Trail overlooking the green, irrigated parts of the park below, a good place for a restful pause.

Complete the circuit by descending past the viewpoint into a picnic area below and then crossing the creekbed via a paved path. Wander among the park's central attractions, clustered around the boating lake, to return to the starting point.

trip 8.7 **Irvine to Santiago Loop**

Distance	4.5 miles (loop)
Hiking Time	2½ hours
Elevation Gain	600'
Difficulty	Moderate
Trail Use	Cyclists, equestrians, dogs
Best Times	All year
Agency	OC Parks: IRP
Permit	OC Parks parking fee required

see maps on p. 90 and p. 95

DIRECTIONS From Interstate 5 in Irvine, exit north on Jamboree Road, and follow it 6 miles to the end. Stay right onto Irvine Park Road into the park. After passing the entrance gate (request a park map), veer left at the first junction, and curve around for 0.3 mile to Parking Lot #2, the first lot on your right.

Alternatively, the park can be reached from either of the eastern toll roads (241 or 261) by exiting at Santiago Canyon Road and taking it 1 mile northwest, then turning right on Jamboree Road and proceeding 0.25 mile. Or from the 55 Freeway in Orange, take Chapman Avenue east 4.2 miles, then turn left on Jamboree and proceed 0.25 mile.

This scenic loop tours the diverse riparian and sage scrub habitats along Santiago Creek and the ridges overlooking them between Irvine and Santiago Oaks Regional Parks. Plenty of groundwater nourishes dense growths of willows and underbrush alongside the creek in this area, providing excellent bird habitat. Bring binoculars! At present, a maze of illegal trails forks off the main path. Rangers are planning to mark the official trail better, but be prepared for possibly confusing junctions. In a wet winter, the trails south of the Villa Park flood-control dam could be inundated and impassable.

From Lot #2, look for the Roadrunner Loop trailhead on the north side of the park road. Take the trail north into the canyon, and make an immediate right onto a trail crossing the creek. In 0.1 mile, the Roadrunner Trail splits. The right fork is a fire road, but this trip takes the more attractive left fork through the oaks and sage scrub. In 0.4 mile, pass a signed path on the left cutting across the canyon floor to the Willows Trail. In another 0.1 mile, rejoin the fire road at a turnaround. Stay left and continue north to a kiosk at the end of the Roadrunner Trail.

Two trails continue north across the wash at the mouth of Weir Canyon, then rejoin at the start of the Chutes Trail. The Chutes Trail again splits, with a graded path switchbacking up onto the hillside and a much steeper Chutes Ridgeline path leading straight up the ridge. Pick your preference and make the stiff climb. The trails cross once along the way and rejoin atop Barham Ridge. You are rewarded with expanding views and a lovely cactus garden.

You are now in Santiago Oaks Regional Park, and your next goal is to descend the ridge and loop back west and south past the Villa Park flood-control dam. Turn left, then make an immediate right onto the Mountain Goat Trail leading west down the ridge. The trail forks, rejoins, forks again, and rejoins; choose either the graded equestrian option or the steep, rutted path straight down the ridge favored by mountain bikers.

When you reach the floor of the canyon, you need to pick a path on the west side of Santiago Creek to pass the dam by its spillway. The most direct path along a dirt road beneath the dam is closed to public access, so you instead veer onto the Santiago Creek Trail that leads west and

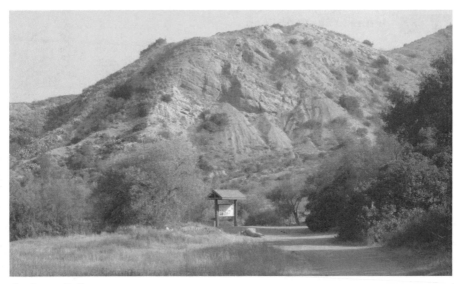

Roadrunner Trail

north. Stay left at the next three junctions in quick succession to join the Pony Trail, which fords the often dry Santiago Creek and reaches a staging area near a corral. Pick up the Santiago Creek Trail (here, it's a road) that resumes on the south side and climbs steeply to pass the dam.

A network of parallel trails leads south back to Irvine Regional Park. At your first opportunity, veer left onto the Egret Trail. Pass a junction with a trail cutting back across the wash to the Roadrunner Loop, and then shortly after veer left onto the (possibly unsigned) Willow Trail. Pass through an attractive grove of willows, and then make the easy but somewhat dull walk along the canyon. At a confusing junction just before the road, veer left on the Horseshoe Loop Trail to reach the trailhead where you began.

---

trip 8.8 El Modena Open Space

see map on p. 90

Distance	2.4 miles (loop)
Hiking Time	1½ hours
Elevation Gain	700'
Difficulty	Moderate
Trail Use	Cyclists, equestrians, dogs, good for kids
Best Times	All year
Agency	OC Parks: SORP

DIRECTIONS Exit Highway 55 at Chapman Avenue in Orange. Drive 2 miles east to Cannon Street. Turn north and drive 1.3 miles north to Patria Court, on the left, where curbside parking is available.

The long, narrow El Modena Open Space, a satellite of Santiago Oaks Regional Park in the city of Orange, preserves a steep-sided miniature mountain range, clothed in a tough mixture of drought-resistant cactus and sage scrub vegetation,

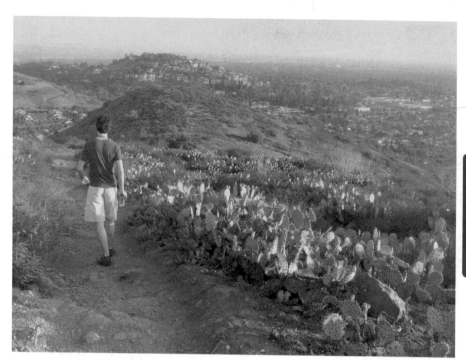

El Modena Ridge

and underlain by colorful andesite and pyroclastic rock—volcanic rock dating back some 15 million years. This type of rock, in colors of brick red, pink, white, gray, green, and beige, is found within Orange County only here and in a couple of spots just south of Chapman Avenue. The small but biologically rich park is also notable for hosting every species of mariposa lily, as well as the rare many-stemmed dudleya.

Pick up a poorly signed trail from Patria Court that leads south into the sage scrub paralleling Cannon Street. Quickly veer right on a steeply ascending trail through a natural garden of California sagebrush, encelia, wild hyacinth, and wild onion. As you wind upward toward the top of the ridge, dense thickets of prickly pear cactus appear. The large number of coastal cholla cactus are also notable, especially this far inland.

At the ridgeline, turn left and follow it to the highest summit, elevation 806 feet.

Enjoy a spacious, pseudoaerial view of the flat LA Basin, wrapping around more than 180 degrees, and the rim of the mountains to the east and north—the Santa Anas and the San Gabriels—a mind-blowing view on days of crystalline atmospheric conditions.

From the high point, descend south and pass over two more summits in the next mile. A very steep path goes down the west side of the southernmost hill and meets a dirt path leading back to the intersection of Cannon Street and Stillwater Avenue. Use the bicycle path or sidewalk along Cannon to complete the mile-long return to Patria Court. Done this way, the entire loop measures 2.4 miles.

Two shortcut trails link the ridgeline to Cannon Street, and either one of those can be used to shorten the hike. Beware that other potentially confusing use trails sometimes form as hikers cut the official trail. Stay on the official trails to avoid exacerbating this problem.

trip 8.9 Peters Canyon Regional Park

Distance	2.2–4-plus miles (loop or semiloop)
Hiking Time	2 hours
Elevation Gain	At least 200'
Difficulty	Moderate
Trail Use	Cyclists, equestrians, dogs, good for kids
Best Times	All year
Agency	OC Parks: PCRP
Permit	OC Parks parking fee required

see map on p. 90

DIRECTIONS From either of the two eastern toll roads (Highways 241 and 261), exit at Santiago Canyon Road. Drive 1 mile northwest to Jamboree Road, and turn left (south). Drive 0.5 mile to Canyon View Avenue, turn right, and then go left into the regional park.

Deeded to Orange County by the Irvine Company in 1992, Peters Canyon Regional Park has, like other newly declared open-space areas, gained almost instant popularity among lovers of the outdoors. Expect to see plenty of hikers, bikers, and joggers on the busy trails. The park features the 55-acre Upper Peters Canyon Reservoir, several natural habitats (freshwater marsh, riparian woodland, grassland, and coastal sage scrub), and about 6 miles of trails. The shallow reservoir is not open to fishing, but birding is fine here. Mats of marsh vegetation and water-loving trees (willows, cottonwoods, and sycamores) hug most of the shoreline, attracting egrets, grebes, herons,

Peters Canyon Reservoir

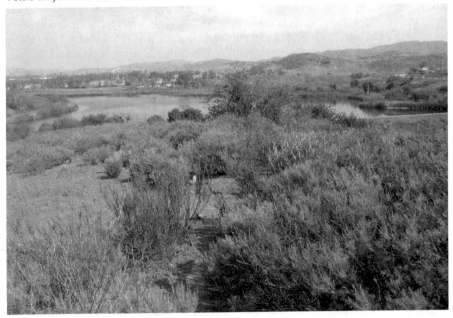

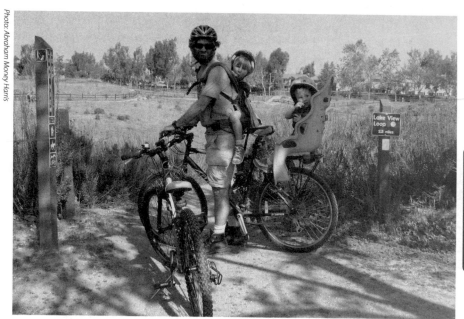

Photo: Abraham Money Harris

Happy riders

and other birds. The park is open from 7 a.m. to sunset daily. It may be closed for up to 72 hours after rains.

From the park's northern (main) entrance and parking lot, off Canyon View Avenue in the city of Orange, you can start hiking by going west on the Lake View Trail. The shortest circumnavigation of the lake measures 2.2 miles, while side trips to the south, below the reservoir dam, can easily add 1.5 or more miles.

Pass several side trails, but stay on the main path, which climbs steeply to a vista point on the south side of the lake, then descends below the dam. When Lake View Trail meets Peters Canyon Trail just beyond, turn right (south) and proceed down the wide Peters Canyon Trail until you reach Creek Trail, which diverges on the right about 300 yards south of the dam. Mountain bikers must stay on the main trail, but hikers can follow the paralleling, relatively primitive Creek Trail. On it, you duck under the limbs of willow, black cottonwood, and

sycamore; inhale the humid odors of riparian vegetation and the pungent scent of eucalyptus; and sometimes (depending on the season) splash through shallow water or squish through mud in the canyon bottom. Footbridges are provided at some of the creek crossings.

At the end of the Creek Trail, you come up out of the shady canyon bottom to rejoin the main Peters Canyon Trail. By turning left and continuing all the way north on the same trail, you end up circling the reservoir's east side and returning to the starting point. Alternatively, you can make a more strenuous loop by turning east up the Scout Trail and following the steep East Ridge View Trail back to rejoin Peters Canyon Trail near the dam.

As you approach the north end of the lake, don't miss the narrow shortcut trail—through a dense growth of willows—on the left. This "Willows Trail" is closed March–September to protect the nesting rights of certain birds.

chapter 9

Whiting Ranch Wilderness Park

In 1991, Orange County opened the 1,500-acre Whiting Ranch Wilderness Park (now grown to 2,500 acres), which sprawls across the foothills of the Santa Ana Mountains just east of the communities of Lake Forest and El Toro. Whiting Ranch's rounded hills look a bit dry and nondescript when viewed from the suburbs below, but up close they reveal some pleasant surprises. One can be found in the upper reaches of a narrow ravine called Borrego Canyon: strangely weathered outcrops of red-tinted sandstone, rising a sheer 100 feet or more. The park is also noteworthy for its dense riparian and oak woodland vegetation, which smothers the bottoms of the park's larger ravines.

In 1885, Dwight Whiting acquired parts of two huge Mexican land grants and established a ranch. In 1959, most of the ranch was sold to build subdivisions, but a portion was subsequently granted to Orange County as a wilderness park.

Whiting Ranch's most popular entrance stands alongside a shopping center on Portola Parkway, opposite Market Place and between Alton Parkway and Bake Parkway, east of the Foothill Transportation Corridor Toll Road in the city of Lake Forest. Look for a trailhead parking lot here, open from 7 a.m. to sunset. Another staging area serving the park is located on Glenn Ranch Road. The ranger station is oddly located at the historic McFadden Ranch House, which is discontiguous from the rest of the park and effectively isolates rangers from visitors.

This chapter offers a sampling of hikes in the park, but you can spend many enjoyable days exploring the web of trails.

Borrego Canyon

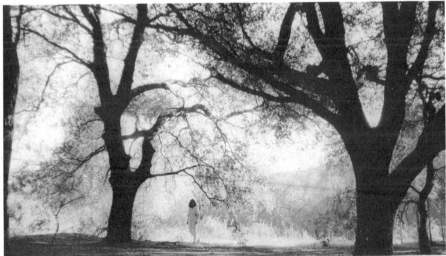

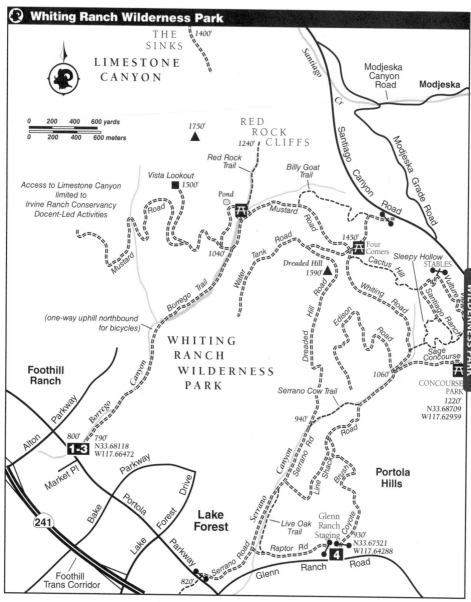

Whiting Ranch Wilderness Park

THE SINKS

LIMESTONE CANYON

1400'

Santiago Cr

Modjeska Canyon Road

Modjeska

Modjeska Grade Road

0   200   400   600 yards
0   200   400   600 meters

1750'

RED ROCK CLIFFS

1240'

Vista Lookout
1500'

Red Rock Trail

Billy Goat Trail

Access to Limestone Canyon limited to Irvine Ranch Conservancy Docent-Led Activities

Pond

Mustard Road

Mustard

Borrego Trail

1040'

Tank Road

Water Road

Dreaded Hill
1590'

Road

Cactus

1450'
Four Corners

Sleepy Hollow STABLES

Whiting Road

Santiago Ranch

View

Vulture

(one-way uphill northbound for bicycles)

Foothill Ranch

Canyon

WHITING RANCH WILDERNESS PARK

Dreaded Hill Road

Edison Road

Road

1060'

Sage Concourse

CONCOURSE PARK
1220'
N33.68709
W117.62959

Serrano Cow Trail

Borrego Parkway

Alton Parkway

800'   790'
N33.68118
W117.66472

1-3

Market Pl

Parkway

Portola Forest Drive

Bake

Lake

Parkway

241

Foothill Trans Corridor

820'

Lake Forest

940'

Serrano Rd

Serrano Canyon

Road

Line Shack

Brush

Live Oak Trail

Glenn Ranch Staging

Raptor Rd

Serrano Road

Glenn   Ranch   Road

Coyote

Portola Hills

930'
N33.67521
W117.64288

4

WHITING RANCH WILDERNESS PARK

Generally expect splendid oak groves in the canyons and interesting views on the ridges. A park brochure and trail map is available at either trailhead, and maps or directional signs posted at critical trail junctions help make navigation easy. All of the trails except Red Rock Canyon are open to equestrians and mountain bikers as well as hikers. Whiting Ranch has earned a reputation as a world-class mountain biking destination, and cyclists easily outnumber hikers on the trails south and east of Four Corners.

In October 2007, an arsonist started the Santiago Fire, which burned more than 30,000 acres, including 90% of Whiting

Ranch. Fortunately, chaparral has evolved to recover rapidly after fire, and the park remains beautiful.

The park is officially known as Limestone Canyon and Whiting Ranch Wilderness Park, but the Limestone Canyon portion to the north of Whiting Ranch remains closed to the public except through guided activities. More details for Limestone Canyon are given in Trip 10.1.

trip 9.1 Borrego and Red Rock Canyons

see map on previous page

Distance	4.4 miles (out-and-back)
Hiking Time	2 hours
Elevation Gain	500'
Difficulty	Moderate
Trail Use	Good for kids
Best Times	October–June
Agency	OC Parks: WRWP
Permit	OC Parks parking fee required

DIRECTIONS Exit the Foothill Transportation Corridor Toll Road (Highway 241) at Alton Parkway in Lake Forest. Go east on Alton 0.5 mile, then turn right on Portola Parkway. At the first traffic light (for Market Place), turn left into a strip mall parking area. There is a fee for parking by the trailhead to the left.

From Whiting Ranch's Portola Parkway trailhead, the Borrego Trail leads straightway toward Red Rock Canyon, where sandstone cliffs banded with layers of ancient sand and mud rise into the air. The best illumination of the cliffs usually occurs late in the day, when the sun's warm glow brings out the ruddy tint of oxidized iron on the surface of the rock.

Like most trails in the Whiting Ranch Wilderness Park, the Borrego Trail is open to mountain biking and horseback riding, as well as hiking. Mountain bikers, however, are not allowed to ride all the way to Red Rock.

At the beginning, you immediately plunge into densely shaded Borrego Canyon, alongside a stream that happily trickles through during winter and spring. For a while, suburbia rims the canyon on both sides, but soon enough it disappears without a trace. The trek up the canyon feels Tolkienesque as you pass under a crooked-limb canopy of live oaks and sycamores and sniff the damp odor of the streamside willows. Often in late fall and winter, frigid air sinks into these shady recesses overnight, and by early morning, frost mantles everything below eye-level.

After about 40 minutes of walking and 1.5 miles, you come to Mustard Road, a fire road that ascends both east and west to ridgetops offering expansive views of the ocean on clear days. Turn right on Mustard Road, pass a picnic site, and take the second trail to the left (the Red Rock Trail—for hikers only), into an upper tributary of Borrego Canyon. The trail starts up the wash but in 20 yards veers right at a post.

Out in the sunshine now, you meander up the bottom of a sunny ravine that becomes increasingly narrow and steep. In 0.7 mile, you reach the base of the eroded sandstone cliffs, a part of the Sespe Formation made of sediment deposited on a shallow sea bottom about 20 million years ago. This type of rock containing the fossilized remains of shellfish and marine mammals underlies much of Orange County. Rarely is it as well exposed as it is here.

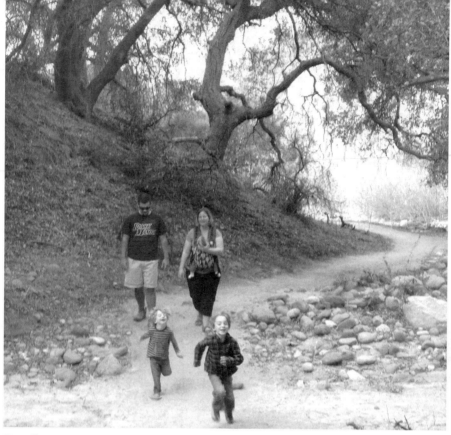

Boundless energy in Borrego Canyon

trip 9.2 Vista Lookout

Distance	4.8 miles (out-and-back)
Hiking Time	2½ hours
Elevation Gain	800'
Difficulty	Moderate
Trail Use	Cyclists, equestrians
Best Times	October–April
Agency	OC Parks: WRWP
Permit	OC Parks parking fee required

see map on p. 107

DIRECTIONS Exit the Foothill Transportation Corridor Toll Road (Highway 241) at Alton Parkway in Lake Forest. Go east on Alton 0.5 mile, then turn right on Portola Parkway. At the first traffic light (for Market Place), turn left into a strip mall parking area. There is a fee for parking by the trailhead to the left.

Vista Lookout is a hill at the north end of Whiting Ranch with superb views. The hike to the top up a steep fire road offers an excellent workout and escapes the crowds teeming in the rest of the park.

Go on a cool day because the climb can be a sweaty affair.

Follow the lovely Lower Borrego Canyon 1.5 miles to its junction with Mustard Road. Turn left and ascend the steep road across

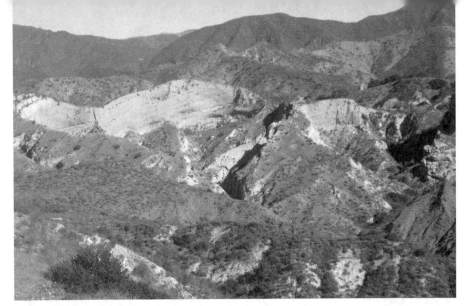

Red Rock Canyon views

slopes smothered in grass and invasive black mustard, which produces an attractive yellow flower in spring but soon dries to become a fire hazard. In 0.5 mile, veer right at a fork onto the Vista Lookout Trail, and take it 0.4 mile to the top of the hill, where a small oak may shade a picnic bench.

The lookout is notable as one of the few places outside of Limestone Canyon where you can glimpse the dramatic Sinks (take Trip 10.1 to visit them). It also offers a stunning aerial view of Red Rock Canyon and much of Whiting Ranch. Look west over the San Joaquin Hills to see Catalina and San Clemente Islands, or swivel your head for views of the San Gabriel and Santa Ana Mountains.

trip 9.3　**Whiting Ranch Loop**

see map on p. 107

Distance	6 miles (loop)
Hiking Time	3 hours
Elevation Gain	650'
Difficulty	Moderately strenuous
Trail Use	Cyclists, equestrians
Best Times	October–May
Agency	OC Parks: WRWP
Permit	OC Parks parking fee required

DIRECTIONS Exit the Foothill Transportation Corridor Toll Road (Highway 241) at Alton Parkway in Lake Forest. Go east on Alton 0.5 mile, then turn right on Portola Parkway. At the first traffic light (for Market Place), turn left into a strip mall parking area. There is a fee for parking by the trailhead to the left.

For a more comprehensive survey of Whiting Ranch Park, try this outstanding loop through the park's two largest canyons. You'll travel up Borrego Canyon to a watershed divide, then descend through Serrano Canyon. The basic loop is a little less than 6 miles (including a mile on the sidewalk along Portola Parkway at the end), though

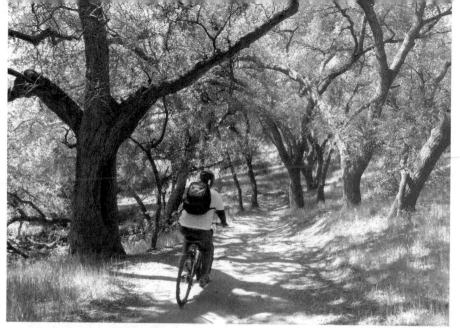

Mountain-biking in Whiting Ranch

numerous side trips and extensions are possible if you want to lengthen your hike. If you're mountain biking, you must follow the loop in the direction described below—the initial stretch through Borrego Canyon is designated one-way uphill for bikes.

Start by heading up Borrego Trail from Portola Parkway. At 1.5 miles, you meet Mustard Road. Turn right. Continue on Mustard Road, going north and later steeply east, up the main tributary of Borrego Canyon to Four Corners (2.3 miles), where four road segments join at a saddle. (A more scenic but strenuous way of reaching Four Corners,

for hikers only, involves the Billy Goat Trail, a rough path to the north with constant and often severe ups and downs, and little shade.)

At Four Corners, go across to Whiting Road and start descending—gradually at first along a ridge, then more steeply off the ridge and into an oak-lined valley (upper Serrano Canyon). Simply maintain your descent at all junctions, following the Serrano Cow Trail through a sublime tunnel of live oaks and finally the Serrano Road out to Portola Parkway. From there, follow the sidewalk a mile back to your starting point.

trip 9.4 **Dreaded Hill**

Distance	5 miles (loop)
Hiking Time	3 hours
Elevation Gain	1,000'
Difficulty	Moderately strenuous
Trail Use	Cyclists, equestrians
Best Times	October–April
Agency	OC Parks: WRWP
Permit	OC Parks parking fee required

see
map on
p. 107

DIRECTIONS Exit the Foothill Transportation Corridor Toll Road (Highway 241) at Portola Parkway. Go north on Portola for 0.3 mile, then turn right onto Glenn Ranch Road. In 0.6 mile, find the large Glenn Ranch staging area on the north side of the road. Be sure to pay your parking fee at the kiosk.

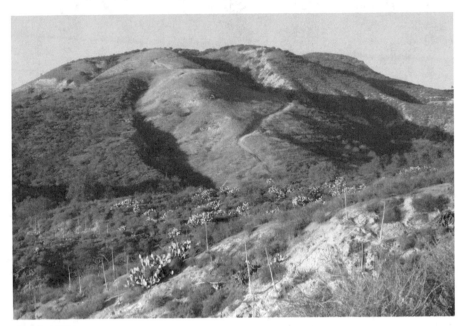

Dreaded Hill

Dreaded Hill is the highest point in Whiting Ranch, and the fire road leading to the summit offers a vigorous workout. Although the name may seem overly dramatic to hikers, it is quite appropriate for mountain bikers grunting their way up the path.

From the kiosk at the Glenn Ranch staging area, head west on the signed Raptor Road toward a transmission line tower. Descend into the cool Serrano Creek Canyon, and meet the Live Oak Trail in 0.3 mile. Follow it 0.4 mile through the oaks, then merge onto Serrano Road. In another 0.3 mile, reach the signed Dreaded Hill Road on the left.

Your workout now begins as you make the mile-long ascent of the hill. The plaque on the bench at the top, which has great views, commemorates Mark Reynolds: "He was doing what he loved." The 36-year-old amateur mountain bike champion was fixing his chain while on a solo ride in January 2004 when he was attacked and killed by a young mountain lion. A female ex-Marine was attacked by the same lion while biking later in the day but was saved by her companions, and the lion was shot as it went to retrieve Reynolds's corpse.

Descend northwest to a junction with the Water Tank Road, and make a hairpin turn to the right to reach Four Corners, where you can find shade and a drinking fountain. Start south down Whiting Road, but promptly veer left onto the Cactus Hill Trail, which has few cacti remaining after the Santiago Fire. In 0.5 mile, stay right as you join the Santiago Ranch Trail. In 0.2 mile, turn onto the aptly named Sleepy Hollow Trail, where the canopy of oaks creates a mysterious feel. In another 0.3 mile, merge onto the wide Whiting Road. Follow it downhill for 0.4 mile to a junction where you stay left and climb Line Shack Road to a transmission line tower. From this ridge, you have good views back to Dreaded Hill. In 0.4 mile, veer left again onto the signed Coyote Brush Road, and follow it 0.8 mile down to the staging area.

chapter 10

Irvine Ranch Open Space

Thanks in part to the efforts of countless Orange County conservationists, the Irvine Company has set aside more than half of the 93,000 acres of the vast historic Irvine Ranch as permanently protected open space or wilderness while the City of Irvine has grown up in the center. In 2006, a 37,000-acre swath was designated as the Irvine Ranch National Natural Landmark for their biological and geological significance. The protected lands include the 20,000-acre Irvine Ranch Open Space abutting the Cleveland National Forest, owned by OC Parks, and the City of Irvine's 5,200-acre Irvine Open Space Preserve area around Bommer Canyon and abutting Crystal Cove State Park (see Chapter 11). The land serves dual functions as a nature preserve where animals can live mostly undisturbed and as an outdoor recreation area.

To balance the needs of wildlife and humans, this open space is accessible to hikers, mountain bikers, and equestrians exclusively through regularly scheduled activities, organized primarily by the Irvine Ranch Conservancy. Many of the trails in this area are the wilderness equivalents of the nearby gated communities, providing excellent opportunities for local residents and frequent users while establishing

Limestone Canyon

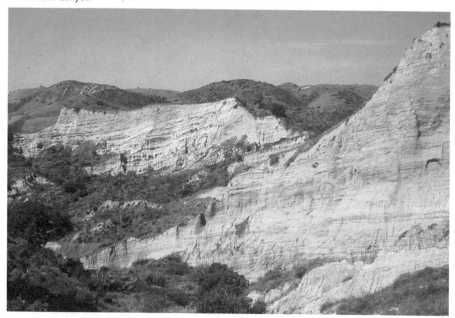

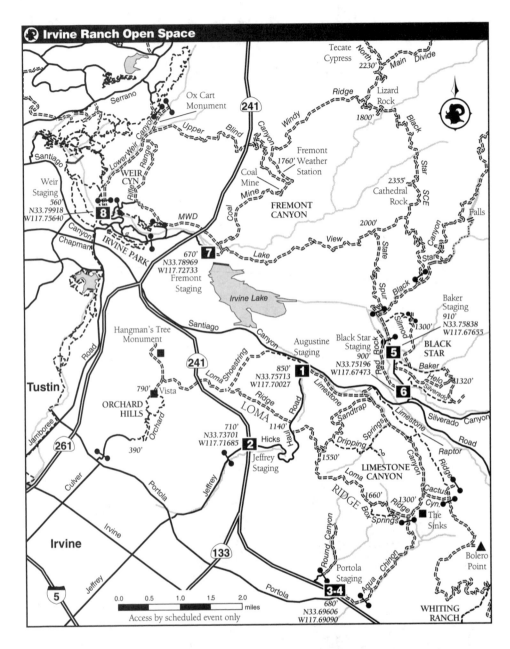

Irvine Ranch Open Space

Tecate
Cypress

North

Main Divide

2230'

Ridge

Lizard
Rock

Windy

1800'

Serrano

Ox Cart
Monument

Upper

Blind

241

Canyon

Fremont
1760' Weather
Station

Black

Star

2355'
Cathedral
Rock

SCE

Falls

Lower Weir Canyon

Coal
Mine

Santiago

WEIR
CYN

Range

Rifle

8

MWD

Mine

Coal

FREMONT
CANYON

2000'

View

Weir
Staging
560'
N33.79918
W117.75640

Canyon

Chapman

IRVINE PARK

670'
N33.78969
W117.72733
Fremont
Staging

7

Lake

State

Spur

Black

Star

Baker
Staging
910'
N33.75838
W117.67655

Irvine Lake

Silmod

1300'

Red Rock

5

BLACK
STAR

Hangman's Tree
Monument

Santiago

Canyon

Augustine
Staging

Black Star
Staging
900'
N33.75196
W117.67473

Baker

Helo

Silverado

1320'

Tustin

Road

Loma Shoestring

850'
N33.75713
W117.70027

1

Limestone

6

241

790'

Vista

ORCHARD
HILLS

Orchard

LOMA

Ridge

Hani

Road

1140'

Limestone

Silverado Canyon

Sandtrap

Springs

Road

261

390'

710'
N33.73701
W117.71685

2

Hicks

Dripping

Raptor

Ridge

Culver

Portola

Jeffrey

Jeffrey
Staging

1550'

Loma

Canyon

LIMESTONE
CANYON

RIDGE

1660'

1300'

Cactus
Cyn.

Irvine

1300'

Ridge

Box Springs

The
Sinks

Jamboree

Irvine

133

Round Canyon

Agua

Chinon

Bolero
Point

Jeffrey

5

Portola
Staging

Jeffrey

Portola

3-4

680'
N33.69606
W117.69090

WHITING
RANCH

0.0   0.5   1.0   1.5   2.0
miles
Access by scheduled event only

barriers to casual visitors who don't plan ahead. The trails are accessible only via free docent-led trips or on monthly wilderness access days; advanced registration is required through letsgooutside.org. With help from many volunteers, the Irvine Ranch Conservancy also restores native habitat and builds and maintains trails.

Irvine Ranch dates back to the 1837 Rancho San Joaquin land grant from Mexico to Don José Andrés Sepúlveda. Sepúlveda built a successful ranch but fell into debt through gambling. When a severe drought hit in 1864, he was forced to sell the 48,803-acre ranch to James Irvine and partners for $18,000. Irvine, who had become a wealthy San Francisco merchant serving gold miners, built a ranch house that was the first permanent structure between Anaheim and San Diego. He took over the ranch in 1876, and his son James Harvey Irvine took over in 1886. James improved the water supply and built the Irvine Ranch into a tremendously successful agricultural enterprise, including oranges and the world's leading lima bean fields. World War II marked the beginning of the ranch's decline, when the prized lima bean field was converted into El Toro Marine Corps Air Station. After

James's death in 1947, the ranch came into control of the James Irvine Company. The prime land soon became too valuable for farming. University of California–Irvine was established in 1964, and the master planned city of Irvine was incorporated in 1971.

This chapter provides brief summaries of the major attractions, accessible during scheduled activities or on open-access days. Beware that Orange County traffic can be highly variable on weekdays and that latecomers will be shut out of scheduled events.

trip 10.1 Limestone Canyon: The Sinks

Distance	8 miles (out-and-back)
Hiking Time	4 hours
Elevation Gain	500'
Difficulty	Moderate
Trail Use	Cyclists, equestrians
Best Times	October–April
Agency	OC Parks: IROS
Permit	By docent-led activities or on open-access days only, letsgooutside.org

DIRECTIONS Parking is available at the Augustine Staging Area only during scheduled events. Exit from either of the eastern toll roads (Highway 241 or 261) at Santiago Canyon Road; you can also get to this point from Highway 55 via Chapman Avenue. Head southeast on Santiago Canyon Road for 3.5 miles to the gated lot on the south side.

Limestone Canyon is only open for scheduled events. At the time of this writing, the canyon has scheduled open-access days every other month. Reservations are not required for open-access days, but with preregistration, you can join a variety of other docent-led activities including interpretive nature walks, bike rides of all levels, equestrian rides, and fast-paced "extreme cardio" hikes.

The Sinks in Limestone Canyon are the most dramatic natural formation in Orange County and a must-do trip for OC hikers. Catastrophic erosion of the soft sandstone here has led to the formation of a receding cliff—most dramatically sheer on the north side, where it exhibits a relief

of about 150 feet. The scene is impressive under mid-morning sunlight, and spectacular in bright moonlight. The sandstone cliffs are part of the Sespe Formation, approximately 30 million years old. Ironically, Limestone Canyon was named for the far less conspicuous deposits that are found in the area.

The most direct path to the Sinks is to walk up the gently sloping oak-lined 4-mile Limestone Canyon Trail to the viewpoint. Wildlife is relatively plentiful in the canyon. In late summer and fall, this is a great place to watch for tarantulas who emerge from their burrows seeking a mate. More strenuous options loop up Loma Ridge or Limestone Ridge.

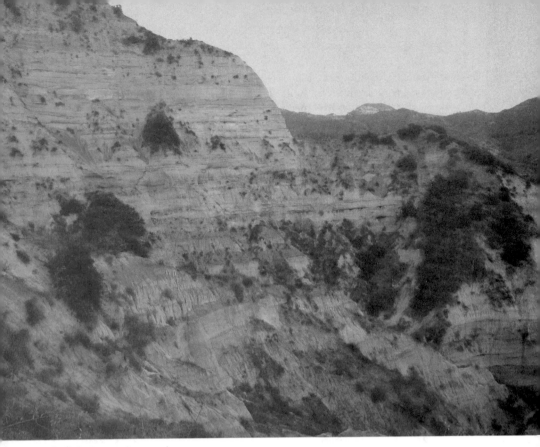

The Sinks (see previous page)

see map on p. 114

trip 10.2 Hicks Haul Road

Distance	3.5 miles (out-and-back)
Hiking Time	1½ hours
Elevation Gain	400'
Difficulty	Moderate
Trail Use	Cyclists
Best Times	October–April
Agency	OC Parks: IROS
Permit	By docent-led activities only, **letsgooutside.org**

DIRECTIONS From Interstate 5 or 405 in Irvine, exit north on Jeffrey Road. North of Portola Parkway, it becomes private and the name changes to Hicks Haul Road. During scheduled events, disregard the private signs, and continue 1.5 miles to a metal gate where you will meet your docent. Turn right through the gate, and continue to park under the 241 Toll Road.

Several mornings and evenings a week, docents open the Hicks Haul Road for a fitness hike up the paved road to Loma Ridge. Although walking a paved road may not sound like much of a hike, the closed road leads through attractive sage scrub country near sheer sedimentary cliffs and offers excellent views of Orange County. The easy footing is also appealing on dark winter evenings and for parents pushing jogging strollers. Expect a vigorous walk. Bring a flashlight for night hikes.

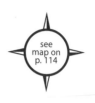
see map on p. 114

trip 10.3 Agua Chinon

Distance	5 miles or more (out-and-back)
Hiking Time	2 hours or more
Elevation Gain	800' or more
Difficulty	Moderate
Trail Use	Cyclists, equestrians
Best Times	All year
Agency	OC Parks: IROS
Permit	By docent-led activities only, **letsgooutside.org**

DIRECTIONS From the 241 Toll Road, take the northern Portola Parkway (Irvine) exit east. Immediately pass through a gate, and turn left to reach the Portola Staging Area. Alternatively, from Interstate 5 or 405 in Irvine, exit northeast on Culver Drive. Turn right on Portola Parkway, and proceed 5.2 miles to the gate at the end.

Agua Chinon Canyon is the short way into The Sinks. An old ranch road ascends the wash, gently at first, and more steeply as it approaches the sinks. The trail is lined with diverse sage scrub and occasional live oak and sycamore, and the wash it parallels supports riparian vegetation and more wildlife. OC Parks has been removing the invasive plants and restoring the native vegetation.

Agua Chinon is only open to the public during scheduled docent-led programs. Activities include hikes to The Sinks or beyond to Box Springs (about 8 miles), short full moon hikes and nature walks, bike rides, and restoration projects. Note that Agua Chinon is inaccessible on Limestone Canyon Open Access days.

Agua Chinon Canyon

Photo: © Irvine Ranch Conservancy. Reprinted with permission.

IRVINE RANCH OPEN SPACE

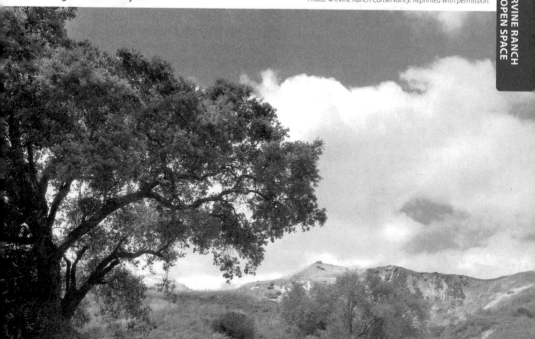

trip 10.4 **Round Canyon**

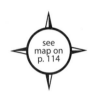
see map on p. 114

Distance	2.4 miles (out-and-back)
Hiking Time	1½ hours
Elevation Gain	300'
Difficulty	Easy
Trail Use	Good for kids
Best Times	All year
Agency	OC Parks: IROS
Permit	By docent-led activities only, letsgooutside.org

DIRECTIONS From the 241 Toll Road, take the northern Portola Parkway (Irvine) exit east. Immediately pass through a gate and turn left to reach the Portola Staging Area. Alternatively, from Interstate 5 or 405 in Irvine, exit northeast on Culver Drive. Turn right on Portola Parkway and proceed 5.2 miles to the gate at the end.

Round Canyon is an unassuming canyon at the base of Loma Ridge. The quiet canyon is a good place to observe coastal sage scrub, live oak, and sycamore, as well as the animals who dwell in such habitat.

Round Canyon is open to the public only during scheduled docent-led programs.

From the staging area, you will carpool to a smaller parking area at the mouth of the canyon. Common trips include birding and family-friendly nature walks. The knowledgeable and engaging naturalists make up for the lack of dramatic natural features in this canyon.

trip 10.5 **Black Star Canyon**

see map on p. 114

Distance	Various loops of 3–4 miles
Hiking Time	2 hours
Elevation Gain	Up to 500'
Difficulty	Easy
Trail Use	Cyclists, equestrians, good for kids
Best Times	October–April
Agency	OC Parks: IROS
Permit	By docent-led activities or on open-access days only, **letsgooutside.org**

DIRECTIONS Parking is available at the Baker Staging Area. Exit from either of the eastern toll roads (Highway 241 or 261) at Santiago Canyon Road; you can also get to this point from Highway 55 via Chapman Avenue. Drive 6 miles east to Silverado Canyon Road, turn left, and turn left again in 0.1 mile onto Black Star Canyon Road. Park on the side of the road in 0.8 mile.

The Irvine Ranch Open Space portion of Black Star Canyon is open only for scheduled events. At the time of this writing, the canyon has open-access days (registration not required) every other month that include nature activities for kids. Black Star also has regular docent-led hikes and bike rides. Don't mix up this area with

the popular Black Star Canyon Falls hike in Cleveland National Forest (Trip 15.5), which is open all the time and does not require registration.

The most popular loop hike uses the Baker, Helo, and/or Silverado Creek Trails. The SilMod Loop trail climbs onto a ridge with views, then returns via the Black Star

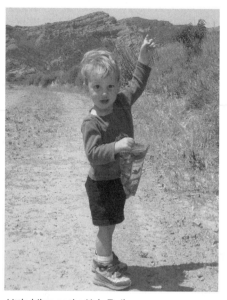

Little hiker on the Helo Trail

Canyon Road. The Red Rock Trail (see next trip) follows the bright cliffs on the west side of Black Star Road, but it's not always accessible during open-access days.

Of historical interest, Baker Canyon was named for Deputy Charles Baker. In 1857, Baker and Sheriff Barton were ambushed and killed in Santiago Canyon by the notorious bandit Juan Flores (see Trip 15.9). A posse soon captured Flores and his gang. Two of the banditos were hanged right away at the north end of Loma Ridge. The 2007 Santiago Fire cleared the brush off the hill and revealed a long-hidden monument marking Hangman's Tree. The Irvine Ranch Conservancy occasionally leads trips to the monument from Limestone Canyon. Flores was taken to Los Angeles and publicly hung on Fort Hill, which is now the site of the Los Angeles Board of Education.

trip 10.6 **Red Rock Trail**

see map on p. 114

Distance	Up to 2.6 miles (out-and-back)
Hiking Time	2 hours
Elevation Gain	Negligible
Difficulty	Easy
Trail Use	Good for kids
Best Times	October–April
Agency	OC Parks: IROS
Permit	By docent-led activities only, **letsgooutside.org**

DIRECTIONS Parking is available at the Black Star Staging Area. Exit from either of the eastern toll roads (Highway 241 or 261) at Santiago Canyon Road; you can also get to this point from Highway 55 via Chapman Avenue. Drive 6 miles east to Silverado Canyon Road, turn left, and turn left again in 0.1 mile onto Black Star Canyon Road, then left again in another 0.1 mile into the gated Black Star Staging Area. Do not confuse this staging area with the Black Star Canyon trailhead (Trip 15.5) farther north on the same road.

Red Rocks

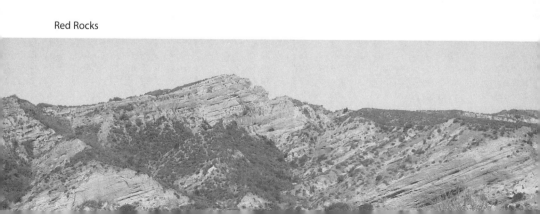

The Irvine Ranch Conservancy offers interpretive hikes for adults and families beneath a stunning formation of red rocks above Santiago Creek. This is a good place to learn about the wildlife, botany, and geology of the region, as well as its early human history.

The Red Rock Trail, a dirt road, leads through buckwheat and other sage scrub and mulefat, which takes advantage of the seasonal water. After crossing the usually dry wash, the trail reaches the base of the sandstone cliffs, which are part of the Sespe formation and get their red color from traces of iron. Watch for an abandoned eagle's nest high on the wall. Beyond, the trail crosses sandy soil rich with animal tracks, including large mountain lion prints. The trail ends ingloriously near the property boundary, and you return the way you came.

trip 10.7 Fremont Canyon

Distance	Various hikes up to 14 miles
Hiking Time	Varies depending on chosen route
Elevation Gain	Varies depending on chosen route
Difficulty	Moderate–strenuous
Trail Use	Cyclists, equestrians
Best Times	October–April
Agency	OC Parks: IROS
Permit	By docent-led activities only, **letsgooutside.org**

see map on p. 114

DIRECTIONS The Fremont Staging Area is open only during scheduled events. From the north end of Jamboree Road, enter Irvine Regional Park. Turn right and follow the park loop to parking area #15, where docents will open a gate to the staging area.

Fremont Canyon is a large and wild portion of Irvine Ranch Open Space with excellent opportunities for long-distance hikes and mountain bike rides. It is open only during scheduled docent-led events. If you are interested in Southern California geology, don't miss the outstanding geology hike.

The complete 14-mile loop follows a network of powerline service roads. Spurs branch off the loop into Weir Canyon and Black Star Canyon.

The weather station on Fremont Ridge is a worthy destination for a 6-mile out-and-back hike with 1,200 feet of elevation gain. During Santa Ana wind conditions, the station regularly measures 100 mile-per-hour winds blasting over the shoulder of the mountains.

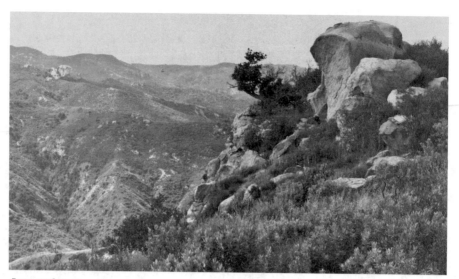

Fremont Canyon

Photo: © Irvine Ranch Conservancy. Reprinted with permission.

trip 10.8 **Weir Canyon**

Distance	Various hikes up to 8.5 miles
Hiking Time	Varies depending on chosen route
Elevation Gain	Varies depending on chosen route
Difficulty	Moderate
Trail Use	Cyclists, equestrians
Best Times	October–April
Agency	OC Parks: IROS
Permit	By docent-led activities only, **letsgooutside.org**

see map on p. 114

DIRECTIONS Weir Canyon is accessed from Irvine Regional Park. From the north end of Jamboree Road, enter Irvine Regional Park. Turn left and follow the park loop 0.5 mile to parking area #3.

The Irvine Ranch Open Space portion of Weir Canyon is only open for scheduled events, including moderate and cardio hikes, mountain bike rides, and equestrian trips. Don't mix this area up with the adjoining Weir Canyon Trail in Santiago Oaks Regional Park (see Trip 8.5), which is open to the public during regular park hours.

Weir Canyon is noted for its oak woodlands and vibrant wildlife. Native Americans once lived here and ground acorns in bedrock metates. Later, ranchers carried cowhides down the canyon by oxcart. In the late 19th century, a small dam was built on the creek, giving the canyon its present name.

The Rifle Range Loop is a commonly scheduled 5-mile hike, passing through a World War II training range before descending the canyon. Longer loops climb onto the slopes above the canyon or link to Fremont Canyon.

IRVINE RANCH OPEN SPACE

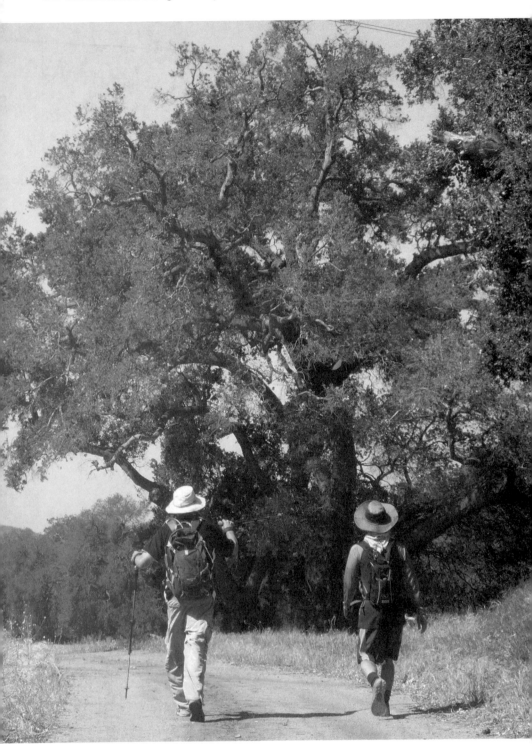

Oak woodland in Weir Canyon

chapter 11

Irvine Open Space Preserve

The planned community of Irvine was established on the historic Irvine Ranch in 1971. In 1988, Irvine voters approved the Open Space Initiative, which boosted protected open space to 12,300 acres in exchange for development rights in other parts of the city. The Irvine Open Space Preserve, centered on Bommer Canyon, borders Crystal Cove State Park and Laguna Coast Wilderness Park. Collectively, these parks are informally known as the South Coast Wilderness.

The core of Bommer Canyon is protected wildlife habitat, open only during open-access days once every other month or on scheduled trips led by Irvine Ranch Conservancy docents. Trails on the periphery of the canyon are open for daily access. Moreover, one public-access trail threads its way through the canyon, allowing hikers to loop from Bommer Canyon through Turtle Ridge or Crystal Cove any day of the year. Trip 11.1 has limited access, while the other trips are accessible daily. The map highlights trail restrictions.

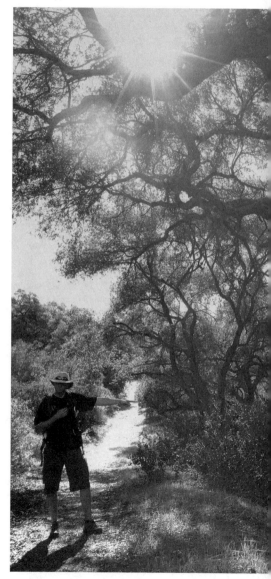

Docent walk in Bommer Canyon

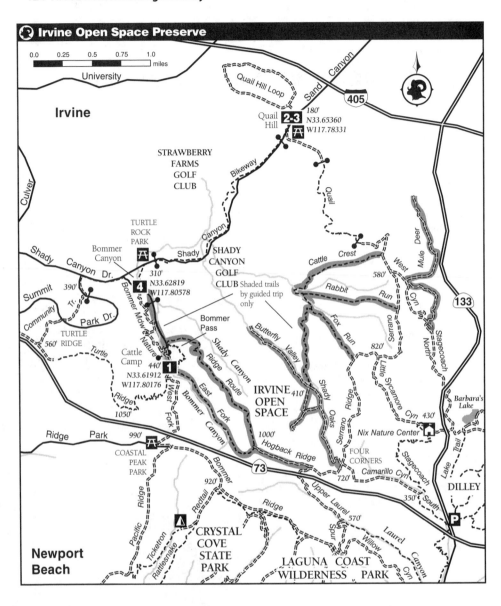

Irvine Open Space Preserve

0.0   0.25   0.5   0.75   1.0
miles

University

Irvine

Quail Hill Loop

Sand Canyon

405

Quail Hill **2-3** 180'
N33.65360
W117.78331

STRAWBERRY
FARMS
GOLF
CLUB

Bikeway

Quail

Culver

TURTLE
ROCK
PARK

Bommer
Canyon

Shady Canyon Dr.

Shady Canyon

SHADY
CANYON
GOLF
CLUB

310'
4 N33.62819
W117.80578

Shaded trails
by guided trip
only

Cattle   Crest

580'

Rabbit

West   Deer

Mule

Cyn

133

Summit   390'

Tr.

Park Dr.

Community

TURTLE
RIDGE   560'

Turtle

Bommer Mdw Nature

Cattle
Camp   440' **1**
N33.61912
W117.80176

Bommer
Pass

Shady Canyon

Butterfly Valley

Fox Run

Run

Serrano

Little Sycamore Cyn

820'

Stagecoach North

Barbara's
Lake

Ridge   1050'

West Fork

East Fork

Bommer Canyon

IRVINE
OPEN
SPACE   410'

Shady Oaks

Serrano Ridge

430'

Ridge   Park   990'

COASTAL
PEAK
PARK

1000'
Hogback Ridge

73

FOUR
CORNERS

Nix Nature Center

Camarillo Cyn   720'

Stagecoach

Lake Trail

DILLEY

P

920'

Bommer

Redtail

Ridge

Upper Laurel

350'

South

Pacific Ridge

Ticketron

Rattlesnake

CRYSTAL
COVE
STATE
PARK

Spur   570'

Willow

Laurel Canyon

Cyn

Newport
Beach

LAGUNA COAST
WILDERNESS PARK

trip 11.1   **Bommer Canyon and Ridge Loop**

Distance	3.2 miles (loop)
Hiking Time	2 hours
Elevation Gain	700'
Difficulty	Moderate
Trail Use	Cyclists, good for kids
Best Times	October–April
Agency	City of Irvine: IOSP
Permit	By docent-led activities or on open-access days only, letsgooutside.org

DIRECTIONS From the 405 Freeway in Irvine, exit south on Culver Drive. In 2.6 miles, turn left on Shady Canyon Drive. In 1.2 miles, turn right on Bommer Canyon Road into the Bommer Canyon parking area. During scheduled programs, you can continue through the gate for 1 mile to the large grassy Cattle Camp parking area. Alternatively, from the 73 Toll Road, exit east on Bonita Canyon Road, and turn right onto Shady Canyon Drive to join the directions above.

This hike and most of Bommer Canyon are open only during scheduled programs. At the time of this writing, Bommer Canyon open-access days are generally scheduled from 8 a.m. to 2 p.m. on a Saturday every month. See **letsgooutside.org** for a list of events.

The loop through the heart of Bommer Canyon starts at the old Irvine Ranch Cattle Camp. Walk south to the end of the road near a volleyball court, where the trail begins at a gate. Just past the gate, turn left onto the signed East Fork Trail, which leads up Bommer Canyon through coastal sage scrub. Singed oaks remind you that a fire burned through the canyon, but the scrub has fully recovered. Watch for sandstone outcrops, some of which have been carved into caves. Prickly pear and coastal cholla cactus grow on the dry exposed slopes.

The lampposts visible on the ridge line the 73 Toll Road. This area was once under the sea before being uplifted. When the freeway was built in the 1990s, archaeologists unearthed an astonishing variety of fossils, including duck-billed dinosaurs, megalodon sharks, baleen whales, and mammoths.

In 1 mile, the trail begins to climb and undulate. Families with young kids may prefer to enjoy the view and turn around before the very steep climb ahead. The views get even better at a sandstone outcrop at the top of the hill, and then the trail tops out at a three-way junction, 1.3 miles from the start.

Turn left and follow the Ridge Route 1.7 miles back to the staging area. This trail has terrific views as it weaves along the ridge before dropping.

Bommer Canyon

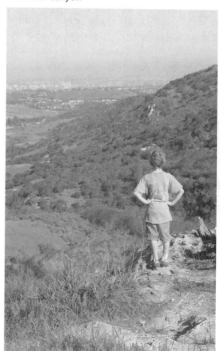

Hikers looking for a longer walk can loop through the remote eastern canyons. Stay right at the Ridge Route junction, and continue down Hogback Ridge to Serrano Ridge. At the next junction, known as Four Corners, turn left down the Shady Oaks service road. In 1 mile, turn right as Shady Oaks turns into a narrow path, climbs over a low ridge with interesting sandstone outcrops, and drops into the next canyon. From here, you can climb back up to Serrano Ridge via Fox Run, Rabbit Run, or Cattle Crest, all of which are steep. Turn right and follow Serrano Ridge, Hogback Ridge, and Ridge Route back. The Fox Run option is 9 miles with 1,700 feet of elevation gain.

---

trip 11.2 **Big Bommer Loop**

Distance	14 miles (loop)
Hiking Time	7 hours
Elevation Gain	1,600'
Difficulty	Strenuous
Trail Use	Cyclists, equestrians
Best Times	All year
Agency	City of Irvine: IOSP

see map on p. 124

DIRECTIONS From the 405 Freeway in Irvine, exit south at Sand Canyon Avenue. Follow the road southwest (here called Shady Canyon Drive) through a traffic circle. Shortly beyond, 0.4 mile from the freeway, turn right into the large signed Quail Hill Trailhead parking area. A study of the map will show many other possible trailheads along the loop, including Bommer Canyon and Coastal Peak Park.

Although most of the Irvine Open Space Preserve is accessible only on guided trips or special open-access days, one perimeter trail network through the preserve and the Laguna Coast Wilderness Park is open to the public year-round. This trip makes a grand loop around the preserve on this path through diverse country, ranging from a neighborhood path in Irvine to an intimate trail through Bommer Canyon to the Bommer Ridge fire road with expansive views over coastal sage scrub to the sea. This trip is especially enjoyable in the spring, when the sage scrub is in bloom. The coastal cactus flower from April to July. The first part of this trip is heavily used by mountain bikers, but you are more likely to find seclusion in Laurel Canyon and on Serrano Ridge.

From the Quail Hill Trailhead, pick up the unsigned Shady Canyon Bikeway leading southwest alongside Shady Canyon Drive (closed to nonresident motor vehicles). The trail leads over a low pass between the hills and down past a gated community and two golf courses. Emerging from a gate near Turtle Rock Community Park, it reaches the Bommer Canyon Trailhead in 2.6 miles.

Pick up the Bommer Meadow Trail behind the restrooms, and follow it through the meadow and over a bridged seasonal creek. In 0.4 mile, pass a junction with the Nature Loop Trail, but the most direct choice is to stay on the Bommer Meadow Trail that parallels the gated access road to reach the Irvine Ranch Cattle Camp in 0.3 mile. The road through the camp is normally closed to the public, so you must bypass it on the oddly named Bommer Pass Trail, which gratuitously climbs 120 feet onto the east slope of the canyon before dropping to meet the road again near the junction with the East Fork Trail in 0.5 mile. Along the way, you can enjoy an elevated view of the canyon and close-up views of coastal cholla and prickly pear cactus.

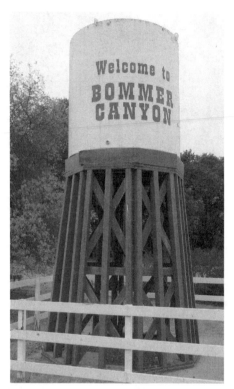

Historic Bommer Canyon Cattle Camp

Stay on the broad West Fork Trail leading south up Bommer Canyon as you pass a junction with the Turtle Ridge Trail. After a vigorous climb, cross under the 73 Toll Road underpasses, and continue up to a trailhead at Coastal Peak Park atop the San Joaquin Hills in 1.1 miles. Mountain bikers favor this trailhead because of the free streetside parking and good access to challenging trails in Crystal Cove State Park. The hills got their name from José Sepúlveda's 1842 Rancho San Joaquin. The sedimentary rock was once beneath the sea floor but has likely been uplifted by a fault laying deep below. During the toll road's excavation, 5-million-year-old fossilized whales were unearthed.

From here, join the Bommer Ridge fire road leading southeast parallel to the toll road. You are now in the Laguna Coast Wilderness Park. You'll see many spurs

branching south into Crystal Cove State Park, plus some stretches of singletrack trails, popular among mountain bikers, paralleling the fire road. The ridge cuts through coastal sage scrub, especially buckwheat and laurel sumac, and provides views all the way out to the Pacific Ocean. In 1.8 miles, stay left on to Bommer Spur. In 0.2 mile, it ends at the Willow Canyon Road, where you turn left and immediately left again onto Laurel Spur, which drops down into pleasantly wooded Laurel Canyon. Reach the canyon floor in 0.5 mile, and turn left onto the Upper Laurel Canyon Trail. Gently climb for 0.7 mile to a second toll road underpass. These underpasses are not only important for hikers, but also for deer, coyote, and bobcats, which require free passage across larger tracks of land to find food and a mate.

Changing names to Serrano Ridge as you reenter the Irvine Open Space Preserve, the ridgeline trail has sweeping views over interesting sandstone formations. Santiago Peak is the high point of the Santa Ana Mountains to the east, while Mt. Baldy is the high point of the San Gabriel Mountains to the north. Turkey vultures love to circle on the thermals, perhaps hoping to pick the bones of a hiker who neglects to bring enough water on this long shadeless ridge.

Pass a series of signed trails. Those on the west side lead into Bommer or Shady Canyons in the open space preserve and are accessible only during scheduled programs. Those on the east reach the Nix Nature Center in the Laguna Coast Wilderness Park.

After 3.7 miles, switchback down to cross a paved road near a cluster of hilltop mansions. The Quail Trail resumes on the far side and curves on or east of the ridge past more huge homes and above the Quail Hill subdivision. It passes two spurs accessing the Quail Hill neighborhoods and finally reaches Shady Canyon Road at an unsigned intersection on the south edge of a sports park in 1.8 miles. Cross the street, turn right, and follow the bikeway the last 0.2 mile north to the Quail Hill Trailhead where the loop began.

trip 11.3 Quail Hill Loop

Distance	1.7 miles (loop)
Hiking Time	45 minutes
Elevation Gain	150'
Difficulty	Easy
Trail Use	Cyclists, equestrians, dogs, good for kids
Best Times	All year
Agency	City of Irvine: IOSP

see map on p. 124

DIRECTIONS From the 405 Freeway in Irvine, exit south at Sand Canyon Avenue. Follow the road southwest (here called Shady Canyon Drive) through a traffic circle. Shortly beyond, 0.4 mile from the freeway, turn right into the large signed Quail Hill Trailhead parking area.

The Quail Hill Loop tours the grassy open space on the south side of the freeway. Oddly, it does not loop around a hill but stays on the north slope. This is a pleasant place to take a stroll, especially in winter and spring when the country is verdant. An unusual feature of the loop is its cell-phone audio tour. At five posts along the way, you can dial the phone number on the post (949-743-5943) and enter the post number to get a recorded narration about that point of interest. Alternatively, you can listen online at **goo.gl/Wcw5p**.

Two wide dirt trails diverge from the trailhead. The Shady Canyon Bikeway leads south paralleling the road, but you should be sure to pick up the Quail Hill Loop Trail that starts at the back of the parking lot to the right of the restrooms. The trail passes through a fence and promptly forks. Turn right and make a counterclockwise loop. Pass a vernal pool near the north end that fills up after heavy winter rains. Fairy shrimp live through a short lifecycle while the pool is full, then lay their hardy eggs in the mud, where they lay dormant until the next rains. Near the end of the loop, reach a vista point where views range the skyscrapers of Los Angeles to the San Gabriel and Santa Ana Mountains. The wooden hangars in Tustin housed blimps that were used in World War II to patrol for submarines off the Pacific coast.

Irvine Ranch Conservancy hike at Quail Hill

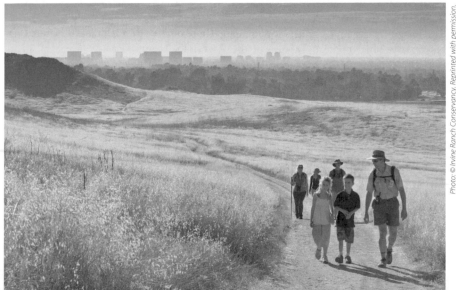

Photo: © Irvine Ranch Conservancy. Reprinted with permission.

trip 11.4   ## Turtle Ridge Loop

Distance	5.5 miles (loop)
Hiking Time	2½ hours
Elevation Gain	900'
Difficulty	Moderate
Trail Use	Cyclists, equestrians
Best Times	All year
Agency	City of Irvine: IOSP

see map on p. 124

DIRECTIONS From the 73 Toll Road in Irvine, exit east onto Bonita Canyon Drive. In 1 mile, turn right (southeast) onto Shady Canyon Drive. Alternatively, from the 405 Freeway in Irvine, exit south on Culver Drive, and follow it 2.6 miles to a left turn onto Shady Canyon Drive. In either case, follow Shady Canyon Drive 1.2 miles, and then turn right into the Bommer Canyon parking area. This trailhead closes at 6 p.m., so if you plan to take a summer-evening walk, you're better off continuing on Shady Canyon Drive to Turtle Rock Community Park and walking 0.5 mile back to Bommer.

Although much of Bommer Canyon is closed outside of scheduled programs, the scenic Turtle Ridge Loop is open to the public daily from 7 a.m. until sunset. It threads a scenic path through Bommer Meadow, up onto Turtle Ridge, and down through a gated community.

Pick up the signed Bommer Meadow Trail behind the restroom at the Bommer Canyon Trailhead. If you are coming from Turtle Rock Park, you can reach Bommer Canyon via the Shady Canyon Trail on the south side of the road, starting at the entrance to the gated community. The Bommer Meadow Trail leads through the meadow, crossing a seasonal creek on bridges. Although you are close to Irvine's endless subdivisions, you quickly gain a feeling of seclusion.

In 0.4 mile, reach Bommer Canyon Road (closed to public access). The shortest option is to continue on Bommer Meadow Trail alongside the road, but a more scenic option is to veer right onto the Nature Loop Trail, which rejoins the road and Meadow Trail in 0.6 mile at the Irvine Ranch Cattle

Turtle Ridge Trail

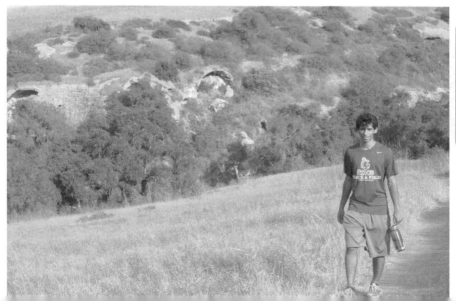

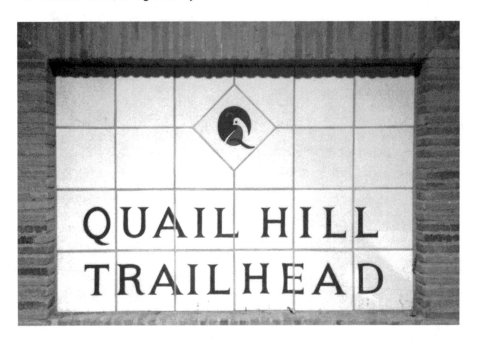

Camp staging area. The camp is also closed except during scheduled programs, but you can cross the road and continue on the oddly named Bommer Pass Trail, which climbs through coastal sage scrub onto the hillside and then returns to the canyon floor in 0.5 mile. Pass the gated East Fork Trail on the left, then the gated road coming from the cattle camp, and continue onto the West Fork Trail. In another 0.1 mile, veer right onto the Turtle Ridge Trail.

The Turtle Ridge Trail has good views of the oak-lined canyon floor and the odd sandstone caves across the canyon. As it steadily climbs via a series of switchbacks, views open up to the Santa Ana and San Gabriel Mountains and the toll road, which cuts across the head of the otherwise quiet canyon. In 1.1 miles, top out on Turtle Ridge, and follow it northwest to the Turtle Ridge gated community. At a split, stay to the right. Soon after, continue straight at a four-way junction and then cross Summit Park Drive. Regain a trail on the far side that hugs the east edge of a hill and drops through a greenbelt to the Turtle Ridge entrance gate. Follow the sidewalk down to Shady Canyon Drive, where you turn right and continue 0.4 mile back to the Bommer Canyon Trailhead.

chapter 12

O'Neill and Riley Regional Parks

Encompassing more than 4,000 acres of riparian bottomlands, oak woodlands, grassy meadows, and scrub-covered hills, O'Neill Regional Park is one of the oldest parks in Orange County. Starting with 278 acres donated in 1948 by the descendants of the O'Neill family (owners of what was once a vast ranching empire stretching across southern Orange County), the park grew steadily to accommodate the needs of the expanding county population. A nice complement of recreational facilities was developed: picnic tables, a playground, nature center, small arboretum, and camping areas for equestrians and motorists. Later additions to the park west of Live Oak Canyon Road made possible the development of an extensive trail system for hikers, horseback riders, and mountain bikers.

The most recent acquisition, the 935-acre Arroyo Trabuco Wilderness, lay off-limits for more than a decade before it opened for public use in 1995. Its long, curvilinear form, stretching almost 6 miles through the suburban landscape of Mission Viejo, serves as an important wildlife corridor between the Santa Ana Mountains and the remaining open spaces of coastal Orange County. This and other long, narrow strips of open space throughout this growing part of the county are being preserved in perpetuity as greenbelts.

South of O'Neill Park, another patch of open space, laden with trails, welcomes you. This 540-acre parcel, Thomas F. Riley Wilderness Park, was deeded to the county in 1983 by the developers of the adjacent community of Coto de Caza. Not until easy access was assured (by way of the east extension of Oso Parkway) was the park opened for public use in December 1994.

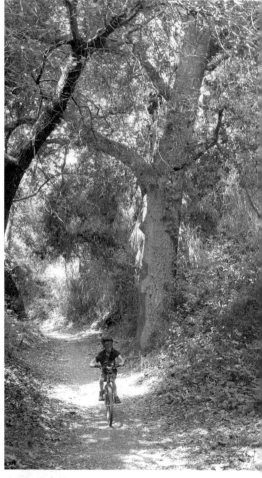

Arroyo Trabuco

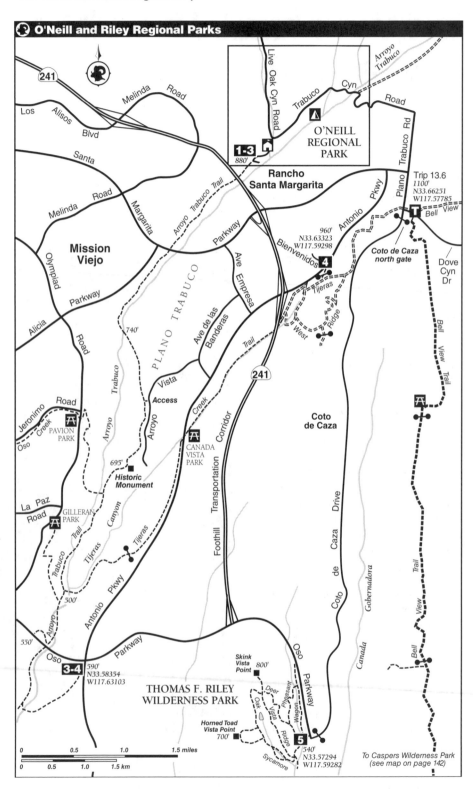

O'Neill and Riley Regional Parks

O'Neill Regional Park (inset)

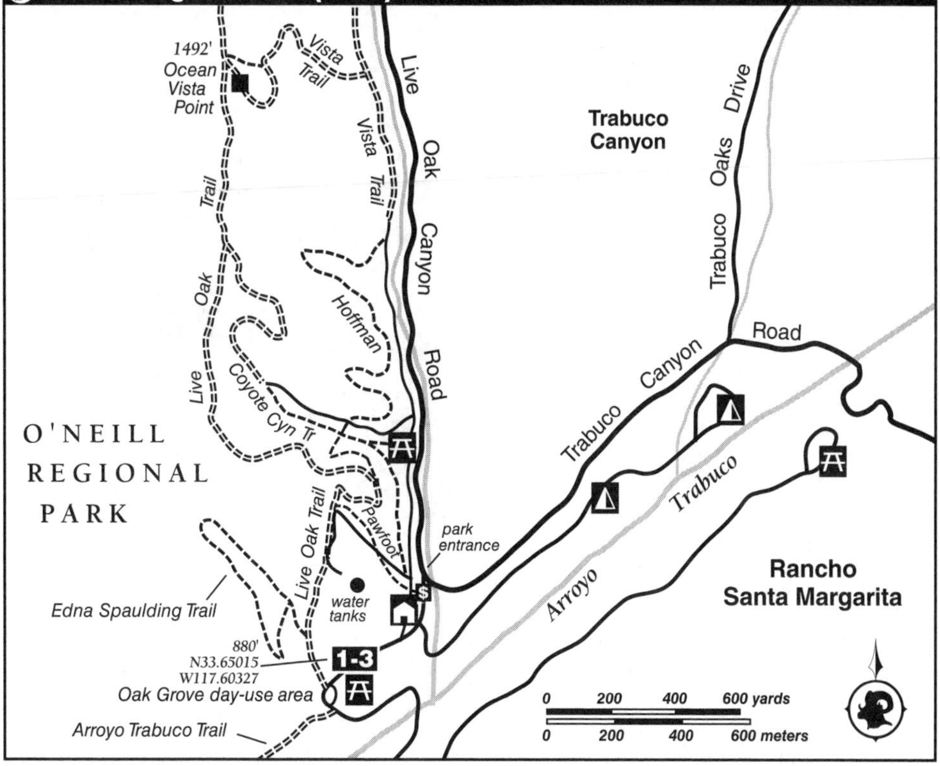

1492'
Ocean
Vista
Point

Vista Trail

Vista Trail

Oak Trail

Live Oak Canyon Road

Hoffman

Coyote Cyn Tr

Live

Trabuco Canyon

Trabuco Oaks Drive

Road

Trabuco Canyon

Trabuco

Rancho Santa Margarita

O'NEILL REGIONAL PARK

Edna Spaulding Trail

Live Oak Trail

Pawfoot

park entrance

water tanks

880'
N33.65015
W117.60327

1-3

Oak Grove day-use area

Arroyo Trabuco Trail

Arroyo

| 0 | 200 | 400 | 600 yards |
| 0 | 200 | 400 | 600 meters |

trip 12.1   **Ocean Vista Point**

Distance	3.5 miles (loop)
Hiking Time	1½ hours
Elevation Gain	700'
Difficulty	Moderate
Trail Use	Cyclists, equestrians, good for kids
Best Times	All year
Agency	OC Parks: ONRP
Permit	OC Parks parking fee required

DIRECTIONS From Interstate 5, take El Toro Road 7.5 miles northeast to a Y-junction at Cooks Corner. Turn right onto Live Oak Canyon Road, and proceed 3 miles to the O'Neill Regional Park entrance on the right. Pay your fee at the kiosk, then turn right and promptly left into a large parking lot at the Oak Grove day-use area.

An inspiring vista of sea on one side and chaparral- and sage-covered mountains on the other awaits you at the midpoint of this hike, a 1,492-foot-high overlook in O'Neill Regional Park. Don't forget your binoculars and perhaps a county map to familiarize yourself with Orange County's urban and natural geography.

From the Oak Grove day-use area, continue west toward a traffic circle where you can pick up the signed Live Oak Trail, which heads north and upward onto a dry slope. Ignoring the Edna Spaulding Trail on the left, pass under a couple of hilltop water tanks, and for a moment, touch upon the paved driveway going to them. Stay left on the ascending Live Oak Trail, swing around two hairpin turns, and stay left at the next fork, remaining on Live Oak Trail. You climb up to and then along the top of a viewful ridgeline with a bench. Soon after, pass the Coyote Canyon Trail on the right. Your destination, a 1,492-foot bump on the ridge ahead called the "Overlook" on park maps, may be identified from afar by a spiky cellular telephone antenna structure near its top. Just past the antenna, veer right onto the Vista Trail, and follow it up to Ocean Vista Point.

Breezy days from late fall to early spring are best for the view. Often visible above the layer of low haze or smog are San Clemente and Santa Catalina Islands, the Palos Verdes Peninsula, and the Santa Monica Mountains. To the east, the Santa Ana Mountains rise impressively—so much more so because you look down on their lower flanks, as well as up to their summits.

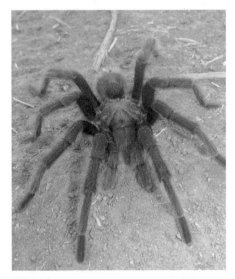

Tarantula

To make this hike a loop trip and return quickly, drop east on the Vista Trail toward shady Live Oak Canyon. Bear right at the bottom on the Hoffman Homestead Trail, which soon meets an old service road paralleling Live Oak Canyon Road. Continue south on the road (very gradually downhill) until you reach your starting point.

see maps on pages 132–133

trip 12.2 Edna Spaulding Nature Trail

Distance	1 mile (loop)
Hiking Time	½ hour
Elevation Gain	250'
Difficulty	Easy
Trail Use	Good for kids
Best Times	All year
Agency	OC Parks: ONRP
Permit	OC Parks parking fee required

DIRECTIONS From Interstate 5, take El Toro Road 7.5 miles northeast to a Y-junction at Cooks Corner. Turn right onto Live Oak Canyon Road, and proceed 3 miles to the O'Neill Regional Park entrance on the right. Pay your fee at the kiosk, then turn right and promptly left into a large parking lot at the Oak Grove day-use area.

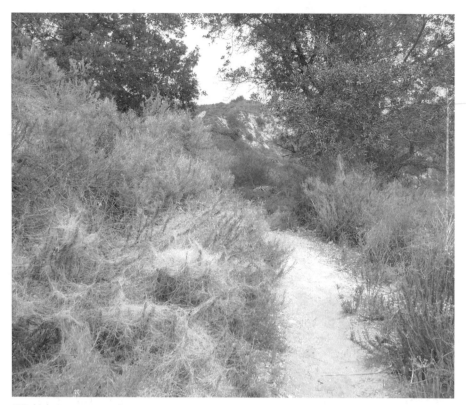

Witch's hair on sage scrub

The Edna Spaulding Nature Trail is a fine way to become acquainted with the coastal sage scrub plant community that is widespread across Orange County. The trail was named for a local botany teacher who developed it for school trips in 1953. Although this loop is short and good for most families, it has a sustained uphill climb and may be unsuitable for very young children.

From the Oak Grove day-use area, continue west toward a traffic circle where you can pick up the signed Live Oak Trail, which heads north and upward onto a dry slope. In 0.1 mile, veer left onto the signed Edna Spaulding Trail. You may find a pamphlet at the start describing its points of interest. The trail soon forks; turn left and hike clockwise up onto the hillside to follow the interpretive posts in order. In spring, you can expect plentiful wildflowers, including blue dicks, flowering prickly pear cactus and whipple yucca, and California buckwheat. The yellow stringlike parasite growing on many plants is dodder, more vividly known as witches hair.

If the interpretive pamphlet is unavailable, watch for the following signposts: (1) coastal sage scrub habitat, (2) California sagebrush, (3) scrub oak, (4) prickly pear cactus, (5) views of Santiago Peak, the high point of the Santa Ana Mountains, (6) laurel sumac, (7) view of a sandstone outcrop across the canyon, and (8) coast live oak.

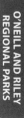

see
maps on
pages
132–133

trip 12.3   **Arroyo Trabuco**

Distance	6 miles (one-way)
Hiking Time	3 hours
Elevation Gain/Loss	170'/500'
Difficulty	Moderately strenuous
Trail Use	Cyclists, equestrians
Best Times	October–June
Agency	OC Parks: ONRP
Permit	OC Parks parking fee required

DIRECTIONS This is a one-way trip with a car, bicycle, or bus shuttle. To reach the south end, or pick-up point: From Interstate 5, take Oso Parkway 2.3 miles east. The trip ends on the west end of Oso Parkway's long bridge over Arroyo Trabuco. There is no parking available at the trailhead, but plenty can be found 0.3 mile further east at the corner of Antonio Parkway.

To reach the starting point at the north end, turn left on Antonio Parkway, and go north for 5.6 miles. Turn right on Santa Margarita Parkway, then in 0.2 mile, turn left onto Plano Trabuco. In 0.6 mile, the road turns left and becomes Trabuco Canyon Road. Continue 1.8 miles, then turn left into O'Neill Regional Park. After the entrance station, turn right, then park in the first lot on the left (the Oak Grove day-use area).

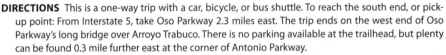

The somewhat long but easygoing trek down the Arroyo Trabuco is most adventurous after winter rainy periods, when turbid water dances over a wide, gravelly bed and there's no way to avoid a good foot-soaking at each of four fords you encounter along the trail. Be aware, however, that for most county park trails, there's usually a drying out period (about three days) during which all visitation is prohibited. You will pass many unmarked and unmapped paths on both sides; stay on the wide main trail, which is marked every mile.

By early April, waist-high green grass pokes upward from the soft ground, and the emerging leaves on the sycamores flutter on the marine air that persistently pushes its way inland. Blooming mustard and poppies appear as April grades into May—just as the grass bleaches to yellow or brown. By summer, the arroyo creekbed is usually dry, and the midday heat can be oppressive. The scenery improves greatly in November and December as the sycamore leaves turn crispy and yellow and drift earthward on capricious puffs of Santa Ana winds.

This one-way downhill trip is also particularly well suited to mountain biking for kids. The path is continually interesting, with forest, creek crossings, sandy areas, and rocky patches, yet easy enough that those without bulging calves can come through successfully.

From the Oak Grove day-use parking area, walk west along the park road for 0.1 mile to a traffic circle, and look for the signed Arroyo Trabuco Trail to the left, just south of the circle. You soon pass under a massive twin bridge (Foothill Transportation Corridor Toll Road) and later pass under another equally huge bridge (Santa Margarita Parkway). As an environmental mitigation for the construction of these bridges, county workers and volunteers have planted thousands of native trees and shrubs—live oak, sycamore, toyon, mulefat, and willow—on the arroyo banks. Barring huge floods, this upper stretch of the arroyo will look more lush with the passage of time.

At 1.9 miles, well past the second bridge, the trail swings left across the creek and ascends moderately toward the lip of the shallow gorge and toward a subdivision built upon the sloping plain to the east, called Plano Trabuco. The plano ("plain" in English) is a broad terrace made up of alluvial deposits cast off of the Santa Ana

Mountains. Over recent geologic time, the abrasive floodwaters of Arroyo Trabuco have cut about 100 feet deep into Plano Trabuco's soft sediments. Plano Trabuco acquired its name in 1769, when a soldier traveling with the Portolà expedition (led by Gaspar de Portolà) lost a blunderbuss (trabuco) there. A string of contemporary place-names are descended from the original: Arroyo Trabuco, Trabuco Canyon, and the Trabuco Ranger District (the part of Cleveland National Forest that encompasses the Santa Ana Mountains).

In 0.7 mile, after a moderate ascent, the Arroyo Trabuco Trail sidles up to a residential street called Arroyo Vista, where there is a signed access point for the trail. Plenty of curbside parking is here, if you want to plan a shorter trip up or down the arroyo. In another 0.7 mile, notice a small structure on the left accompanied by a historical plaque. It marks the campsite, designated San Francisco Solano, used by the Portolà expedition on the night of July 24–25, 1769.

Continue on the main trail, not the path on the right, which drops steeply to the creek. Eventually, the Arroyo Trabuco descends back into the canyon and continues for another 2 miles down alongside the wide floodplain, always staying close to the streambed. This is perhaps the most agreeable part of the arroyo, with gnarled sycamores and oaks alternating with grassy clearings. After a stream crossing, pass the Tijeras Creek Trail on the left. Make two more stream crossings, and pass under the Oso Parkway bridge high overhead. Just beyond it, you can pick up a powerline access road up the right (west) slope of the arroyo and ascend to reach the shoulder of Oso Parkway.

If you wish to return to the trailhead via public transportation, the Orange County Transportation Authority #82 bus stops at the corner of Antonio and Oso Parkways roughly every hour and a half (except on Sundays) and can carry a pair of bicycles. Take the bus north, and ask to be let off at the corner of Santa Margarita Parkway and Avenida de Las Flores. Go up Las Flores, make the first left onto Via Con Dios, and follow the curving street around to an O'Neill Regional Park entrance on the left. Take the service road steeply down to the Featherly day-use area and continue along the road to your vehicle.

Boy Scouts in Arroyo Trabuco

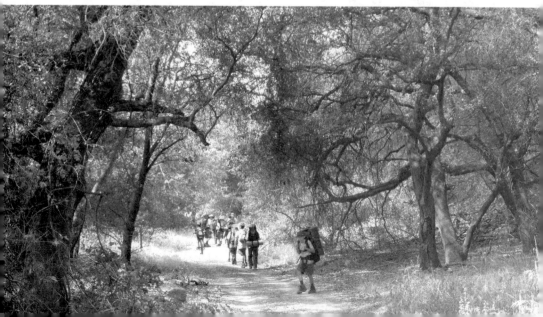

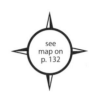

see
map on
p. 132

trip 12.4   Tijeras Creek

Distance	6 miles (one-way)
Hiking Time	3 hours
Elevation Gain/Loss	300'/600'
Difficulty	Moderately strenuous
Trail Use	Cyclists, equestrians
Best Times	October–June
Agency	OC Parks: ONRP

DIRECTIONS This is a one-way trip with a car, bicycle, or bus shuttle. To reach the south end, or pick-up point: From Interstate 5, take Oso Parkway 2.6 miles east, then turn right and leave your getaway vehicle at the plaza at the corner of Antonio Parkway. To reach the starting point at the north end, turn left on Antonio Parkway and go north for 4.3 miles. Then turn left onto Bienvenidos, and find street parking near the intersection.

The most farflung trail in O'Neill Regional Park follows Tijeras Creek, a tributary of the Arroyo Trabuco. The creek, lined with tall sycamores, is most appealing in spring when it flows and the wildflowers are in bloom. This trip describes a one-way descent. You'll need to make your way 4.3 miles back up Antonio Parkway afterward. If you don't want to set up a second car, Antonio is conveniently served by the Orange County Transportation Authority #82 bus line (except on Sundays) and also has a bike lane the full way. Another option for a 13-mile loop is to return via Arroyo Trabuco and then work your way out of O'Neill Park on winding neighborhood streets.

The signed Tijeras Creek Trail begins on the southeast side of Antonio Parkway opposite Bienvenidos. Walk south to an intersection with a fire road, then veer right and descend to the canyon bottom. Ford the creek and hike past lovely live oaks. The narrow path briefly hugs the lip of a cliff above the creek before dropping back down and fording the creek again. On the far side, stay right where you meet a path coming down from the West Ridge Trail. Soon, pass under the 241 Toll Road, 0.5 mile from the start.

The next 1.5 miles is especially scenic, following a narrow path close by Tijeras Creek. The canyon is home to huge sycamores heavily laden with mistletoe. Pass the Canada Vista Sports Park (another

alternative trailhead) just before crossing under Antonio Parkway.

The trail is now squeezed between Antonio Parkway and the Tijeras Creek Golf Club. In 1.1 miles, it is briefly forced onto the sidewalk along Antonio Parkway to bypass a ravine, then it veers right behind a neighborhood and reaches a gated dirt service road in 0.4 mile.

Pass through the gate, and descend the road into Arroyo Trabuco. In 0.6 mile, ford its broad gravelly bed just below the confluence with Tijeras Creek, then walk through an elfin glen completely overhung with sycamores where you meet the Arroyo Trabuco Trail.

Turn left on Arroyo Trabuco, and follow it downstream with repeated creek crossings. In 0.4 mile, cross under Oso Parkway, where you could take a path on the right up to the street. Instead, continue downstream, ford the creek yet again, and climb to a junction with paved service roads. Continue straight as your path turns back to dirt, and watch for a narrow trail on the left in 0.6 mile. Take this narrow trail, which curves back northeast and ascends another canyon. Near the top, veer right at an unmarked junction to reach Antonio Parkway by the Santa Margarita Water District parking lot. Head north up the sidewalk for 0.1 mile to the corner of Oso Parkway where this hike ends.

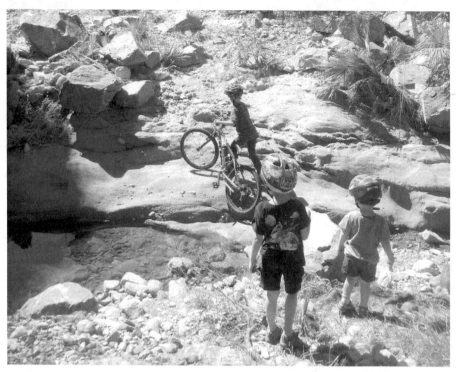

Fording Tijeras Creek

VARIATION

You could start farther up at the beginning of the Tijeras Creek Trail at the corner of Plano Trabuco and Dove Canyon Road. This option adds 1.8 miles on rolling fire roads before you join the creek.

---

trip 12.5 ## Riley Wilderness Park

Distance	2.8 miles (loop)
Hiking Time	1½ hours
Elevation Gain	500'
Difficulty	Moderate
Trail Use	Cyclists, equestrians, good for kids
Best Times	All year
Agency	OC Parks: RWP
Permit	OC Parks parking fee required

see map on p. 132

DIRECTIONS From Interstate 5, take Oso Parkway east for 5.8 miles to its end, where you'll see the Riley Park entrance on the right. If you are coming from the 241 Toll Road, take Oso Parkway 2 miles east.

Thomas F. Riley Wilderness Park, a wilderness in name only, spreads across 540 acres of rolling hills and oak-lined ravines and includes about 5 miles of trails open to hikers, equestrians, and mountain bikers. Like much of Orange County's foothills, this area was until recently home to far more cattle than people. Hardly pristine

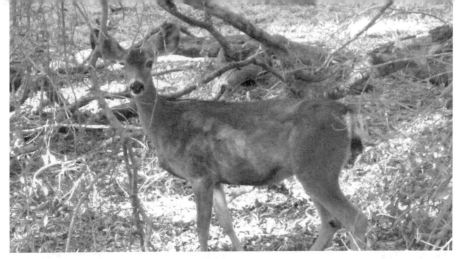
Mule deer

in a biological sense, the park nonetheless preserves a pleasant pocket of open space that will permanently resist the bulldozer blade used to develop the surrounding hills and canyons.

The Spanish first marched through Wagon Wheel Canyon in this area in 1769 when Captain Gaspar de Portolà led his expedition seeking sites for missions to subjugate the local Native Americans. In a fine example of nepotism, Governor Pio Pico granted 47,000 acres in this area to his brother-in-law in 1845. Ranchers James Flood and Richard O'Neill subsequently acquired the land and established a huge ranch.

Brigadier General Thomas F. Riley was the retired commander of Camp Pendleton Marine Base who served for two decades on the Orange County Board of Supervisors starting in 1974. On the board, he presided over rapid and controversial development of open spaces into subdivisions across the county—some people consider it ironic that this park was named in his honor.

The following moderately easy trek around the perimeter gives you a good feel for the park. From the parking lot, head north on oak-shaded Wagon Wheel Canyon Trail, which runs parallel to Oso Parkway. After 0.4 mile, turn left, cross the shallow bottom of Wagon Wheel Creek, and double back south on the narrow Pheasant Run Trail. After a gentle rise and fall, you arrive at the Mule Deer Trail, nearly back at the starting point.

Make a sharp right and start climbing again. Early spring brings forth a good display of wildflowers on the grassy hillsides ahead: shooting stars, lupine, wild hyacinth, and monkeyflower. Later in the spring, blooming mustard paints yellow patches across these slopes. Prickly pear cactus and jimson weed also dot the fields.

The crooked climb on the Mule Deer Trail leads toward a ridgetop trail junction. Skink Vista Point, offering a somewhat wider view of the park and the Santa Ana Mountains, lies on the bald ridgeline a little higher and 0.2 mile farther north of that junction. Continue straight onto the Oak Canyon Trail, and make a short, sharp descent into a shallow valley. Proceed south down the valley past an old stock pond, noting the sign for Horned Toad Vista Point on the right. The short, steep side trip up through aromatic sage scrub vegetation is worth it; from the top of the trail, you can gaze down on the most secluded parts of the park.

Back on the Oak Canyon Trail, descend toward the oak- and sycamore-dotted floor of the valley. By staying straight on it at all subsequent junctions, you will return to the parking lot, approaching it from the south.

At the south end of the parking area, wander through the well-maintained butterfly garden before returning to your vehicle. The blooms and butterflies are at their peak in May and June.

chapter 13

Caspers Wilderness Park

Ronald W. Caspers Wilderness Park is without a doubt the crown jewel of Orange County's regional park system. It is the largest park established to date in the county, the least altered by human activities, and the most remote from population centers. Its position adjacent to Cleveland National Forest on the east and north and the Audubon Society's Starr Ranch Sanctuary on the north and west integrates it into the only area within Orange County that can truthfully be called a wilderness. Caspers wouldn't qualify as a statutory wilderness area (that is, roadless and primitive) by federal standards, as does nearby San Mateo Canyon Wilderness, but the richness of its wildlife is testimony enough to its de facto primitive state.

Strangely enough, the area encompassing Caspers Park—the former Starr Ranch—narrowly escaped development as a commercial amusement park back in the early 1970s. Fortunately, the owners of the property at the time went bankrupt, and most of the north half of the property was deeded to the Audubon Society in 1973. The south half was purchased by Orange County in 1974 for use as a regional park, largely through the efforts of Board of Supervisors chairman Ronald W. Caspers. Subsequent purchases increased the total park area to its present 8,000 acres.

Caspers Windmill

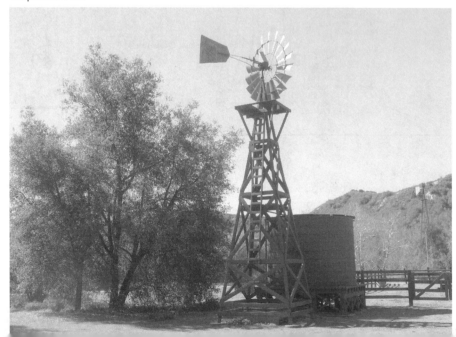

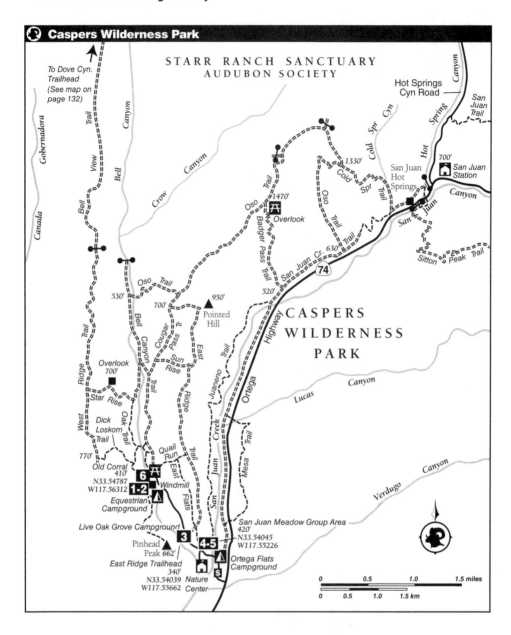

Caspers Wilderness Park

True to the vision of those who foresaw Caspers Park as protecting one of Orange County's last natural areas and being a great recreation resource as well, the park is graced with a fine complement of facilities and improvements. The beautiful visitor center houses a small museum and an open-air loft offering spectacular views of the Santa Ana Mountains. The camping and picnic facilities are second to none in Orange County; a separate campground is devoted to equestrians. Radiating to the outer reaches of the park are 35 miles of riding and hiking trails.

Protection and enhancement of natural habitat are among the park's most important goals. To this end, firebreaks have been constructed on some of the ridges in order to facilitate controlled burns. Periodic burning favors native plants over the nonnative grasses and weedy plants introduced in the past and helps to maintain the natural sage scrub vegetation, which is well adapted to fire. Parts of these firebreaks have been incorporated into the trail system, which also includes dirt maintenance roads and footpaths. A firestorm in October 1993 (one of several simultaneous fires that burned throughout Southern California) swept through the northeastern two-thirds of the park but did not destroy any of the its visitor facilities.

Visitors could spend several days exploring the remainder of the trail system, which visits two basic kinds of environments: the always impressive oak-and-sycamore woodlands along San Juan and Bell Canyons (the two largest drainages in the park) and the sage- and chaparral-covered hillsides offering at times magnificent views stretching from the ocean to the Santa Ana Mountains.

Caspers is sure to delight children who like the outdoors. Its excellent nature center has a platform on top with a telescope commanding a view of the park. Watch for turkey vultures circling overhead. The playground nearby, with boulders for climbing, is a sure hit as well. Stay the night at one of the campgrounds and attend the Saturday evening campfire program. On Sundays, children and the young at heart will enjoy the ranger-led walks on the Nature Trail Loop (the first part of Trip 13.2), which may explain how the native peoples hunted and found food and tools. See **letsgooutside.org** for current schedules.

trip 13.1   **Pinhead Peak**

Distance	1.5 miles (out-and-back)
Hiking Time	1 hour
Elevation Gain	400'
Difficulty	Easy
Trail Use	Equestrians, good for kids
Best Times	All year
Agency	OC Parks: CWP
Permit	OC Parks parking fee required

DIRECTIONS Exit Interstate 5 at Ortega Highway (74) in San Juan Capistrano. Proceed east 7.6 miles to Caspers Wilderness Park on the left at mile marker 74 ORA 7.50. Follow the main park road 1.3 miles to its end at the historic windmill at the Old Corral Picnic Area, where you will find trailhead parking. (If you are staying at the Starr Mesa Equestrian Campground, you can also pick up the trail there via a spur near site 9.)

The view from the nature center is impressive, but from Pinhead Peak it's even better. Here you can look down on the three-way confluence of dry creekbeds—San Juan, Bell, and Verdugo—and spot the toylike visitor center perched atop the knoll between the first two.

The obscure Pinhead Peak Trailhead is marked by a lone signpost behind the smaller metal windmill at the south end of the parking area. Take the trail south across a meadow, passing a spur on the left to the equestrian campground. Cross a grassy cove, then climb onto the scrub-covered

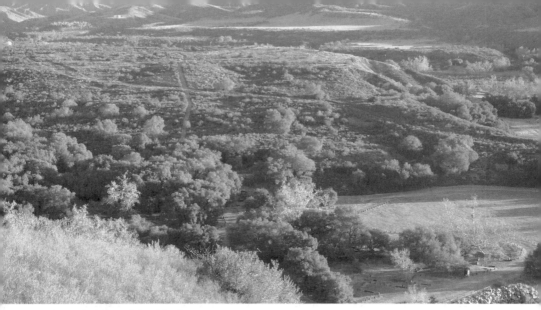

Caspers Park from Pinhead Peak

ridge on the left. After a short but vigorous ascent, you'll reach a high point on the ridge, the 662-foot peak called "Pinhead," next to a wire fence defining the park boundary.

You may wish to follow the trail 300 yards farther down to a saddle and up to a slightly lower bump on the ridge offering a more panoramic view. From both peaks, you can see almost all of the park. Successively higher ridges lead the eye northward and eastward toward the two summits of Old Saddleback and other notable promontories in the southern Santa Ana Mountains.

trip 13.2 West Ridge to Bell Canyon Loop

see map on p. 142

Distance	3.3 miles (loop)
Hiking Time	1½ hours
Elevation Gain	400'
Difficulty	Moderate
Trail Use	Equestrians, good for kids
Best Times	October–June
Agency	OC Parks: CWP
Permit	OC Parks parking fee required

DIRECTIONS Exit Interstate 5 at Ortega Highway (74) in San Juan Capistrano. Proceed east 7.6 miles to Caspers Wilderness Park on the left at mile marker 74 ORA 7.50. Follow the main park road 1.3 miles to its end at the historic windmill at the Old Corral Picnic Area, where you will find trailhead parking.

This hike features a rather dizzying passage across the top of some curious white sandstone formations, rather like the breaks along the upper Missouri River or the barren cliffs of the South Dakota badlands. You'll loop up and over the main ridge defining the west edge of the park, enjoying views of adjacent areas of the county not ordinarily seen from any road.

Start your trip on the hiking and equestrian Nature Trail Loop at a kiosk behind the corral. Follow that path across the wide bed of Bell Canyon past mistletoe-dotted sycamores and into the dense oak woodland on the far side. After 0.3 mile, you'll spot a park bench beneath a gorgeous, spreading oak tree.

Just beyond, veer left on the Dick Loskorn Trail, named in memory of a volunteer naturalist who devoted much effort to the park. This path meanders up a shallow draw and soon climbs to a sandstone ridgeline that at one point narrows to near-knife-edge width. For a step or two, you are within a foot of a modest but unnerving abyss. The sandstone is part of a marine sedimentary formation, called the Santiago Formation (roughly 45 million years old), which crops out along the coastal strip from here down to mid-San Diego County.

After climbing about 350 feet, you come to a dirt road, the West Ridge Trail. Turn north, skirting the fence line of Rancho Mission Viejo, a vast landholding that encompasses much of southern Orange County and formerly included (before World War II) all of Camp Pendleton as well. To the left and right, there are good views of both Bell Canyon and Canada Gobernadora ("Canyon of the Governor's Wife"—though a less literal meaning refers

to the invasive chamise, or greasewood, that used to fill the canyon). Canada Gobernadora is now largely given over to agriculture and to the gated Coto de Caza housing development, which has spread southward in recent years. The confluence of Canada Gobernadora and San Juan Canyon is one of several supposed sites for Mission Vieja, the original San Juan Capistrano Mission, founded in 1776.

After 0.7 mile on the West Ridge Trail, turn right down Star Rise, the dirt road descending toward Bell Canyon. On the left is a flat terrace and a resting bench with a commanding view of almost the entire park. You can look down on the line of oaks and sycamores in Bell Canyon below.

At the bottom of the Star Rise downgrade, veer right onto the beautiful Oak Trail. The limbs and branches of the coastal live oaks are fantastically contorted, but there's an underlying order to the seemingly random pattern. By intricately branching, the tree can support more leaves with less wood. Many of the oaks show fire scars dating back to the Stewart Fire of 1958, which originated in Riverside County. Pushed along by Santa Ana winds, the fire swept across all of what is now Caspers Park,

Nature hike

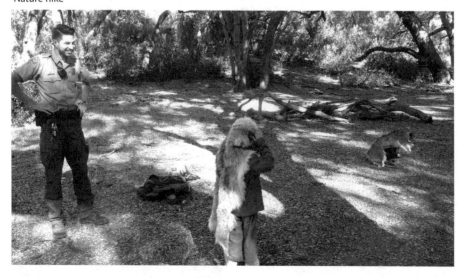

charring a total of 66,000 acres. The 1993 Ortega Fire, which also swept southwest on a Santa Ana, stalled about a mile from here.

In late fall, the tall sycamores along the Oak Trail can be even more attractive than the oaks. Crunch through the crispy leaf litter beneath their spreading crowns, and watch golden sunbeams dance amid thousands of fluttering leaves overhead. In winter, the trunks and branches are ghostly white.

By early spring, new leaves are emerging, and sunlight passing though them bathes the ground shadows in a jungle-green luminance.

The Oak Trail ends at a T-junction with the Nature Trail in the dry wash of Bell Creek. Veer right and continue through another lovely oak glen to the Loskorn Trail junction, and retrace your steps to the trailhead.

---

trip 13.3   **East Ridge to Bell Canyon Loop**

Distance	6 miles (loop)
Hiking Time	3 hours
Elevation Gain	900'
Difficulty	Moderate
Trail Use	Cyclists, equestrians
Best Times	October–May
Agency	OC Parks: CWP
Permit	OC Parks parking fee required

see map on p. 142

DIRECTIONS Exit Interstate 5 at Ortega Highway (Highway 74) in San Juan Capistrano. Proceed east 7.6 miles to Caspers Wilderness Park on the left at mile marker 74 ORA 7.50. Drive up the main park road for 0.7 mile to the East Ridge Trailhead parking area with a restroom and drinking fountain.

On this hike or ride (mountain bikes are welcome on the route described here), you'll pass through two very different kinds of natural habitat: first, a scruffy mix of drought-resistant coastal sage scrub and chaparral plants on the sunny hillsides and ridges; second, the moisture-loving oak-and-sycamore woodlands along Bell Canyon.

Start up the East Ridge Trail, which is a wide fire road. You commence a steady, seldom-steep ascent north along the ridge parallel to and east of Bell Canyon. Dead ahead lies the summit of Santiago Peak, Orange County's high point, some 10 miles north and almost a mile higher.

Aside from the usual California sagebrush, white sage, black sage, and laurel sumac of the sage scrub community, several common chaparral-community plants make their appearance as you climb: chamise, toyon, yucca, deerweed, manzanita, and elderberry. Here and there, you pass some dense thickets of prickly pear cactus.

Promptly cross the East Flats Trail, and later pass signs on the left for the Quail Run and Sun Rise Trails. After 2.5 miles of ascending, the fire road abruptly turns left and descends. Walk 120 yards over to the slightly higher knoll to the east, Pointed Hill, and you'll be treated to a grand view up San Juan Canyon toward the higher Santa Anas.

Back on East Ridge Trail, descend a grassy slope to the west. At the bottom, turn right on the Cougar Pass Trail, and continue 0.2 mile through a cluster of oaks to the intersection of the Oso Trail, where you turn left toward Bell Canyon. After a little climbing, you level off and begin crossing a grassy terrace before dropping again. This flat area is a remnant of one of three or four ancient river terraces exposed on the wall of Bell Canyon. Each terrace represents a stage when Bell

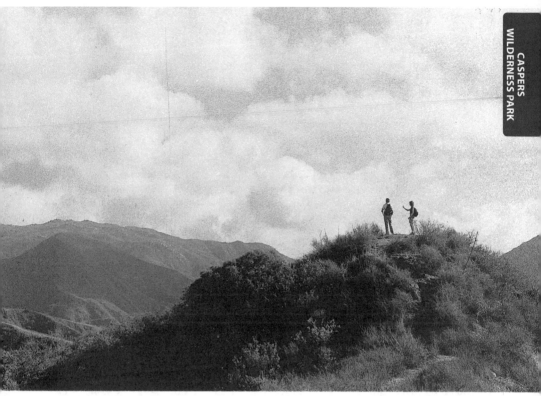

Pointed Hill

Creek became stabilized and used most of its energy to widen its bed rather than cut a deeper channel. Between these quiescent stages, tectonic uplift or other factors, such as a change to a wetter climate, rejuvenated the creek, which then rapidly cut itself to a lower level. The creek is currently engaged in a period of widening, as evidenced by the canyon's broad, flat floor.

Upon reaching the canyon floor, turn left on the Bell Canyon Trail, yet another fire road, and follow it all the way back (2 more miles) to the old corral and windmill. You're unlikely to find water tumbling down the bouldery bed of Bell Canyon, unless it's rained a lot recently—though there's plenty underground to support scattered sycamores and oaks.

In the last mile, where the trail gains a little elevation and sticks to the left side of the canyon bottom, you'll find native coast cholla cactus, prickly pear cactus, and various sage scrub and chaparral plants. Some of the naturalized nonnatives include wild oats and rye grass, filaree, mustard, artichoke thistle, milk thistle, and tree tobacco. Here, in the transition zone between the shady woodland along the creek and the warm, dry slopes, your chances of spotting wildlife and birds are the greatest. Look for deer, coyotes, bobcats, mountain lions, and a host of smaller creatures. When the ground is wet, tracks easily give away their presence. When the trail ends at the historic windmill, continue south on the park road 0.6 mile to the East Ridge Trailhead. Alternatively, use the Quail Run and East Flats trails to avoid the pavement; this option is 0.5 mile longer, but it's more scenic.

trip 13.4   Oso to Juaneno Loop

Distance	9 miles (loop)
Hiking Time	5 hours
Elevation Gain	1,400'
Difficulty	Moderately strenuous
Trail Use	Equestrians
Best Times	November–April
Agency	OC Parks: CWP
Permit	OC Parks parking fee required

see map on p. 142

DIRECTIONS Exit Interstate 5 at Ortega Highway (Highway 74) in San Juan Capistrano. Proceed east 7.6 miles to Caspers Wilderness Park on the left at mile marker 74 ORA 7.50. Follow the park road 0.4 mile. Then make a right into the San Juan Meadow group area, and head to the Juaneno Trail parking area at the north end of the group area.

Pick a clear, cool day, and set aside the better part of it for this hike to one of the highest ridges in Caspers Wilderness Park. You'll have a wonderful view of the higher Santa Anas, Los Angeles Basin, San Joaquin Hills, and ocean. You'll return along San Juan Creek, meandering in and out of the shade of oaks and sycamores.

Continue around the San Juan Meadow road that loops back toward the main park road. Watch for an unmarked path through the oaks on your right that shortcuts 0.1 mile over to the East Flats Trail; if you don't find it, walk west on the road and immediately reach the East Flats Trailhead marker. In any event, turn right on the East Flats Trail, and follow it up onto a terrace overlooking Bell Canyon. Early on a still morning, you're likely to feel the temperature suddenly rise about 10 degrees. A river of cold, dense air flows off the Santa Anas down Bell Canyon, but as soon as you start climbing, you reach the warmer air above.

Cross the East Ridge Road, and continue across the terrace to a T-junction with Quail Run Trail. Turn left and drop down to reach Bell Canyon Road just north of its gate at the Old Corral Picnic Area, 1.5 miles from the start.

Walk north up the dirt Bell Canyon road for one 1.1 miles, then bear right on the Sun Rise Trail. Immediately pass a spur cutting back hard left to Bell Canyon, then turn left onto Cougar Pass Trail in 0.2 mile. Follow Cougar Pass Trail 0.8 mile, up and over a river-terrace remnant, briefly through a cluster of oaks, and to a junction with Oso Trail. A large trailside clearing tempts hikers to have a snack and enjoy the view before the steep climb ahead.

Turn right on Oso Trail, which is a fire road bulldozed directly up the spine of the ridge. Follow it straight up through a blanket of prickly pear cacti. After blooming yellow, orange, or red in the spring and early summer, these cacti grow bulblike fruits called *tuna*, loaded with black seeds, along the edges of their paddle-shaped leaves. The fruits themselves, most conspicuous in October and November, exhibit a variety of bizarre colors best described as shades of purple, magenta, and red. Purple scat along the trail attests to coyotes' fondness for tuna despite its small, vicious spines.

Make a sustained climb for 1.4 miles to where a shade ramada with a picnic table awaits the footsore. Here, you can savor the most panoramic view you're going to get on this hike. The Oso Trail continues farther along the ridgeline (see Trip 13.5), but our way descends south along a crooked firebreak—the Badger Pass Trail—toward San Juan Creek. The huge artichoke thistles along the trail are noxious weeds that infest much of Orange County. The leaves bristle with spines, and the large purple flower becomes a fire hazard when it dries out.

When you reach the bottom, next to the Ortega Highway bridge over San Juan Creek, go right on the San Juan Creek Trail. You could follow this highway-paralleling mountain biking route all the way back, but after just 0.2 mile, you have the option of veering right on the narrow, much more interesting Juaneno Trail.

Follow the Juaneno Trail's winding course downstream for 3.1 miles along the west side of San Juan Creek's usually dry floodplain. Sometimes you're along cobbled banks dotted with riparian vegetation. Other times you swing onto terraces delightfully shaded by oak trees. Bluffs consisting of buff-colored marine sedimentary rock soar dramatically on your right. At one point, you circle a covelike indentation in the cliff reminiscent of the stone amphitheaters in Zion National Park.

After a final detour up and over a wooded slope overlooking the floodplain, the trail emerges at the northeast end of the San Juan Meadow group area where you began.

Deer on Juaneno Trail

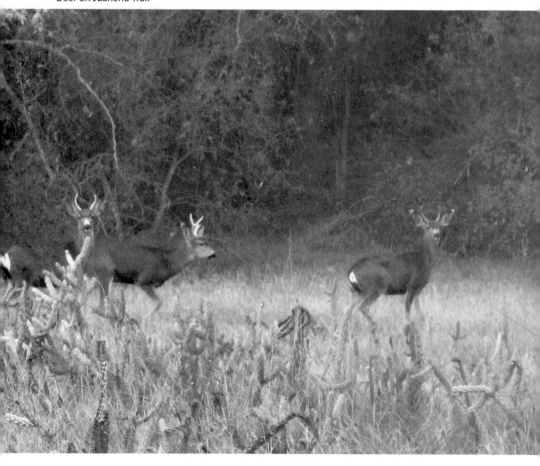

see
map on
p. 142

trip 13.5 Hot Springs Loop

Distance	13 miles (loop)
Hiking Time	6 hours
Elevation Gain	1,500'
Difficulty	Strenuous
Trail Use	Equestrians
Best Times	November–April
Agency	OC Parks: CWP
Permit	OC Parks parking fee required

DIRECTIONS Exit Interstate 5 at Ortega Highway (Highway 74) in San Juan Capistrano. Proceed east 7.6 miles to Caspers Wilderness Park on the left at mile marker 74 ORA 7.50. Follow the park road 0.4 mile. Then make a right into the San Juan Meadow group area, and head to the Juaneno Trail parking area at the north end of the group area.

This trip, essentially a longer variation of Trip 13.4, makes a grand loop around the park, touring many of its most attractive and remote corners, including San Juan Hot Springs. The hot tub resort that once stood at the springs was wiped out in the 1993 Ortega Fire. Caspers Wilderness Park acquired the land and closed the access route from Highway 74, so the only regular access point is via this very long walk. Caspers naturalists occasionally open the east gate for much shorter interpretive hikes to the hot springs; check the schedule of park events at **ocparks.com/parks/ronald** if you are interested.

This trip begins like Trip 13.4. Walk west on the San Juan Meadow loop road for 0.1 mile to pick up the East Flats. Turn left on Quail Run and drop down to the canyon floor, where you turn right on the Bell Canyon Trail. Veer right on Sun Rise, then promptly left onto Cougar Pass Trail. At a T-junction, turn right onto Oso Trail and climb to the picnic bench and lookout at the top of the Badger Pass Trail, 4.9 miles from the start.

Continue northeast on the Oso Trail, passing two unsigned spur roads on the left to Starr Ranch Sanctuary, then curve south and descend to a signed junction with the Cold Springs Trail in 1.6 miles. Take this former jeep road, now a rocky trail, that drops into Cold Springs Canyon, one of Caspers's most pristine and beautiful areas. A creek flows beneath the oaks and sycamores during the wetter months, but copious poison oak discourages close investigation.

At a shady junction with the San Juan Creek Trail in 1.1 miles, turn left and climb 0.2 mile onto a low ridge. As you begin to descend, watch for a path on the right leading to the San Juan Hot Springs at the foot of a palm tree. The park does not permit soaking in the faintly sulphurous, bacteria-laden 122-degree waters, and the bees that frequent the springs discourage close investigation.

San Juan Hot Springs has drawn visitors since the 1870s, and a hotel and resort were constructed here before 1900. The Health Department closed the facilities in 1936. Russ Kiessig reopened a resort here in 1980 but closed it in 1992 after the highway was relocated too close to the facilities, and most of the structures burned the following year. The springs became part of Caspers Wilderness Park, and the rangers closed the nearby gate after thoughtless illegal users damaged the area.

Return to the Cold Springs Trail junction, and continue southwest on the San Juan Creek Trail. The sometimes unmaintained trail surmounts a steep ridge by way of tight switchbacks. At its crest, abruptly turn left, and descend precipitously. Then parallel Highway 74 to a junction at the foot of the Oso Trail.

Continue southwest on the San Juan Creek Trail, which is now a wide dirt park boundary road paralleling the noisy highway. After an unpleasant 0.8 mile, pass a junction with the Badger Pass Trail.

Continue another 0.2 mile to the much more appealing Juaneno Trail on the right, which you follow 3.1 miles back to the start (see Trip 13.4 again).

San Juan Hot Springs

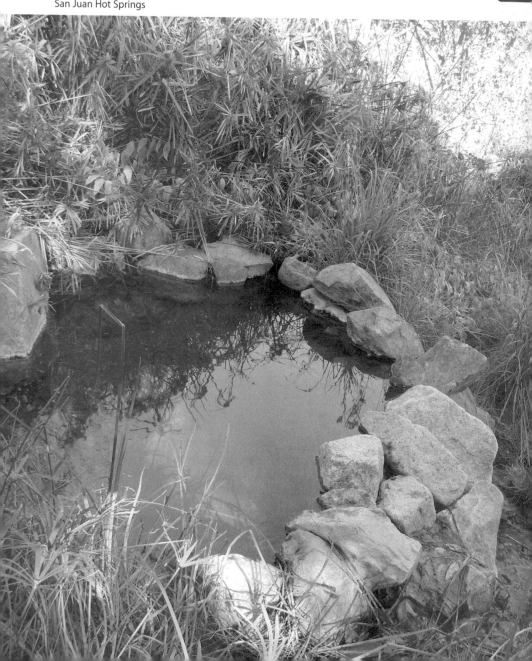

see maps on p. 132 and p. 142

trip 13.6 Bell View Trail

Distance	8 miles (one-way to the windmill at Caspers)
Hiking Time	4 hours
Elevation Gain/Loss	1,000'/1,650'
Difficulty	Moderately strenuous
Trail Use	Cyclists, equestrians
Best Times	November–May
Agency	OC Parks: CWP
Permit	OC Parks parking fee required

DIRECTIONS This trip requires a car or long bicycle shuttle. To reach the south end, or your destination: From Interstate 5 in San Juan Capistrano, take Highway 74 east for 7.5 miles to Caspers Wilderness Park. Follow the main park road 1.3 miles to its end at the historic windmill at the Old Corral Picnic Area, where you will find trailhead parking.

To reach the north end (your starting point, shown on the map on page 132) from the south end: Exit Caspers and go back west on Highway 74 for 5.1 miles. Turn right on Antonio Parkway, and follow it north 10 miles. Turn right on Alas de Paz, then immediately right onto Plano Trabuco and immediately left onto Dove Canyon Drive, where you can park on the street.

The Bell View Regional Trail, for hikers, equestrians, and cyclists, starts as a community trail threading through the suburban-edge communities of Rancho Santa Margarita and Coto de Caza. It then assumes a wilder character as it undulates along a ridge overlooking open land to the east as far as the eye can see. The route ends inside Caspers Wilderness Park, not far from Ortega Highway. For mountain bikers, the out-and-back distance of 16 miles seems reasonable. Hikers, however, will better enjoy the journey as an 8-mile point-to-point hike facilitated by a willing driver-friend. If your friend doesn't want to hike with you, arrange to have him or her to drop you off at the start, the north gate for the private Coto de Caza housing development, and pick you up at the finish at the Old Corral Picnic Area.

The Bell View Trail picks up on a gated, paved service road by a faux waterfall on Dove Canyon Drive. Head south up a short, steep hill on the service road, and then veer right on the dirt path designated the Bell View Trail. You climb toward a broad ridge, with Coto de Caza houses stretching miles ahead down the valley on your right and the Dove Canyon subdivision and golf course to your left (east).

After 2 miles of unexciting travel overlooking densely packed McMansions, you descend past the last of the Dove Canyon housing and continue alongside the east boundary of the spacious (and closed to the public except for special tours) Audubon Society Starr Ranch Sanctuary. You'll also see the first of many private trails on the west side descending into the gated Coto de Caza neighborhood.

At 2.6 miles, you pass an equestrian rest area with a drinking fountain and picnic tables. Continue south, soon passing a gate, on or near the top of the ridgeline, occasionally going steeply up or down. The Coto de Caza development continues on the right side, while the Bell Canyon drainage lies on the left. Note the effect of regional uplift in this area over a period of 1 million years or so. The shelflike fluvial (stream) terraces flanking the canyon represent where the river once flowed across a broad plain. The brooding Santa Ana Mountains rise behind this spacious scene, with no sign of civilization in that direction.

At 3.8 miles, you reach another gate. Go around it, and bear left to stay on the Bell View Trail. The trail briefly follows one of the flat terraces, which at this point lies on the ridgeline, then descends to the west side, passing assorted ruins of the not-long-bygone cattle ranching era.

At 5.2 miles, a bench affords a view down into Bell Canyon at the gated edge of Caspers Wilderness Park. A sign indicates that dogs are prohibited on the trail anywhere south of this point. The name "Bell," incidentally, commemorates an 8-ton granitic boulder that once lay precariously balanced on some smaller rocks in what is now the Audubon Sanctuary. When struck with great force, the boulder resonated like a bell, audible a mile away. Removed from the canyon in 1936, Bell Rock was taken to the courtyard of the Bowers Museum in Santa Ana, where it rests today. The process of excavation ruined the rock's unique acoustic properties.

Continue 1.5 miles down the ridge-running road (now called the West Ridge Trail) to a junction with Star Rise, a fire road descending east into Bell Canyon. Make a left, descend to the bottom, and make a right on Oak Trail. The delightfully woodsy trail meanders through oak and sycamore woodland on the left or west bank of Bell Canyon. At a T-junction with the Nature Trail Loop, stay right and make your way back to the Old Corral Picnic Area. (**Note:** *Mountain bikers must stay on Star Rise as it swings north and connects with Bell Canyon Trail. The Oak Trail and Nature Trail Loop are off-limits to bikes.*)

Resting bench overlooking Bell Canyon

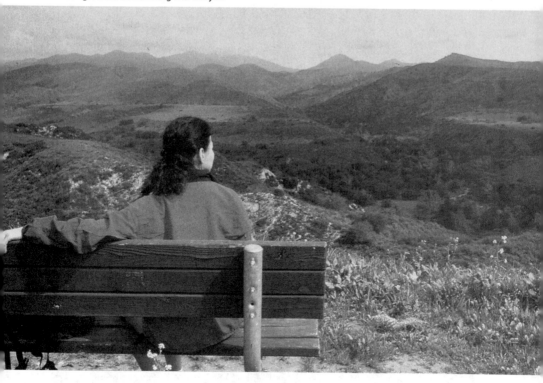

chapter 14

Santa Rosa Plateau Ecological Reserve

The Santa Rosa Plateau, on a southeastern spur of the Santa Ana Mountains, rises over the rapidly expanding suburban communities of southwest Riverside County like a Shangri-la in the sky. In the early 1980s, hardly anyone knew of its existence or ecological significance. Starting with a nucleus of 3,100 acres purchased by The Nature Conservancy from a housing development company in 1983, the current ecological reserve on the plateau now includes more than 9,000 acres—some 14 square miles. The reserve is managed by Riverside County Parks in cooperation with the California Department of Fish and Wildlife. About 40% is classified as a research area with no public access, about 40% is laced with dirt roads and trails for use by hikers only, and the remaining 20% or so has multiuse roads and trails open to hiking, horseback riding, and mountain biking.

A circle, 100 miles in radius, centered on the reserve, encompasses a megalopolis of some 20 million people. File this fact away in your mind, and then try to fathom its truth while walking amid the green and golden hills of this exquisitely beautiful place. Here is a classic California landscape of wind-rippled grasses, swaying poppies, statuesque oak trees, trickling streams, vernal pools, a dazzling assortment of native plants (around 500 at last count), and a variety of animals.

Aerial view of Santa Rosa Plateau

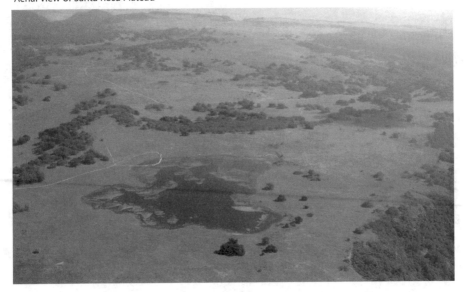

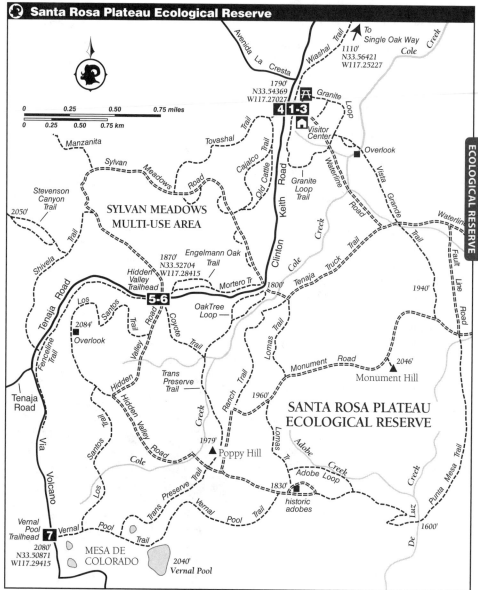

You will be struck by the reserve's timelessness and insularity, and you will quickly realize how important it was to save it.

Every Southern Californian should see the Santa Rosa Plateau Ecological Reserve at its stunning best—during March and April, following a wet winter—at least once. The blooming wildflowers, including California poppies, can be fantastic. Make a note in your calendar now to pay it a visit next spring.

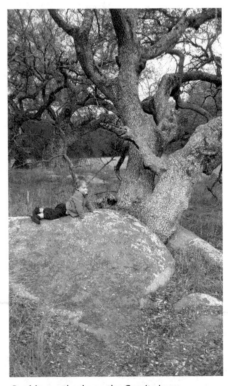

trip 14.1   Granite Loop

Distance	1.6 miles (loop)
Hiking Time	1 hour
Elevation Gain	100'
Difficulty	Easy
Trail Use	Good for kids
Best Times	All year
Agency	SRPER
Permit	Riverside County Parks day-use fee required

see map on previous page

DIRECTIONS Exit Interstate 15 at Clinton Keith Road in Wildomar (Riverside County). Proceed south on Clinton Keith Road 4.1 miles to the Santa Rosa Plateau Visitor Center on the left. Be watchful; the entrance road is easy to miss.

This minitour, circling the visitor center, will introduce you to a variety of contrasting habitats within Santa Rosa Plateau Ecological Reserve. The inclusion of a 0.4-mile side trip to and from the east end of the 1.2-mile Granite Loop route lets you visit some tenajas (pools) along Cole Creek and a nice patch of willow and sycamore woodland.

Start the Granite Loop by going north from the west side of the parking lot (don't take the nearby Wiashal Multi-Use Trail, which also goes north). Right away, a slight drop in elevation results in a big change of habitat. You go from sunny chaparral to shadowy live oak woods in only a couple of minutes. Picnic tables amid the oaks overlook a small ravine. The trail continues down along that ravine, then climbs onto a bouldery, chaparral-clad slope on the right.

At 0.4 mile, you pass a shortcut trail on the right going back toward the visitor center. At 0.6 mile (right before the Granite Loop crosses Waterline Road), you come to the Vista Grande Trail, intersecting on the left. Follow the Vista Grande Trail (out and later back) to visit the Tenajas Overlook, with a view of Cole Creek. An interpretive panel explains how these tenajas, or small basins worn into the granitic bedrock, are instrumental in supporting the web of life in the reserve during times of drought. In a wet year, the waters of Cole Creek form a large, attractive reflective pool here.

Back on the Granite Loop, cross Waterline Road (a dirt road), and enjoy the next 0.3 mile in particular as you stroll through a parklike landscape of spreading live oak trees. Two sites have benches under the oldest, most spectacular oaks. Nearing the end of the loop, you climb just a bit and finish the hike amid sunny chaparral.

Boulders and oaks on the Granite Loop

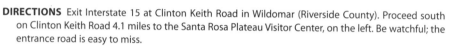

trip 14.2   Punta Mesa Loop

Distance	8 miles (loop)
Hiking Time	4 hours
Elevation Gain	650'
Difficulty	Moderately strenuous
Trail Use	Hiking only
Best Times	December–May
Agency	SRPER
Permit	Riverside County Parks day-use fee required

see map on p. 155

DIRECTIONS Exit Interstate 15 at Clinton Keith Road in Wildomar (Riverside County). Proceed south on Clinton Keith Road 4.1 miles to the Santa Rosa Plateau Visitor Center, on the left. Be watchful; the entrance road is easy to miss.

SANTA ROSA PLATEAU ECOLOGICAL RESERVE

For a comprehensive tour of the Santa Rosa Plateau Ecological Reserve, try this half-day hike, which will introduce you to virtually every attractive feature characteristic of Southern California's foothills. The hike is far too hot and dry for most people during the warmer half of the year, but it's pleasant during the winter and on cool spring days.

Start your journey at the visitor center. Follow dirt Waterline Road southeast. At 0.8 mile, turn right on Tenaja Truck Trail and traverse its flat, straight course across a treeless plain. At 1.7 miles, near the junction of Ranch Trail, make a left on the narrow Lomas Trail. Ascend a slope dotted with Engelmann oaks, jog right for about 0.2 mile on Monument Road, and then find the continuation of Lomas Trail on the left. You now descend into a valley, where the Adobe Loop branches left, and two adobe buildings set amid towering oaks lie just ahead. You won't want to miss these adobes of the former Rancho Santa Rosa. Constructed around 1845, they are Riverside County's oldest standing structures. Your hike has taken you 3 miles so far.

After a look at the adobes and a refreshing pause in the shade, backtrack 0.1 mile north on Lomas Trail, and take the Adobe Loop east, down along an oak-filled canyon. Enjoy

Vista Grande Trail

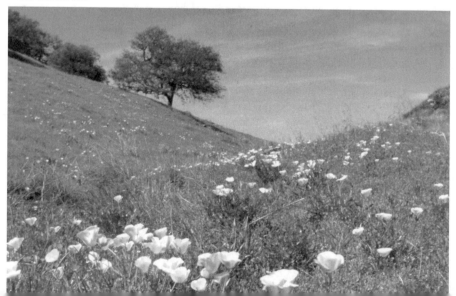

the last deeply shaded stretch of trail you're going to get on this hike. Soon enough, it's back into the sunshine again as you climb up to a junction with the Punta Mesa Trail. Turn left and follow this deteriorating former fire road a total of 2 miles—down across De Luz Creek and back uphill, heading north. Mesa de la Punta rising to the south and Mesa de Burro to the east, both capped with erosion-resistant basalt, are part of the reserve's off-limits-to-the-public research zone.

At the next intersection (a total of 5.8 miles into the hike), turn left on Monument Road, travel 0.2 mile west, and veer right on the aptly named Vista Grande Trail. Follow Vista Grande Trail north to a crest (elevation 1,940 feet), where your gaze takes in hundreds of acres of wind-rippled grass and the distant, winter-snow-capped San Bernardino and San Jacinto Mountains. Curving northwest, the Vista Grande Trail crosses Tenaja Truck Trail and then more or less makes a beeline for the visitor center, traversing nearly flat terrain punctuated with scattered oaks and lichen-encrusted piles of granitic rock.

---

trip 14.3　Wiashal Trail

see map on p. 155

Distance	3.5 miles (one-way) or 6.6 miles (out-and-back)
Hiking Time	2 hours (one-way)
Elevation Gain	600' (one-way down) or 1,700' (out-and-back)
Difficulty	Moderate or strenuous
Trail Use	Cyclists, equestrians
Best Times	October–April
Agency	SRPER
Permit	Riverside County Parks day-use fee required

DIRECTIONS This trip involves a car shuttle if you wish to hike it one-way. From Interstate 15 in Wildomar, exit southwest on Clinton Keith Road. In 1.6 miles, turn left (east) onto Calle del Oso Oro. Then turn right (south) onto Calle Cipres, then immediately left onto Placer Creek Street. At a T-junction, turn right on Single Oak Way. Leave a vehicle here. You will emerge through a gap between the houses. Finding your vehicle at the end of the hike can be confusing, so take some time to familiarize yourself with the trailhead.

Return to Clinton Keith Road, and continue 2.5 miles up to the Santa Rosa Plateau Ecological Reserve Visitor Center on the left side of the road. Park at the visitor center.

The Wiashal (*wee-uh-shawl*) Trail descends from the Santa Rosa Plateau Ecological Reserve to an open-space preserve in Cole Canyon at the edge of Murrieta. It is the steepest trail in the reserve and has some areas with poor traction; a trekking pole and reliable sense of balance are helpful. Remarkably, hard-core mountain bikers love this trail and have nicknamed it the Superman Trail. It features great views and some of the oldest chaparral in Southern California. The route is not marked on the topographic map and mostly falls beyond the edge of the reserve map. (**Note:** *The Wiashal Trail has washed out and is closed until further notice as the reserve develops a plan and secures funding to reroute it on a more suitable path. Check with the visitor center for updates.*)

The signed upper end of the Wiashal Trail starts at the junction of Clinton Keith Road and the dirt road leading to the visitor center parking. The trail leads north parallel to Clinton Keith Road for 0.3 mile to a second trailhead at a dirt lot opposite Avenida la Cresta.

Much of this area burned in the 1981 Turner Fire, but the next stretch has not

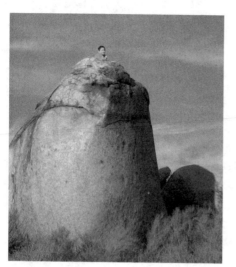

Eagle Rock

SANTA ROSA PLATEAU
ECOLOGICAL RESERVE

a century if not burned. Scrub oak, sugar bush, and many other chaparral species are common along other stretches.

The trail passes along rolling hills with many ups and downs. In another 1.4 miles, a sign indicates a trail leading left for 0.1 mile to an overlook with great views. Another 0.7 mile beyond, reach a junction with a trail leading left for 0.1 mile to where you can look over the town of Murrieta. Adjacent to this junction is a boulder named Eagle Rock. Under the right light, the resemblance is uncanny.

Beyond Eagle Rock, the rolling terrain ends and the trail plunges steeply to town. In 0.9 mile, reach a gate at the preserve boundary, a good turnaround spot for a round-trip hike. Otherwise, continue to a T-junction in Cole Canyon, and turn left. Wander through a maze of paths, generally trending north as much as possible before turning west to reach Single Oak Way in 0.3 mile.

burned in many decades and contains some of the oldest hoaryleaf ceanothus plants in Southern California. This plant requires fire for the seeds to grow and lives for about

trip 14.4 Sylvan Meadows

see map on p. 155

Distance	6 miles (loop)
Hiking Time	3 hours
Elevation Gain	500'
Difficulty	Moderate
Trail Use	Cyclists, equestrians, dogs
Best Times	November–May
Agency	SRPER
Permit	Riverside County Parks day-use fee required

DIRECTIONS Exit Interstate 15 at Clinton Keith Road in Wildomar (Riverside County). Proceed south on Clinton Keith Road 4.1 miles to the Santa Rosa Plateau Visitor Center, on the left. Be watchful; the entrance road is easy to miss.

The Santa Rosa Plateau's Sylvan Meadows Multi-Use Area is open to all nonmotorized means of travel—hiking, jogging, biking, and horseback riding—with the stipulation that all users stay on the designated roads and trails. The comprehensive tour of the whole Sylvan Meadows area, described here, includes an out-and-back side trip into Stevenson Canyon that would seem to be superfluous but should not be missed.

From the visitor center parking lot, cross to the west side of Clinton Keith Road, and descend 0.1 mile to a trail junction in a shady ravine. Turn right on the Tovashal Trail (Cajalco Trail ahead is your return route). After proceeding 0.8 mile up through and eventually out of the shallow ravine, you come to the next junction, Sylvan Meadows Road, on the north edge of an expansive, oak-dotted meadow. This is a part of the

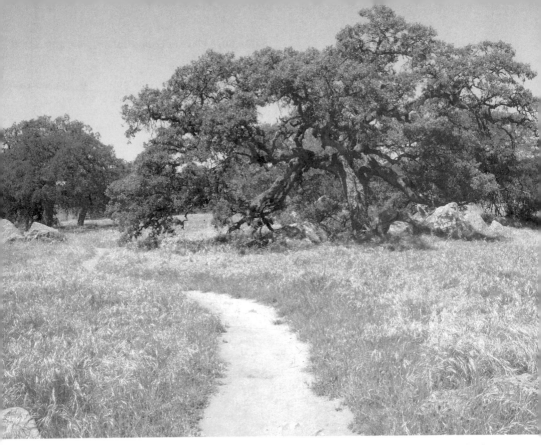

Sylvan Meadows

roughly 3,000 acres of "bunchgrass prairie" in the reserve that is regarded as the finest example of native grassland habitat in California. Ongoing prescribed fires and selective removal of nonnative grasses in such meadows are encouraging the growth of natives, including purple needlegrass, malpais blue grass, and deergrass.

Make a right on Sylvan Meadows Road, continue 0.5 mile along the rim of the meadow, and then begin the highly recommended 1.6-mile side trip, which is included in this trip's mileage. Turn right on the Shivela Trail, continue 0.4 mile, then go right again on the Stevenson Canyon Trail. The trail loops, so you can go up along the brushy slope east of the canyon and back down on a singletrack pathway through the canyon bottom itself. This latter trail segment is arguably the most enchanting passage in the

entire reserve, with inky shadows, a gallery of twisted oak limbs, a trickling stream (in season at least), and luminescent greenery everywhere. Mountain bikers may breeze through here without warning, so those on foot should be alert.

Retrace your steps on Shivela Trail, and then use Sylvan Meadows Road to reach Hidden Valley Trailhead (which has restrooms but no water). Now, head east, more or less along the north-side fenceline of Tenaja Road, first on Engelmann Oak Trail and then on Mortero Trail, to the right-angle bend where paved Clinton Keith and Tenaja Roads join. That's where the east leg of Sylvan Meadows Road intersects. It will take you 0.5 mile north to Cajalco Trail, which will lead you 0.7 mile to the junction you passed at the beginning, just shy of the visitor center.

trip 14.5   **Oak Tree Loop**

Distance	2.1 miles (semiloop)
Hiking Time	1 hour
Elevation Gain	100'
Difficulty	Easy
Trail Use	Good for kids
Best Times	All year
Agency	SRPER
Permit	Riverside County Parks parking fee required

see map on p. 155

DIRECTIONS Exit Interstate 15 at Clinton Keith Road in Wildomar (Riverside County). Proceed south on Clinton Keith Road. Note the turnoff for the Santa Rosa Plateau Visitor Center, 4.1 miles from I-15. Continue (without making any turns but following the curves of the roadway) to the Hidden Valley Trailhead on the left, 1.7 miles from the visitor center.

The Oak Tree Trail loop takes you through one of the few protected, self-reproducing stands of Engelmann oaks remaining on Earth. The Engelmann oak (or mesa oak), native to the coastal foothills of Southern California and far northern Baja California, is rapidly being displaced by urbanization and other forms of habitat degradation. These trees are easily distinguishable from their botanical cousins and frequent neighbors—coast live oaks—by their grayish scaly bark (especially on young specimens) and grayish-blue-green leaves. Ranging in age up to about 300 years, these particular thick-trunked Engelmanns have real character. Their multifarious, wandering limbs divide into innumerable branches, and their dense foliage spreads outward to cast black pools of shade upon the ground.

There's much more to see along this little trail than just oaks. Cole Creek trickles alongside one leg of the trail, its bed sculpted with small tenajas that support frogs, pond turtles, and newts. California sycamores twine upward among the oaks. One of the oaks in this section has a hollow interior, providing nesting habitat for birds, such as woodpeckers and screech owls.

Touring the short (0.6-mile) Oak Tree Trail requires that you hoof it a while before you reach it. From the Hidden Valley Trailhead, walk 0.5 mile southeast on the Coyote

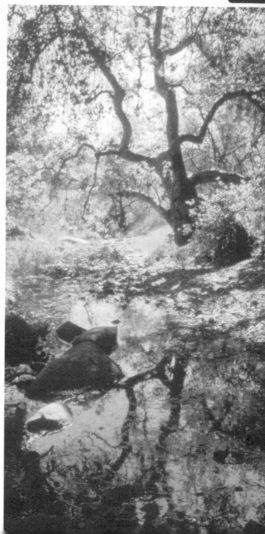
On the Oak Tree Trail

Trail, and then make a left on the Trans Preserve Trail to connect with the Oak Tree Loop. Along the way, over gently rolling, grassy terrain, take note of purple needlegrass, a native, fire-resistant, and drought-resistant bunchgrass that survives by sending down roots several feet deep. The landscape here, partially restored by such techniques as prescribed burning, is a rare facsimile of what much of coastal Southern California looked like centuries ago.

After you've walked fully around the Oak Tree Loop, retrace your footsteps on the Trans Preserve and Coyote Trails.

trip 14.6   Los Santos to Trans Preserve Loop

see map on p. 155

Distance	4.8 miles (loop)
Hiking Time	2½ hours
Elevation Gain	500'
Difficulty	Moderate
Trail Use	Hiking only
Best Times	November–May
Agency	SRPER
Permit	Riverside County Parks day-use fee required

DIRECTIONS Exit Interstate 15 at Clinton Keith Road in Wildomar (Riverside County). Proceed south on Clinton Keith Road. Note the turnoff for the Santa Rosa Plateau Visitor Center, 4.1 miles from I-15. Continue (without making any turns but following the curves of the roadway) to the Hidden Valley Trailhead on the left, 1.7 miles from the visitor center.

This loop hike traverses the open meadows, grassy hillsides, and shady recesses of the reserve's southwest corner. You'll enjoy superb views throughout, plus excellent opportunities for bird and wildlife watching.

Begin at Hidden Valley Trailhead by heading uphill (south) on the wide Hidden Valley Road. After only 0.2 mile, make a right on the narrow Los Santos Trail. This delightfully primitive path crookedly ascends some bald hillsides, gains a ridgetop, and passes a resting bench just south of a 2,084-foot knoll. From this overlook point, the bulk of the reserve's sensuously rolling terrain lies in full view. This may be the ideal spot to break out your high-powered binoculars to scan for deer in the meadows below and track raptors gliding in the sky above.

Beyond the overlook, the Los Santos Trail drops into an upper tributary of Cole Creek and bends left to follow the tributary's tiny (and usually dry) brook. After just 0.1 mile, the path ahead assumes the proportions of a dirt road and continues southeast to join Hidden Valley Road. Don't miss the sign on the right, which directs you onto the sharply ascending, again delightfully primitive, south branch of the Los Santos Trail.

You climb to the lip of an oak-dotted plateau, a northward extension of the nearby Mesa de Colorado. Underfoot, there are small outcrops of basalt, a dark-colored volcanic rock. It once covered the entire area but is now isolated atop these elevated mesas, and its tough, erosion-resistant character is responsible for the plateau's flat topography. The softer, marine sedimentary rocks associated with the terrain behind you have eroded to form all those sensuously rolling hills and valleys.

In spring, look for the coy dark brown blossoms of chocolate lilies under the semi-shade of the oaks.

The Los Santos Trail continues south, dipping into and out of a shady ravine, then enters Mesa de Colorado proper, where you arrive at a junction with the Vernal Pool Trail. You've now come 2.4 miles, exactly halfway around the loop.

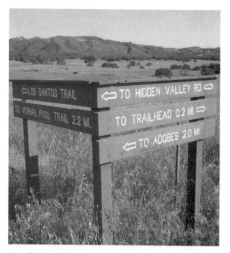

Los Santos Trail

Turn left on the Vernal Pool Trail, proceed 0.3 mile, and turn left on the Trans Preserve Trail. (**Note:** *The large vernal pool lies just ahead on the Vernal Pool Trail; don't miss it, especially if you haven't seen it before.*)

On the Trans Preserve Trail, you meander northeast, descend off the plateau rim by way of an oblique course down a gorgeously oak-draped hillside, and strike a nearly level, northward course alongside Poppy Hill, one of several good sites in the reserve for viewing California poppies in the springtime. On ahead, you gently curve and descend along another Cole Creek tributary ravine, and 4.3 miles into the hike, you reach the Coyote Trail. Turn left and complete the remaining half-mile to Hidden Valley Trailhead.

SANTA ROSA PLATEAU ECOLOGICAL RESERVE

trip 14.7 Vernal Pool Trail

Distance	1.2 miles (out-and-back)
Hiking Time	1 hour
Elevation Gain	50'
Difficulty	Easy
Trail Use	Good for kids
Best Times	January–May
Agency	SRPER
Permit	Riverside County Parks day-use fee required

see map on p. 155

DIRECTIONS Exit Interstate 15 at Clinton Keith Road in Wildomar (Riverside County). Proceed south on Clinton Keith Road. Note the turnoff for the Santa Rosa Plateau Visitor Center, 4.1 miles from I-15. Continue (without making any turns but following the curves of the roadway) to the Vernal Pool Trailhead on the left, 3.7 miles from the visitor center.

One of the largest vernal pools in California (39 acres at maximum capacity) lies in a shallow depression atop nearly flat Mesa de Colorado on the south side of the Santa Rosa Plateau Ecological Reserve. Getting there is very simple. Walk due east on the wide, nearly flat Vernal Pool Trail for 0.6 mile to reach the north edge of the large pool, where a boardwalk allows you to approach the shoreline. On winter and spring weekends, this is far and away the most popular trail in the reserve.

The hard-pan surface underneath vernal pools is generally impervious to water, so once winter storms fill them, the pools dry only by evaporation. Unusual, sometimes unique species of flowering plants have evolved around the perimeter of many vernal pools, including this one. As the pool contracts during the steadily lengthening and warming days of spring, successive waves of annual wildflowers bloom along its moist margin. By July or August, there's nothing to be seen but a desiccated depression, its barren surface glaring in the hot sun. The large pool is also home to two species of fairy shrimp and the spadefoot toad, whose egg clusters may be quite conspicuous.

chapter 15

Santa Ana Mountains: Main Divide

Most of the higher Santa Ana Mountains, along with their extensions to the southeast and east (the Elsinore and Santa Margarita Mountains), lie within the overall boundary of Cleveland National Forest, fixed by Congress in 1908. The administrative subunit covering this area is called the Trabuco Ranger District. Of the 255 square miles encompassed by the district, the federal government manages about 210 square miles. Private inholdings make up the difference.

We divide the Trabuco District into three parts—northern, middle, and southern—because of their distinctly different characters. In most of the Main Divide of the Santa Ana Mountains, visitor facilities are almost nil, but an extensive dirt road system, along with a few trails, makes it relatively easy for hikers to get around. The middle section (Chapter 16) along Ortega Highway has camping facilities, many trails, and easy access to them. The southern section (Chapter 17), the San Mateo Canyon Wilderness, has an extensive trail system that receives varying degrees of maintenance.

Geographically, the Main Divide is an important watershed divide, featuring several of the Santa Ana's highest peaks, including (from north to south) Sierra Peak, Pleasants Peak, Bedford Peak, Bald Peak, Modjeska and Santiago Peaks (together forming the familiar "Old Saddleback"), and Trabuco Peak. These rounded summits (except Modjeska) serve, in a connect-the-dots fashion, as benchmarks for the Orange–Riverside county line.

East of the Main Divide, water flows down steep canyons to Temescal Valley, a shallow depression on the far side of the Elsinore Fault, where it usually percolates into the water table. During times of exceptional flood, the runoff may make its way north to Corona and the Santa Ana River.

West of the divide, water flows down canyons steep in their upper reaches, narrow and rather straight in their midsections, and broad and gently meandering through the foothills. If unclaimed by percolation or not detained by dams, the water makes its way across Orange County's coastal plain—typically in concrete-lined channels—to the sea.

The Main Divide appears treeless and rather austere from a distance, yet it holds many surprises. The ubiquitous chaparral and sage scrub cover that appears half-dead in summer's blazing heat turns bright green and pleasingly pungent at the touch of late autumn's first steady rain. Early spring sunshine brings forth a profusion of blossoms and perfumelike aromas.

On both sides of the Main Divide, coniferous trees cling to moist pockets of soil, and scattered springs feed perennial and seasonal creeks that in turn sustain willows, sycamores, maples, bay laurels, and centuries-old oaks in the bottom of the deepest ravines and canyons.

The Main Divide's existing road system, which consists largely of unpaved roads, serves purposes as diverse as fire control, access to utility and telecommunications facilities, recreational driving, hiking, and mountain biking. In the recent past, these roads have been closed to vehicles (part time or all the time) for reasons ranging from storm damage to fire danger to the protection of endangered species, such as the arroyo toad. The gate at the south end of Main Divide Road is usually open, but the road has steep and rocky sections that may require a high-clearance four-wheel-drive vehicle. The gate on Maple Springs Road is also often open. The gates on Skyline Drive, Black Star Canyon, Harding Road, Santiago Trail, and Coal Canyon are permanently closed to recreational users. Bedford Road and Indian Truck Trail are sometimes open when weather and fire danger permit, although heavy construction at the east ends may affect access. For the latest information on road closures in the Santa Ana Mountains, call the Trabuco

Ranger District office in Corona or search online for "Cleveland National Forest Road Status." Hikers and mountain bikers usually have the privilege of unrestricted travel on the Main Divide's roads and trails, but not when the US Forest Service declares an emergency fire closure during extremely dry weather or when an order is issued to protect endangered species. Again, you can find out the latest information from them by calling them or checking the ranger district's website.

At all times and in all seasons, fires and camping are prohibited in the Main Divide area—though you may hike before dawn and after sunset.

Harding Falls

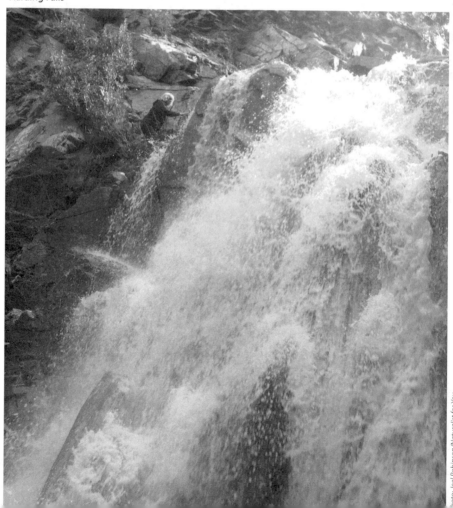

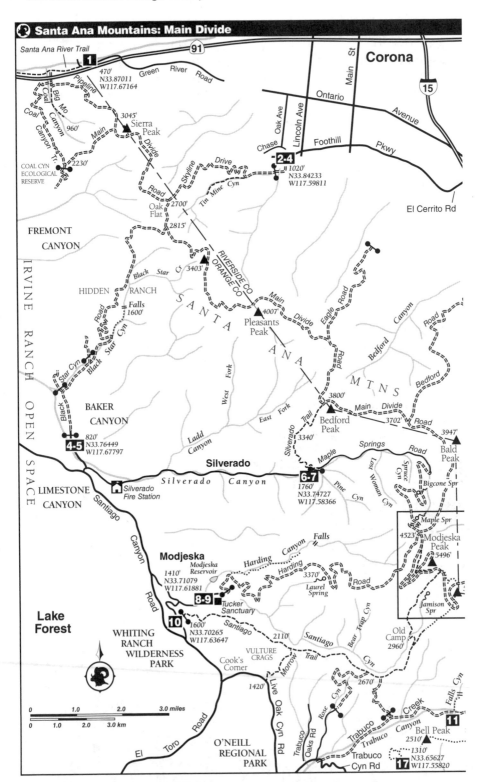

Santa Ana Mountains: Main Divide

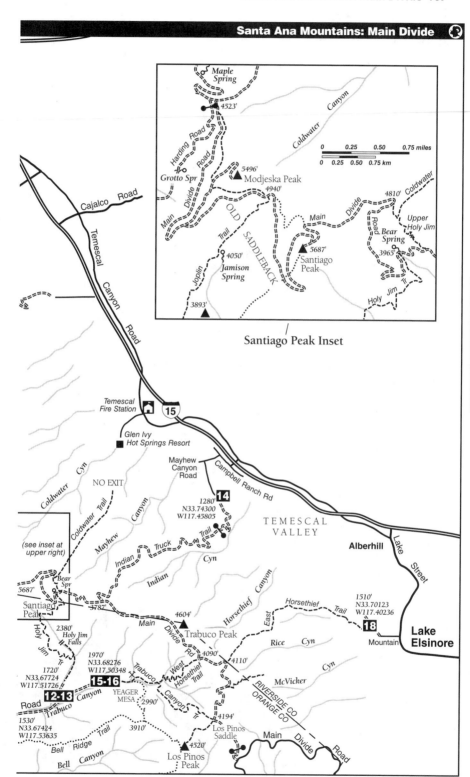

Santiago Peak Inset

SANTA ANA MOUNTAINS

trip 15.1 **Tecate Cypress Preserve**

Distance	9.5 miles (out-and-back)
Hiking Time	5 hours
Elevation Gain	1,900'
Difficulty	Strenuous
Trail Use	Cyclists, equestrians, dogs
Best Times	November–March
Agency	CDFW
Recommended Map	*Cleveland National Forest Visitor Map*

DIRECTIONS From the 91 Freeway in Corona, take Exit 44 for Green River Road, and turn west. After 1 mile, park on the right side of Green River Road near the turnoff for the Green River Golf Club.

The Tecate cypress is one of California's rare conifers, with a few groves in San Diego County and one in the Santa Ana Mountains on the north flank of Sierra Peak. The California Department of Fish and Game established the Coal Canyon Ecological Reserve in 1994 to protect the Sierra Peak stand and to provide a vital wildlife corridor for large mammals to move between the Santa Ana Mountains and the Chino Hills. This trip makes a steep climb from the Santa Ana River Canyon high onto the ridge of Sierra Peak to visit the cypress trees.

Unfortunately, the Tecate forest burned in the 1982 Gypsum Fire, the 2002 Green Fire, and the 2006 Sierra Fire. While the cypress depends on periodic wildfires to open its hard, woody cones and spread seeds, fires that happen too often kill seedlings before they have a chance to mature. Another wildfire in the near future could wipe out this forest. For now, however, you can see seedlings regrowing and a few mature trees that have survived the repeated burns.

From the trailhead, take the Santa Ana River Trail (a paved path popular with cyclists) west as it parallels the noisy 91 Freeway. After this inauspicious start, cross under the freeway at the former Coal Canyon offramp, and walk south on a dirt road into the canyon. Promptly reach a fork, where you veer right and begin climbing.

The next 3.5 miles offer an unrelenting climb onto the west shoulder of Sierra Peak. In the final mile, you'll stroll through the cypress grove. The trees have scalelike leaves reminiscent of a juniper. The mature trees burned but are easily recognized by their spherical cones, about an inch in diameter. Seedlings are growing at their feet amidst the chamise and other scrub. Off-trail exploration is prohibited, but you have plenty of good views from the trail.

When you reach the ridge at a junction with a powerline service road, you can veer right 100 feet to a vista point marked with a huge cairn. Several mature trees here escaped the infernos. Enjoy the sweeping views before returning the way you came.

Alternatively, if you are looking for even more exercise, you can continue up the road to antennae-studded Sierra Peak. This ascent is 2.4 miles with 800 feet of gain.

Tecate cypress

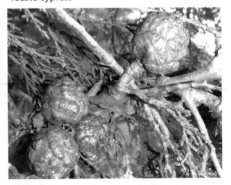

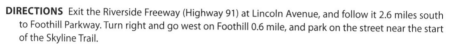

trip 15.2 Tin Mine Canyon

Distance	5 miles (out-and-back)
Hiking Time	3 hours
Elevation Gain	700'
Difficulty	Moderate
Trail Use	Cyclists, equestrians, dogs, good for kids
Best Times	October–May
Agency	CNF: TD

see map on pages 166–167

DIRECTIONS Exit the Riverside Freeway (Highway 91) at Lincoln Avenue, and follow it 2.6 miles south to Foothill Parkway. Turn right and go west on Foothill 0.6 mile, and park on the street near the start of the Skyline Trail.

Tin Mine Canyon is named for an unsuccessful mining operation that took place between 1860 and 1890. The canyon now has a popular and delightful trail leading past some of the old adits and along a creek to a small waterfall. Poison oak is plentiful in the upper part of the trail, so wear pants and long-sleeved shirts. Although dogs, horses, and bikes are permitted, they are not recommended because the trail is short and has so much poison oak.

Walk up the paved path behind a residential neighborhood for 0.6 mile. Then pass the forest gate at the base of Skyline Drive, and continue up the dirt fire road for 0.5 mile. When the road makes a hard switchback to the right, leave it and start up the Tin Mine Canyon Trail at a trailhead kiosk.

The canyon is lined with sage scrub on the southern exposures and chaparral on the cooler northern-facing slopes. Coastal live oak and sycamore grow on the canyon floor. The cold-sensitive laurel sumac bushes indicate that the canyon does not suffer from regular frosts; this bush was an important indicator for early citrus growers evaluating where they could safely plant. In the spring, the canyon erupts with wildflowers, including matilija poppy (resembles a large fried egg), heart-leaf penstemon (long red flowers favored by hummingbirds), soda pop lupine, bush mallow (a delicate pink cup), and several colors of monkeyflowers.

In 0.3 mile, pass an unmarked spur on the left toward a steep ravine. Sometimes, kids

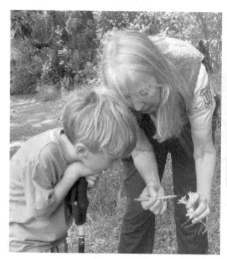

Naturalist walk in Tin Mine Canyon

illegally place nylon ropes on game trails in this canyon, and the Riverside Mountain Rescue Unit has frequently responded to calls from groups who have become stuck or injured. Stay on the main trail in Tin Mine Canyon.

In another 0.3 mile, the trail turns left and the canyon narrows. Watch for a prominent adit on the left. The US Forest Service has sealed the mouth with a bat gate to allow animals access but keep out foolish hikers. (Entering old mines is never safe; resist any temptation to explore the unsealed shafts you may see higher in the canyon.)

Watch for wild blackberry, gooseberry, and grape, as well as dense poison oak, along the narrow trail in the heart of the canyon. Riparian trees, including bay laurel, cottonwood, alder, bigleaf maple, and willow, line the creek. In 0.4 mile, pass another gated adit on the right. You might stop near here to look for California newts in the creek. Soon after, the official trail ends. Shortly beyond, you can find a grotto with a small waterfall and pool. Although it is possible to continue up-canyon, this is a good turnaround point.

trip 15.3 Sierra Peak via Skyline Drive

Distance	14.5 miles (out-and-back)
Hiking Time	7 hours
Elevation Gain	3,200'
Difficulty	Strenuous
Trail Use	Cyclists, equestrians, dogs
Best Times	November through March
Agency	CNF: TD
Recommended Map	*Cleveland National Forest Visitor Map*

see map on pages 166–167

DIRECTIONS Exit the Riverside Freeway (Highway 91) at Lincoln Avenue in Corona, and follow it 2.6 miles south to Foothill Parkway. Turn right and go west on Foothill 0.6 mile, and park on the street near the start of the Skyline Trail.

Wait for a winter storm to clear the air, then try this viewful hike to Sierra Peak, the rounded promontory anchoring the north end of the Santa Ana Mountains. Because the route follows well-graded service roads throughout and the climbing is quite gradual, it is an ideal route for energetic runners and mountain bikers, as well as hikers.

Around the winter solstice, an afternoon and evening trek to and from Sierra Peak can be very rewarding. Plan to reach it in time to watch the sun drop into the Pacific (before 5 p.m. from early November through early January). Then stroll back down under the stars, arriving at your car before 8 p.m. Nights lit by a full or nearly full moon are best; otherwise, the glare of the city lights below makes it hard to see the ground underfoot. Don't forget extra warm clothes and a flashlight.

Geologically, this is an interesting area. About 2 miles up from the trailhead, you'll cross the Elsinore Fault zone, with crumbly 150-million-year-old metavolcanic rock to the southwest and colorfully banded marine sedimentary rocks half that age to the northeast. Near Sierra Peak are some nice exposures of sandstone with embedded cobbles.

Begin hiking (or mountain biking) on Skyline Drive. The first 0.6 mile is a paved path behind a neighborhood. After passing a locked gate, Skyline becomes a dirt road. In 0.5 mile, reach a signed trailhead for Tin Mine Canyon (see Trip 15.2), where Skyline Drive swings back and begins climbing in earnest.

As you curl upward along the ridge north of Tin Mine Canyon, views open up of nearby Corona and the more distant cities of Riverside and San Bernardino, backed up by the towering summits of the San Gabriel and San Bernardino Mountains. Some orange groves remain, but new subdivisions are replacing them—a symptom of the phenomenal growth of the region known as the Inland Empire.

Oak Flat, 4.8 miles from the start, is marked by grassland dotted with a few oaks and a radio communications complex. At the road junction, turn right (Black Star Canyon Road goes left, south), and continue along the main divide of the Santa

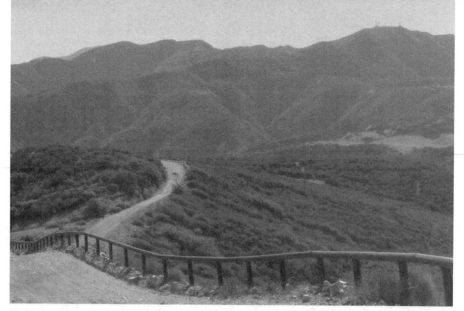

Santa Ana Mountains Main Divide

Anas toward Sierra Peak, the antennae-bristling summit to the north. Shortly before the summit, watch for a small grove of Tecate cypress beside the trail. These are some of the last mature cypress trees in Orange County; the main grove north of the mountain burned in 2002 and 2006. The top has a great view of the Chino Hills and Pomona Valley to the north, the broad trough of lower Santa Ana Canyon to the west, and endless miles of LA Basin suburbia stretching toward the Pacific Ocean.

trip 15.4 North Main Divide Traverse

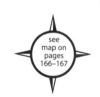

see map on pages 166–167

Distance	13.5 miles (one-way)
Hiking Time	6½ hours
Elevation Gain/Loss	1,950'/2,150'
Difficulty	Moderately strenuous
Trail Use	Cyclists, equestrians, dogs
Best Times	November–April
Agency	CNF: TD
Recommended Map	*Cleveland National Forest Visitor Map*

DIRECTIONS This trip requires a half-hour car shuttle. First, leave a vehicle at Black Star Canyon, the west end. Exit from either of the eastern toll roads (Highway 241 or 261) at Santiago Canyon Road. Drive 6 miles east to Silverado Canyon Road, turn left, proceed 0.1 mile, and turn left on Black Star Canyon Road. Go 1.1 miles to the forest gate. Leave one vehicle here, observing parking restrictions. From there to reach the east end: Return to Highway 241 (toll required), and take it north 6 miles to Highway 91 east, then exit in 8 miles at Lincoln Avenue, and follow Lincoln 2.6 miles south to Foothill Parkway. Turn right and go west on Foothill 0.6 mile, and park on the street near the start of the Skyline Trail.

Incorporating parts of Trips 15.3 and 15.5, this trek over the northern crest of the Santa Ana Mountains is perfect for fit runners, walkers, and mountain bikers. Relatively easy grades, generally smooth dirt and gravel surfaces, and little or no interference from motor vehicles are yours all the way—though the 13-mile distance is

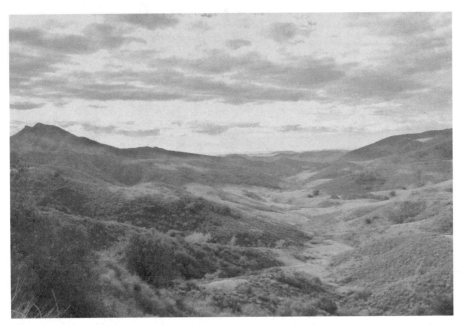

Upper Black Star Canyon

far from trivial. The aftermath of heavy rains, however, can prove to be a serious hindrance, especially for cyclists. This is no problem on the Skyline Drive side, but Black Star Canyon Road in the vicinity of Hidden Ranch can turn into one big mudhole.

Because of elevation differences, it's a little easier to begin on the east near Corona and end by way of Black Star Canyon in Orange County. After taking care of your transportation arrangements, proceed up the moderate but steady incline of Skyline Drive, starting from that road's vehicle gate in Corona.

Skyline Drive is initially a paved path behind a residential neighborhood. After a second gate by a cul-de-sac, it becomes a dirt road. It makes a hard right near the signed trailhead at the mouth of Tin Mine Canyon, then begins climbing in earnest. Only one brief downhill stretch, about 0.3 mile long, interrupts the climb from the gate to Oak Flat. As you cross the county line just before reaching Oak Flat, you'll spot the first of the many BLACK STAR CANYON ROAD—USE AT YOUR OWN RISK signs posted by Orange County.

At 4.8 miles (the Oak Flat intersection), turn left (south) and continue uphill toward the next junction, 5.4 miles, where the Main Divide Road forks left. The tumbledown rock houses nearby, called Beeks Place, are surrounded by an unkempt but still-thriving grove of planted trees—natives like Coulter pine, knobcone pine, and Tecate cypress, plus some nonnatives. Little shade can be found ahead until you reach scattered oaks and sycamores at Hidden Ranch. Joseph Beek was the Secretary of the California Senate for nearly 50 years and owned the Newport Ferry. He built the main cabin in the 1930s and used it on weekends, but vandals eventually destroyed the property. The golf ball–shaped tower on Pleasants Peak to the south is a Doppler weather radar tower installed by the National Weather Service.

From Beeks Place, bear right on Black Star Canyon Road, and begin the long, winding descent into the grassy bowl occupied by Hidden Ranch. This former privately owned cattle ranch (acquired by the Wildlands Conservancy in 2005, designated the Mariposa Reserve, and therefore protected from development) is truly hidden from the sights and sounds of the city below. Hidden Ranch is renowned for its human history. Bedrock mortars here tell of its use as a major Tongva-Gabrieliño village. A single slab of sandstone in a grove of oaks near the trail has at least 32 mortar holes, some as deep as 6 inches, attesting to centuries of labor grinding acorns into flour. Please stay off the rock to help preserve this priceless piece of history.

Two historical incidents fuel ghost stories set in Black Star Canyon. Hidden Ranch was the site of an 1831 raid against Tongva horse thieves. In a notorious murder of 1899, James Gregg was shot over a few dollars in a disputed horse trade. His killers turned themselves in but were unexpectedly acquitted. As the winds howl down the canyon, you can imagine restless spirits crying for vengeance.

Past Hidden Ranch, Black Star Canyon Road continues its leisurely descent down sun-blasted, sage-covered slopes. At 8.7 miles, the road swings close to the gorge concealing Black Star Canyon falls. Finally, at 10.7 miles, you reach the cool bottom of Black Star Canyon, and the remaining miles to the Black Star Canyon Road vehicle gate are pleasantly shaded. The southern portion is lined with private property; please stay on the road.

trip 15.5 Black Star Canyon Falls

Distance	7 miles (out-and-back)
Hiking Time	5 hours
Elevation Gain	800'
Difficulty	Moderately strenuous
Trail Use	Hiking only
Best Times	November–May
Agency	CNF: TD

see
map on
pages
166–167

see map on pages 166–167

SANTA ANA MOUNTAINS: Main Divide

DIRECTIONS Exit from either of the eastern toll roads (Highway 241 or 261) at Santiago Canyon Road; you can also get to this point from Highway 55 via Chapman Avenue. Drive 6 miles east to Silverado Canyon Road, turn left, proceed 0.1 mile, and turn left on Black Star Canyon Road. Go 1.1 miles to the forest gate and park.

Good timing is the key to catching the waterfall in Black Star Canyon at its best. Because only about 3 square miles of drainage area lie above it, it takes persistent rain to get more than a dribble of water over the fall. Whether the water is flowing or not, the canyon bottom itself is delightful to explore any time the weather is mild.

This trip begins up the gated Black Star Canyon Road, a public easement crossing private land; please stay on the road and respect the property owners' rights. After an uninteresting 0.6 mile along the dry, open bed of Santiago Creek, the road abruptly turns east into Black Star Canyon. Scattered oaks, sycamores, and willows and rows of planted eucalyptus trees provide shade as the road meanders gently uphill along the creekbed. The canyon was named after the nearby Black Star Coal Mine (on private land), which was worked briefly more than a century ago during a silver- and coal-mining boom in the Silverado Canyon area. Look for seams of poor-quality coal in the roadcuts you pass. Edwards Ranch owns much of the land on both sides of the road near the bottom of the canyon and has strikingly fortified their property lines with an electric fence and razor wire.

At 2.5 miles, the road doubles back in a hairpin turn to ascend the sage-covered slopes to the north. Two trails depart the road here. You want the lower one into the creekbed; the upper path starts off deceptively well but makes a nasty bushwhack up to the upper road rather than leading to the falls. It's time to put on pants and a long-sleeved shirt to do battle with poison oak and other shrubbery up the canyon. Sometimes you will find a use trail, while other times you must walk right up the creekbed. The poison oak is plentiful but can be avoided with care. Watch for sedimentary rocks heavily laden with shellfish fossils.

After passing a major tributary on the right, the rock obstacles become larger and more challenging. At least 1 hour (0.8 mile) of boulder-hopping, bushwhacking, and increasing hands-and-feet scrambling up the trenchlike confines of the canyon will take you to the base of the falls.

Marine sedimentary rocks are in evidence here. Bold outcrops of stratified, buff-colored siltstone rise hundreds of feet above the canyon bottom, giving safe quarters to nesting raptors and other birds. The creek slides around great blocks of conglomerate rock and pools up in shady grottoes concealed amid large oak, alder, sycamore, and bay trees.

The semicircular siltstone headwall that forms the falls fairly drips with mosses and maidenhair ferns, if not water. When the flow is great enough, water cascades 50 feet down a polished chute and also exits

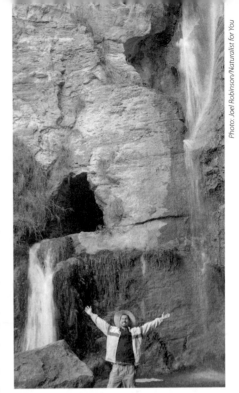

Black Star Falls

through an old mine shaft cut into the headwall about 15 feet above the falls' base.

On your return about 200 yards down-canyon, you may see evidence of a path leading up a very steep ravine full of loose rocks. Don't be tempted to try it; the path ends at a dangerously crumbling band of cliffs. Instead, return the way you came, making your way down the creekbed over now-familiar obstacles.

trip 15.6 **Silverado Trail to Bedford Peak**

Distance	7 miles (out-and-back)
Hiking Time	4 hours
Elevation Gain	2,000'
Difficulty	Moderately strenuous
Trail Use	Cyclists, equestrians, dogs
Best Times	October–May
Agency	CNF: TD
Recommended Map	*Cleveland National Forest Visitor Map*

see map on pages 166–167

DIRECTIONS Exit from either of the eastern toll roads (Highway 241 or 261) at Santiago Canyon Road. Drive 6 miles east to Silverado Canyon Road, and turn left (east). Proceed 5.8 miles to the forest gate (which is sometimes closed to motorized traffic) at the east end of the community of Silverado.

This no-nonsense climb to one of the principal summits of the Main Divide is scenically rewarding and physically demanding enough to serve as an excellent conditioning hike. From the Main Divide's west-side trailheads, there's no faster way to reach the crest by foot.

On foot now, continue up-canyon past the vehicle gate. In 0.2 mile, just after crossing the alder-shaded bottom of the canyon, turn sharply to the left (west) on the trail that climbs up the north wall of the canyon. At the time of this writing, the trail sign was missing. This is the Silverado Trail (Silverado Motorway on older maps), built originally for fire control, then used for a while by four-wheel-drive enthusiasts. Erosion and encroaching shrubs have narrowed it to a single-file path, ideal for hiking.

An excellent view of the whole of Silverado Canyon unfolds as you swing around several hairpin turns. In the roadcuts, a well-stratified, often sharply folded metasedimentary rock (the Bedford Canyon Formation) is exposed. The sediments making up these rocks were deposited on the sea floor more than 150 million years ago, buried and metamorphosed by heat and pressure, and finally elevated to their present position high above sea level. They are now among the oldest rocks remaining in Orange County.

The trail remains in primitive shape until you reach the shoulder of a ridge overlooking Ladd Canyon to the northwest. You bend to the right, staying on top of that ridge striking northeast, toward the Main Divide.

Upon reaching Main Divide Road (3.3 miles from the start), turn right and continue 0.2 mile. When the trail veers slightly left to bypass the rounded, grassy summit of Bedford Peak, step over the steel pipe rail, and follow a short use trail to the high point. There's no place to rest comfortably on the open summit, but the view—from the Pacific coast to the high points of four counties—can be stupendous on a clear day.

Bedford Formation metamorphic rocks

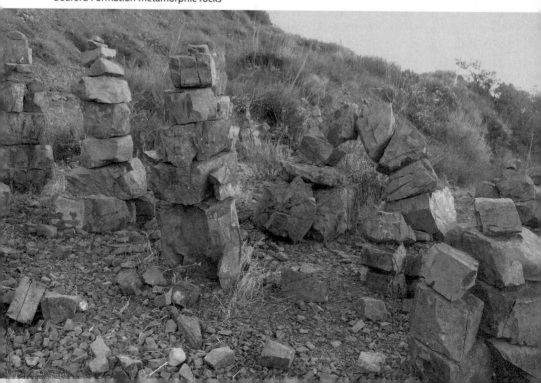

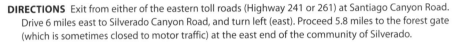

trip 15.7 **Silverado to Modjeska Peak Loop**

Distance	19 miles (loop)
Hiking Time	9 hours
Elevation Gain	4,400'
Difficulty	Strenuous
Trail Use	Cyclists, equestrians, dogs
Best Times	November–May
Agency	CNF: TD
Recommended Map	*Cleveland National Forest Visitor Map*

see map on pages 166–167

DIRECTIONS Exit from either of the eastern toll roads (Highway 241 or 261) at Santiago Canyon Road. Drive 6 miles east to Silverado Canyon Road, and turn left (east). Proceed 5.8 miles to the forest gate (which is sometimes closed to motor traffic) at the east end of the community of Silverado.

The goal of this hike, looping up and over the Main Divide, is to reach the summit of Modjeska Peak, the lower, north summit of Old Saddleback. Omitting the out-and-back leg to the peak, however, shortens the trip by 2.5 miles. Either way, it is an all-day trek on foot. During the clear, crisp weather characteristic of certain periods from November through March (and assuming you won't be sharing the roads with any vehicles), this hike can be among the most rewarding and peaceful in Southern California.

Walk up Silverado Canyon Road for 0.2 mile, then turn sharply left onto the Silverado Trail (the sign may be missing), and follow it 3.1 miles as it climbs vigorously to Main Divide Road. Turn south past Bedford Peak, and follow Main Divide Road for several undulating miles, passing several small summits along the way. Just north of Bald Peak, a big power line barely clears the ridge. This 500-kilovolt line, completed in 1987, links the Palm Springs area and Orange County.

There are clear lines of sight in most directions, and most of Southern California's highest mountain ranges are in view. Below and to the west, a scant mile away, you can trace the zigzag path of Maple Springs Road (your return route) across a sparsely timbered slope and down to the bottom of upper Silverado Canyon.

After 8.7 miles, Main Divide Road comes to an intersection north of, and about 1,000 vertical feet below, imposing Modjeska Peak.

Swing left, staying on Main Divide Road, and continue 75 yards. Then, just beyond a gate, turn onto the obscure trail that angles steeply up the roadcut on the left, and continue climbing across a slope. After a half-mile, you plunge into the shade of some tall chaparral shrubs and small oak trees.

After another 0.3 mile, you reach the access road leading to Modjeska Peak. Go left and continue 0.5 mile to Modjeska's open summit. On a clear day, the 360-degree view of the surrounding mountains, basins, and ocean is obstructed only slightly by

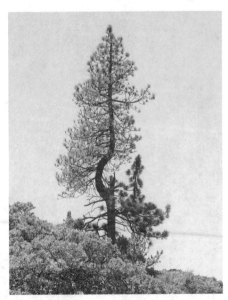

Bent Coulter pine, Upper Silverado Canyon

the antennae-bristling summit of Santiago Peak, a mile southeast. (**Note:** *Mountain bikers headed to Modjeska Peak may want to avoid the trail shortcut to the peak and instead go the long way around using the gradually ascending Main Divide Road.*)

Your return to the starting point is now entirely downhill. Retrace your steps to Main Divide Road and continue north very briefly to the road intersection, where you turn left on Maple Springs Road. The next several miles on it are a botanist's delight. On the upper slopes, huge Coulter pines soar above thick carpets of manzanita shrubs. Bigcone Douglas-fir, bigleaf maple, bay, and live oak trees crowd together in the larger ravines, casting dense pools of shade over trickling streams.

On the sixth sharp hairpin turn from the top, 4 miles down from Main Divide Road,

you finally reach the bottom of Silverado Canyon. Maple Springs Road becomes paved at this point. During the last 3 miles, the stream flows merrily along next to the road, flanked by sycamores, alders, and more maples. In spring, California poppies and golden yarrow brighten the roadside, while the celebrated snowy-white matilija poppy, the "queen of the California wild-flowers," blooms atop swaying stems taller than most adults.

Midway down the final stretch is the mouth of Lost Woman Canyon, a tributary draining into Silverado Canyon from the south. When the wind whistles down this canyon, so the old-timers say, it evokes the plaintive sounds of a woman calling for help. Treading softly down the road, possibly mildly hallucinating after many long miles, you may hear her cries.

trip 15.8   Harding Road to Main Divide

see
map on
pages
166–167

Distance	18.5 miles (out-and-back)
Hiking Time	9 hours
Elevation Gain	3,650'
Difficulty	Strenuous
Trail Use	Cyclists, equestrians, dogs
Best Times	November–March
Agency	CNF: TD
Recommended Map	*Cleveland National Forest Visitor Map*

DIRECTIONS Exit from either of the eastern toll roads (Highway 241 or 261) at Santiago Canyon Road. Drive 9 miles east and south to Modjeska Canyon Road, on the left, which you follow 2 miles to Tucker Wildlife Sanctuary and the start of the Harding Road, just short of the end of Modjeska Canyon Road. Parking is limited and often fills up.

This challenging cool-weather trip is ideal for the exercise-minded, be they long-distance hikers, mountain runners, or mountain bikers. Since well over half this route stays on the north side of the ridgeline dividing Santiago and Harding Canyons, the long shadows of late fall and winter provide plenty of welcome shade. In spring, blue-flowering ceanothus and matilija poppies put on a great show. Harding Road (formerly called Harding Truck Trail) is passable for fire trucks but

is normally closed to motorized traffic, with gates at both the bottom (Modjeska Canyon) and top (Main Divide Road).

Early risers will appreciate this hike, especially in fall and early winter, when late sunrises make it convenient to hit the trail in time to enjoy a bit of stargazing before dawn's first light. Before the sun cleared the horizon one November morning, I ran into two other groups of hikers on the Harding Road with just that idea in

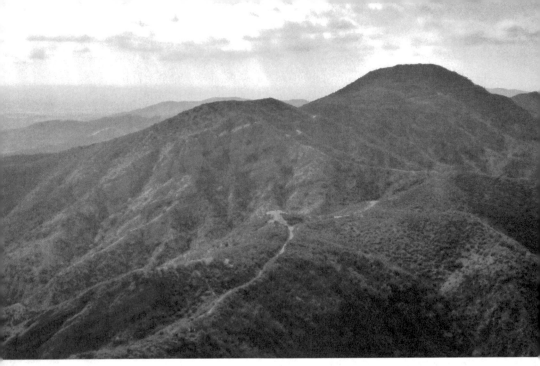

Harding Road

mind. There is also the distinct possibility, perhaps once every year or two, of skiing the upper part of Harding Road immediately following a cold, wet winter storm. (You would, of course, have to carry your cross-country skis perhaps 3 or more miles up the road to the first snow.)

The 2007 Santiago Fire, started by arson, burned 28,445 acres on the west face of the Santa Ana Mountains, including nearly all the vegetation along this trail. The chaparral has recovered quickly, but the beautiful trees that once graced the slopes will take generations to return. The third edition of this book described a hike to Laurel Spring, but nothing appealing remains after the fire.

Across from the Tucker sanctuary, the gated fire road signed 5S08 HARDING TRUCK TRAIL begins curling up a hillside. Heading up this road on foot or by mountain bike, you soon pass into Cleveland National Forest. Ahead is a bold outcrop of conglomerate rock, consisting of sediments laid down in a marine environment roughly 80 million years ago. You will see more of

this erosion-resistant, cliff-forming layer on ridges to the north and south as you climb a little higher.

At a road fork in 0.4 mile, stay right; the left road goes down to Modjeska Reservoir and the mouth of Harding Canyon (see Trip 15.9). At 0.7 mile, a ridgetop clearing next to a hairpin turn provides a view straight up the tree-choked bottom of Harding Canyon, a tributary of Santiago Canyon. The upper reaches of this seemingly impenetrable canyon were the scene of a short-lived mining boomlet shortly following the bigger boom in Silverado Canyon.

After 1 mile, Harding Road descends about 100 feet (the only reversal in the steady ascent) to edge around a couple of steep ravines. Climbing again, you round the nose of a ridge and come upon (at 1.6 miles) a viewpoint with picnic tables overlooking the whole of Modjeska Canyon. To the east, a trenchlike section of Santiago Canyon winds upward toward Old Saddleback.

The road continues generally east on or near the ridgeline dividing Harding and Santiago Canyons. In early morning, the view behind is often that of cottony layers of fog or low clouds obscuring the coastal plain.

At 4.9 miles, a large landslide lies on the left. Just beyond, the road bends around the head of a ravine densely choked with bay laurel. Laurel Spring emerges about 50 vertical feet down the ravine, but the spring is no longer an inviting destination in the aftermath of the Santiago Fire.

At 6 miles, Harding Road curls over to the north-facing side of the ridgeline and thereafter sticks to the slopes overlooking Harding Canyon. Dense chaparral, made up of manzanita, scrub oak, mountain mahogany, and blue-flowering ceanothus (wild lilac), mantles these slopes, but the Coulter pines, bigcone Douglas-firs, sycamores, and canyon live oaks are now gone.

Grotto Spring, at 8.6 miles, is usually completely dry. At 9.5 miles, you reach Main Divide Road at a saddle overlooking the big drainage to the north, upper Silverado Canyon.

VARIATION

Options for further exploration include climbing Modjeska and Santiago Peaks, which lie 1.3 miles and 2.4 miles away, respectively, via the shortest routes. Mountain bikers can piece together a superb 27-mile ride by stringing together Harding and Maple Springs Roads, then closing the loop via the paved Silverado Canyon, Santiago Canyon, and Modjeska Canyon Roads.

trip 15.9   Harding Canyon

Distance	5 miles (out-and-back)
Hiking Time	4 hours
Elevation Gain	900'
Difficulty	Moderately strenuous
Trail Use	Dogs allowed
Best Times	December–May
Agency	CNF: TD

see map on pages 166–167

DIRECTIONS Exit from either of the eastern toll roads (Highway 241 or 261) at Santiago Canyon Road. Drive 9 miles east and south to Modjeska Canyon Road, on the left. Proceed 2 miles to Tucker Wildlife Sanctuary and the start of the Harding Road, just short of the end of Modjeska Canyon Road. Parking is limited and often fills up.

In 1878, a pair of prospectors discovered some nodules containing lead and silver ore about 3 miles up Harding Canyon from the present-day Modjeska Reservoir. Soon miners swarmed so thickly throughout the canyon that, according to a newspaper account of the day, a man could hardly swing a pick without "perforating his neighbor."

Harding Canyon has more recently been famous for its crystalline Seven Pools, but they were wiped out by mudslides after the 2007 Santiago Fire. Nevertheless, some pools remain, floods scoured new ones in 2010, and the canyon remains a beautiful destination.

The canyon bottom features potentially ankle-busting terrain, so wear boots with ankle support. Also, poison oak grows in fair abundance along the banks of the stream, so consider applying a cream to block poison ivy to any exposed areas of your skin. You should budget four hours of moderate hiking and strenuous boulder-hopping for the round-trip—and more time than that if water levels are high.

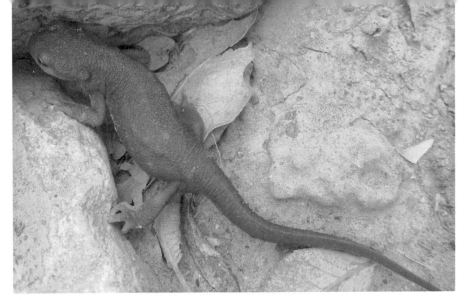
California newt

As for Trip 15.8 to the Main Divide, you begin by starting upward on Harding Road from Modjeska Canyon. Climb toward prominent Flores Peak. Juan Flores escaped from San Quentin Prison in 1855 and formed a gang of Mexican-American bandits who resented and preyed upon US settlers in the newly established state of California. When the gang wreaked mayhem on San Juan Capistrano and murdered a German shopkeeper in January 1857, Los Angeles County Sheriff James Barton formed a posse to arrest Flores. He found out about the plan and ambushed and killed Sheriff Barton and several of his deputies. A large posse of merchants, ranchers, and Native Americans pursued Flores and his gang to the summit of Flores Peak. According to legend, Flores escaped again by executing a daring leap on horseback. However, he was soon caught again and hanged in Los Angeles.

After 0.4 mile, in a saddle along a ridge, Harding Road curves right to follow that ridge upward, and a spur road descends left. Make the descent and soon reach the broad floodplain of Harding Canyon, just below its mouth. Turn right, go upstream alongside the tumbling (or trickling, as it may be) creek, and enter the canyon proper within about 0.2 mile.

Abandon the notion of trying to keep your feet dry if the water level is high. A surprisingly good use trail darts along either the right or the left bank, but you'll encounter plenty of ankle- to knee-deep stream crossings in between the trail segments. After periods of heavy rain, every ravine of any consequence along both sides of the canyon supports a lively brook rushing down to join the main stream. Live oaks, willows, and sycamores in the lower canyon are joined by aromatic bay laurels and straight-trunked white alder trees as you climb into the canyon's progressively narrower, higher reaches. California newts frequent the moist canyon floor.

At about 1.5 miles into Harding Canyon, notice how the canyon walls morph from tan and beige sedimentary rock to light gray granitic rock. At an abrupt bend to the left, where water sometimes sprays down a cliff-like ravine on the right, notice two mining prospects pocking the canyon wall on the left. The next stretch is especially lovely, with a dense cluster of riparian trees and some pleasing pools and cascades. This is a good place to turn around.

Beyond, the trail deteriorates further, and the poison oak becomes thicker. Harding Falls is another mile up the rugged canyon, but reaching it is a significant undertaking.

trip 15.10 **Santiago Trail**

Distance	16 miles (out-and-back to Old Camp)
Hiking Time	8 hours
Elevation Gain	2,650'
Difficulty	Moderately strenuous
Trail Use	Cyclists, equestrians, dogs
Best Times	November–April
Agency	CNF: TD
Recommended Map	*Cleveland National Forest Visitor Map*

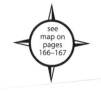

see map on pages 166–167

DIRECTIONS Exit from either of the eastern toll roads (Highway 241 or 261) at Santiago Canyon Road. Drive 9 miles east and south to Modjeska Canyon Road, on the left. Take it 0.9 mile, then turn right onto Modjeska Grade Road. Continue 0.9 mile to the top of the grade and the start of the Santiago Trail. (If you are coming from the south, this starting point is 0.5 mile north of Santiago Canyon Road.) Carefully observe the posted no-parking zones along Modjeska Grade Road when choosing a spot to park; you will have to go several hundred yards in either direction to find legal parking.

Yesteryear, Old Camp was a popular rendezvous point for hunting parties using the Joplin Trail between Rose Canyon and Old Saddleback. The camp and trail fell into obscurity for decades, but mountain bikers and backpackers have revitalized the trail and camp. It is well worth the daylong hike if the weather is cool. In late fall, the maples put on quite a show; by winter or early spring, the adjoining creek, screened by alders, bubbles with a delightfully pure flow of water.

Old Camp is accessible by way of the Santiago Trail, a defunct fire road that has mostly deteriorated into singletrack trail heavily favored by mountain bikers. Sticking close to the original Joplin route over part of its length, it runs for 8 miles along the sunny ridgeline just south of Santiago Canyon, finally dropping abruptly into it. Most of the area burned in the 2007 Santiago Fire, but Old Camp escaped the inferno.

Start by heading east on the now misnamed Santiago Truck Trail; in 1 mile, enter Cleveland National Forest. Initially steep, the climb soon relaxes as you gain the crest of the ridge. At 2.8 miles, you begin skirting the back side of the Vulture Crags. These broken outcrops of conglomerate rock served as a nesting site for California condors more than a century ago. At 3.3 miles, reach a

flag placed to honor America's veterans, where you have the best view back to the crags. Below the crags, layer upon layer of beige to brick-red marine sediments are all spectacularly tilted as a result of the rise of

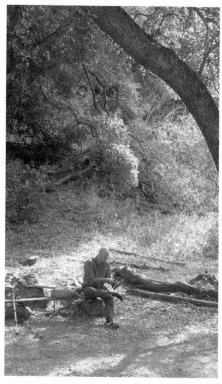

Old Camp

the Santa Ana Mountain crest to the east. An unsigned trail leads south from here to Live Oak Canyon Road. Officially called the Morrow Trail, it is better known as The Luge among mountain bikers who plummet down the narrow curving path.

Continue along Santiago Trail. It was once possible to descend to Santiago Creek and inspect detritus from 1880s-era mining, but the old paths were wiped out in the fire. The US Forest Service asks hikers to stay on the established trail to aid recovery. Watch for a wrecked jeep below the trail in 1.4 miles. In another 1 mile, pass a hilltop viewpoint and then an unsigned

trail leading south just beyond. Then, in 0.4 mile, the trail turns sharply right and becomes Trabuco Creek Road, but you stay straight on the unsigned Santiago Trail.

After 7.5 miles on the Santiago Trail, the road forks. A short spur road continues upward to follow a small power line serving the Santiago Peak antennae, while the Santiago Trail bears left and descends to Old Camp (7.9 miles). In addition to the live oaks, bay laurels, and bigleaf maples that shade the flat, you'll find growths of wild blackberry, buckthorn ceanothus, redberry, coffee berry, and bracken fern in the area.

VARIATION

If you would like to extend this trip to make a strenuous loop, follow the steep Joplin Trail up to the saddle between Modjeska and Santiago Peaks (Old Saddleback). From Old Camp, the trail threads through a shady tributary of Santiago Canyon, then gains a brush-covered slope, passing west of a 3,893-foot knob. Extreme mountain bikers have been keeping this path clear of brush, but watch for the stands of poison oak on both sides. After winding amid some oaks, it angles up a steep slope thickly covered by chamise and buckthorn, a prickly variety of ceanothus.

In 1.5 miles of hard climbing from Old Camp, the trail descends a little; passes through a beautiful thicket of live oaks, bay laurels, and bigcone Douglas-fir; and returns to the bed of Santiago Canyon about 100 yards above Jamison Spring. Another 0.8 mile of ascent brings you to Main Divide Road atop the saddle.

From there, walk east a few paces to find an unmarked trail shortcutting west onto the ridge of Modjeska Peak. You could make an optional detour to the peak via a truck road, then continue north down a trail to rejoin Main Divide Road. Just beyond, you can turn left onto the gated Harding Truck Trail and descend to Modjeska Canyon (see Trip 15.8). From the Tucker Sanctuary, you can meet a getaway vehicle or walk or bike 2 miles back to the Santiago Trailhead. Gonzo mountain bikers will want to do this loop in reverse to ride the Joplin Trail downhill.

---

trip 15.11   ## Falls Canyon

see map on pages 166–167

Distance	0.8 mile (out-and-back)
Hiking Time	30 minutes
Elevation Gain	200'
Difficulty	Easy
Trail Use	Good for kids
Best Times	January–April
Agency	CNF: TD

DIRECTIONS From Interstate 5, take Oso Parkway east for 2.6 miles, then turn left on Antonio Parkway and go 5.5 miles. Jog right on Santa Margarita Parkway for 0.2 mile, then left onto Plano Trabuco Road. In 0.6 mile, the road veers left and becomes Trabuco Canyon Road. In 0.8 mile, turn right onto the rough, unpaved Trabuco Creek Road (normally passable to carefully-driven low clearance vehicles). Proceed 3.4 miles to the unsigned mouth of Falls Canyon. Just beyond, look for a wide spot on the right to park. If the nearby parking is full, more space is available a quarter-mile in either direction along the road.

F alls Canyon is a somewhat obscure jewel in the popular Trabuco Canyon. The falls, when they flow during the winter and spring, are taller than the better-known Holy Jim Falls, and the use trail is shorter, rougher, and more interesting, especially

Falls Canyon

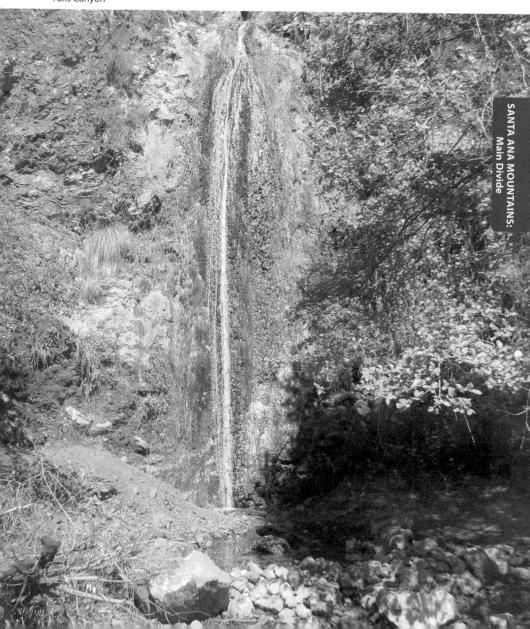

for children. Poison oak is plentiful in the canyon; make sure that everyone in your group knows how to recognize and avoid it.

Falls Canyon lacks a formal US Forest Service trail, but a decent use path has developed over the years. From Trabuco Creek Road directly opposite the mouth of the canyon, find a fisherman's trail dropping down to Trabuco Creek.

Ford the creek and walk north up Falls Canyon, which is lined with lovely sycamores, bay laurels, live oaks, and alders, as well as wild blackberry, gooseberry, and grape. The rough trail avoids heavy vegetation but at one point takes you over a sizable rock. In 0.4 mile, arrive abruptly at your unmissable destination.

trip 15.12 Holy Jim Falls

see map on pages 166–167

Distance	2.8 miles (out-and-back)
Hiking Time	1½ hours
Elevation Gain	650'
Difficulty	Moderate
Trail Use	Cyclists, equestrians, dogs, good for kids
Best Times	November–June
Agency	CNF: TD
Recommended Map	*Cleveland National Forest Visitor Map*

DIRECTIONS From Interstate 5, take Oso Parkway east for 2.6 miles, then turn left on Antonio Parkway and go 5.5 miles. Jog right on Santa Margarita Parkway for 0.2 mile, then left onto Plano Trabuco Road. In 0.6 mile, the road veers left and becomes Trabuco Canyon Road. In 0.8 mile, turn right onto the rough, unpaved Trabuco Creek Road (normally passable to carefully driven low-clearance vehicles). Proceed 4.7 miles to the Holy Jim Trailhead on the left.

Sometimes the intimacy of a tiny, hidden waterfall is more aesthetically rewarding than the thunder of a famous one. Such is the case with Holy Jim Falls. Tucked into a short, steep canyon draining the southeast flank of Santiago Peak, the falls are seemingly remote but relatively easy to reach on foot. The last stretch of trail leading to the falls may be a little overgrown with poison oak, so wear pants and a long-sleeved shirt.

From the Holy Jim Trailhead, proceed up the road heading north into Holy Jim Canyon, passing more cabins beneath the sheltering trees. A century ago, this canyon was home to settlers who eked out a living by raising bees. One beekeeper, James T. Smith, became so famous for his cursing habit that he was popularly named "Cussin' Jim." Other nicknames bestowed on him included "Lyin' Smith," "Greasy Jim," and "Salvation Smith." Dignified government

cartographers invented a new one, "Holy Jim."

After 0.5 mile, you come to a sturdy steel gate. Beyond, a narrow trail continues upstream, crossing the creek seven times in 0.8 mile. Typical moisture-loving native trees, ferns, and chaparral shrubs line the canyon, but you'll also see naturalized fig trees and a purple-flowered ground cover called vinca (or periwinkle), the latter two introduced by the early settlers.

Just after Picnic Rock and the last stream crossing, the trail switches back sharply to the left and begins ascending the west slope of the canyon. Leave the main trail at this point, and continue straight up the bottom of the canyon on an even narrower trail. After about 400 yards, you'll come to the shallow pool and grotto at the base of the falls. Above it, the water cascades perhaps 18 feet over a broken cliff.

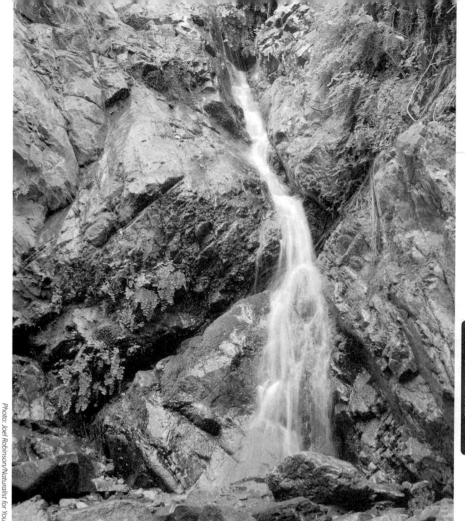

Holy Jim Falls

trip 15.13   **Santiago Peak via Holy Jim Trail**

Distance	16 miles (out-and-back)
Hiking Time	9 hours
Elevation Gain	4,000'
Difficulty	Strenuous
Trail Use	Cyclists, equestrians, dogs
Best Times	November–April
Agency	CNF: TD
Recommended Map	*Cleveland National Forest Visitor Map*

see map on pages 166–167

DIRECTIONS From Interstate 5, take Oso Parkway east for 2.6 miles, then turn left on Antonio Parkway and go 5.5 miles. Jog right on Santa Margarita Parkway for 0.2 mile, then left onto Plano Trabuco Road. In 0.6 mile, the road veers left and becomes Trabuco Canyon Road. In 0.8 mile, turn right onto the rough, unpaved Trabuco Creek Road (normally passable to carefully driven low-clearance vehicles). Proceed 4.7 miles to the Holy Jim Trailhead on the left.

Photo: Joel Robinson/Naturalist for You

To the American Indians, it was Kalawpa ("a wooded place"), the lofty resting place of the deity Chiningchinish. Early settlers and surveyors named it variously Mount Downey, Trabuco Peak, and Temescal Mountain. Finally, mapmakers decided on the name that eventually stuck: Santiago Peak. Today's bulldozer-scraped summit overrun with telecommunications antennae hardly pays sufficient homage to the peak's historic and scenic values. Witness, for example, this record of its first documented ascent in 1853, by a group of lawmen pursuing horse thieves up Coldwater Canyon:

> After an infinite amount of scrambling, danger, and hard labor, we stood on the very summit of the Temescal mountain, now by some called Santiago . . . where we beheld with pleasure a sublime view, more than worth the journey and ascent.

In 1861, while conducting a geologic survey of the Santa Anas, William Brewer and Josiah Whitney reached the same summit on their second try, using the ridge north of Coldwater Canyon. Their impressions echoed the sentiments of the earlier climbers: "The view more than repaid us for all we had endured."

The view so enthusiastically described by these early climbers remains spectacular—given, perhaps, a clearer-than-average winter day. Under good conditions, you can trace the coastline from Point Loma to Point Dume, spot both Santa Catalina and San Clemente Islands, and scratch your head trying to identify the plethora of mountain ranges and lesser promontories filling the landscape inland.

Clockwise around the compass from northwest to southeast, the major ranges on the horizon are the Santa Monica, San Gabriel, San Bernardino, Little San Bernardino, San Jacinto, Santa Rosa, Palomar, and Cuyamaca Mountains. To the south, you might see several of the lower ranges along the US-Mexico border and perhaps glimpse the flat-topped summit of Table Mountain, a few miles inland from the Baja California coast. In the west and northwest, smog permitting, the flat urban tapestry spreads outward, spiked by the glass skyscrapers of downtown Los Angeles.

Don't underestimate the time required to bag Santiago Peak by way of the Holy Jim Trail. In winter, you'll need to start early to ensure you finish before dusk. With summit temperatures roughly 20 degrees cooler than below, you should pack along some extra clothing. Plenty of water is a good idea too: Bear Spring, on the way to the summit, should not be considered a potable source.

From the Holy Jim Trailhead, walk up the road heading north into Holy Jim Canyon past cabins. After 0.5 mile, the route passes a gate and narrows to a streamside trail. In another 0.8 mile, pass Picnic Rock and the last stream crossing to reach a signed junction where the trail switches back sharply to the left and begins ascending the west slope of the canyon. (You may wish to make a brief excursion to Holy Jim Falls on the canyon floor before continuing.)

Switchback up the chaparral-covered west wall of Holy Jim Canyon. Well traveled but minimally cleared of encroaching vegetation, the trail offers intimate glimpses of the immediate surroundings flashing by at eyeball level. Unlike walking on wide fire roads, this trail offers a sense of motion and accomplishment as you ascend.

Soon a few antenna structures atop Santiago Peak come into view; they seem tantalizingly close but are about 3,000 feet higher. At 3.7 miles, the trail crosses the bed of Holy Jim Canyon at an elevation of 3,480 feet, far above the falls. You might be tempted at this point to follow the line of scattered trees that struggle up toward the head of the canyon or to try another shortcut to the summit by way of the scree-covered slopes left or right; however, loose rock and thickets of thorny ceanothus would surely cost you more time, effort, and grief than you ever imagined.

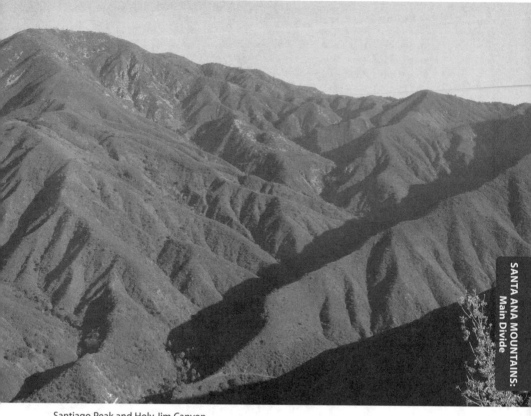

Santiago Peak and Holy Jim Canyon

So continue ahead on the trail, where soon you make a delicate traverse over an old landslide. After another mile on sunny, south-facing slopes, you contour around a ridge and suddenly enter a dark and shady recess filled with oaks, sycamores, bigleaf maples, and bigcone Douglas-firs. By 5 miles, you come to Main Divide Road, opposite Bear Spring.

From here, you can take either the Main Divide Road or Upper Holy Jim Trail; both are 1.4 miles, but the trail is more scenic. Turn left to stay on the road. For the Holy Jim Trail, turn right and walk 0.4 mile. Immediately before reaching a saddle, look for an obscure trail on the left, which switchbacks steeply up the ridge to rejoin the Main Divide Road at a hairpin turn.

Another 1 mile of climbing on the Main Divide Road brings you to a junction north of Santiago Peak. Turn left and take the service road 0.5 mile to Santiago's summit.

You must walk around the antenna farm on the summit to take in the complete panorama. Modjeska Peak, 1 mile northwest and about 200 feet lower, isn't tall enough to block the view of any far-horizon features. Modjeska and Santiago together make up the feature called "Old Saddleback" that appears exactly that shape when viewed from much of urban Orange County.

The fine-grained rock covering both summits of Old Saddleback is the prototype of the Santiago Peak Volcanics exposed on many of the coastal mountain ranges extending south through San Diego County into Baja California. These metamorphosed volcanic rock formations were originally part of a chain of volcanic islands that collided with our continent some 80 million years ago.

trip 15.14 Indian Truck Trail

Distance	14 miles (out-and-back to Main Divide)
Hiking Time	7 hours
Elevation Gain	2,600'
Difficulty	Moderately strenuous
Trail Use	Cyclists, equestrians, dogs (sometimes trucks)
Best Times	November–April
Agency	CNF: TD
Recommended Map	*Cleveland National Forest Visitor Map*

see map on pages 166–167

DIRECTIONS Exit Interstate 15 at Indian Truck Trail south of Corona in Riverside County. Proceed 0.1 mile west, and turn right on Campbell Ranch Road. After 0.4 mile, turn left on Mayhew Canyon Road. Follow it 0.4 mile west, then turn left onto Santiago Canyon Road. In 0.8 mile, turn right onto Indian Truck Trail, and park at the intersection. (**Note:** *These directions may change due to ongoing housing construction throughout the area.*)

The most pleasant, if not shortest, way to hike to the Main Divide Road from the east is by way of Indian Truck Trail. Open intermittently to motor-vehicle traffic, it features easy grades throughout, considerable shade during the fall and winter months, and nice views because of its predominately ridgetop alignment. Hikers and mountain bikers have it all to themselves whenever the vehicle gate down at the bottom end is closed and locked.

On foot (or bike) now, you ascend gradually for 0.6 mile and come to a road fork. A private road into a Korean church camp

Bigcone Douglas-fir

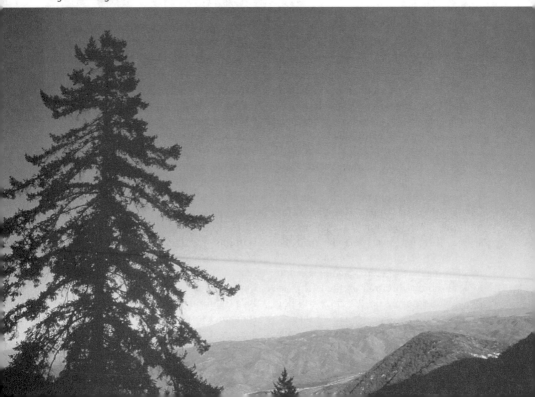

bears left; you stay right on the Indian Truck Trail. A gate, which may or may not be locked shut for vehicles, lies just ahead.

Your ascent quickens as Indian Truck Trail curls up the divide between Indian and Mayhew Canyons. After about 3 miles in the sun, Indian Truck Trail makes a decided switch to the cool, north side of the ridge. Ferns grow in profusion along the shady roadcuts, and the spreading limbs of live oaks and bigcone Douglas-firs frame a beautiful view of the Temescal Valley and the San Bernardino Mountains.

After about 5 miles, Indian Truck Trail traverses somewhat drier slopes, mantled with dense growths of manzanita and ceanothus and dotted with Coulter pines. In the final two switchback legs, the road climbs to a saddle, joining (at 7 miles) Main Divide Road. Here, you can look southwest toward the hills of southern Orange County and the coastline. On clear winter afternoons, the glimmer of sunlight on the ocean's surface is breathtaking.

VARIATION

Indian Truck Trail, the Holy Jim Trail (Trip 15.13), and a short piece of Main Divide Road together make up an excellent transmountain hiking route. The total distance between the foot of Indian Truck Trail on the east side and the Holy Jim Trailhead on the west side is 13 miles.

trip 15.15   Trabuco Canyon

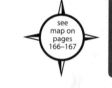

see map on pages 166–167

Distance	3.6 miles (out-and-back)
Hiking Time	2 hours
Elevation Gain	850'
Difficulty	Moderate
Trail Use	Cyclists, equestrians, dogs, good for kids
Best Times	October–June
Agency	CNF: TD
Recommended Map	*Cleveland National Forest Visitor Map*

DIRECTIONS From Interstate 5, take Oso Parkway east for 2.6 miles, then turn left on Antonio Parkway and go 5.5 miles. Jog right on Santa Margarita Parkway for 0.2 mile, then left onto Plano Trabuco Road. In 0.6 mile, the road veers left and becomes Trabuco Canyon Road. In 0.8 mile, turn right onto the rough, unpaved Trabuco Creek Road (normally passable to carefully-driven low clearance vehicles). Proceed 5.7 miles to the end of the road.

Starting from the east terminus of Trabuco Creek Road, an old truck road turned narrow footpath meanders up to some of the most idyllic spots in the Santa Anas. Upper Trabuco Canyon is home to Orange County's biggest alder grove; fine specimens of live oak, bay laurel, and maple; a tiny community of madrones; and a wide variety of spectacular spring wildflowers. Historically, the canyon is significant for its mining activity and as the site of the killing of California's last wild grizzly bear in 1908.

From there the trail passes under some large oaks, squeezes between poison oak and wild blackberry, runs along the creekbed for a stretch, and then decidedly sticks to the sunny slope north of the creek. This slope is botanically best in late March and April when it sports colorful displays of bush lupine, matilija poppy, paintbrush, wild sweet pea, red and sticky monkey-flowers, prickly phlox, mariposa lily, wild hyacinth, penstemon, and other spring wildflowers.

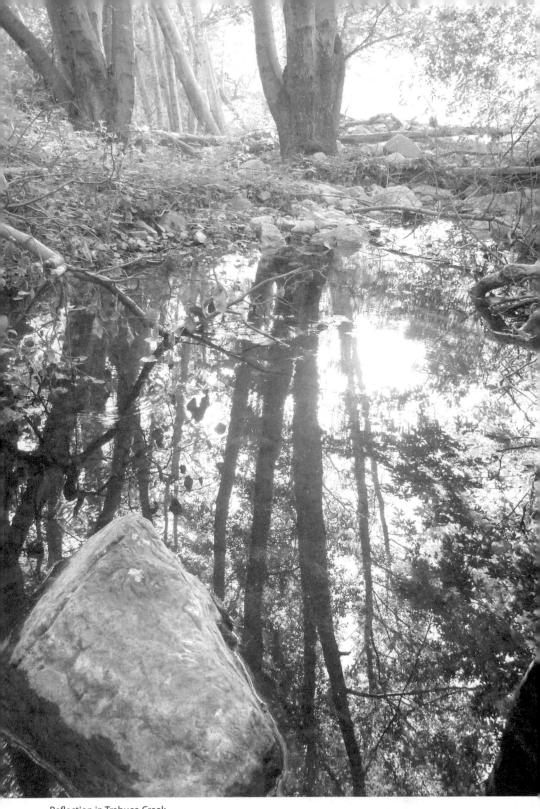

Reflection in Trabuco Creek

At 1 mile, the trail crosses from the south to the north side of Trabuco Creek. Immediately before the crossing, an unmarked trail departs for Yaeger Mesa. The mesa, towering over the trail, is densely forested with bigcone Douglas-fir and coastal live oak. Miner Jake Yaeger built his cabin in the shade of a spreading maple down near the creek as he prospected for gold and silver between roughly 1899 and 1925. Just beyond the crossing, watch for an old adit on the north side of the trail, now covered with a bat gate to give animals access while discouraging humans. Yaeger

also constructed a 2,000-foot-long tunnel through the mesa; it is now gated as well.

At 1.5 miles, the trail climbs, then levels out and veers left. An unsigned spur on the right leads 40 yards to an overlook of the Trabuco Canyon headwaters. In another 0.3 mile, you come to the signed junction of the Horsethief Trail, half-concealed in thickets of brush and poison oak. Down below, the alder-shaded creekbed is a fine place to picnic or rest before heading back along the same trail. Trip 15.16 describes an extended loop hike circling the head of Trabuco Canyon.

VARIATION

Yaeger Mesa was once a private inholding within Cleveland National Forest, but the US Forest Service acquired it in 2009. An unsigned, unofficial trail mentioned earlier leads onto the mesa and makes an interesting but strenuous side trip. It follows the south side of Trabuco Creek past a cliff-side spring, then climbs, very steeply at times, onto the sloping mesa. The mesa is covered with Orange County's largest field of bracken ferns and ringed with oaks and bigcone Douglas-fir. A PT-19 trainer crashed on Yaeger Mesa around 1950, and you can see part of the wreckage in the gully below the trail.

This variation adds 0.7 mile and 600 feet of elevation gain one way. You won't regret bringing sturdy boots and trekking poles. An even steeper use trail continues another 0.7 mile from Yaeger Mesa up to Bell Ridge.

SANTA ANA MOUNTAINS: Main Divide

trip 15.16   West Horsethief to Trabuco Canyon Loop

see map on pages 166–167

Distance	10 miles (loop)
Hiking Time	6 hours
Elevation Gain	2,700'
Difficulty	Moderately strenuous
Trail Use	Cyclists, equestrians, dogs
Best Times	November–April
Agency	CNF: TD
Recommended Map	*Cleveland National Forest Visitor Map*

DIRECTIONS From Interstate 5, take Oso Parkway east for 2.6 miles, then turn left on Antonio Parkway and go 5.5 miles. Jog right on Santa Margarita Parkway for 0.2 mile, then left onto Plano Trabuco Road. In 0.6 mile, the road veers left and becomes Trabuco Canyon Road. In 0.8 mile, turn right onto the rough, unpaved Trabuco Creek Road (normally passable to carefully-driven low clearance vehicles). Proceed 5.7 miles to the end of the road.

The combination of wide-open views atop the Main Divide, and passages through pockets of dense chaparral and timber in the uppermost reaches of Trabuco Canyon make this one of the more varied, interesting hikes in this book.

You begin, as in Trip 15.15, with a steady climb 1.8 miles up Trabuco Canyon to a junction. Take the left branch, the West Horsethief Trail. Earlier, you probably spotted switchbacks carving up the treeless slope that now lies east of you. They replaced the original straight-up-the-ridge route used by American Indians in prehistoric times and by horse thieves in the Spanish days. Traffic by hikers and mountain bikers in recent years has helped keep the trail clear of encroaching vegetation. Nonetheless, some sections are very rough and rocky. After following a canyon bottom for a short while, the West Horsethief Trail begins climbing in earnest, zigzagging through dense chaparral. During the coolness of the morning, diligent effort will get you to the top of this tedious stretch fast enough; later in the day, it could be a hot, energy-sapping climb.

After 1,100 feet of elevation gain, the trail straightens, begins to level out along a ridge, and enters a vegetation zone dominated by manzanita and blue-flowering ceanothus. Cool mountain air washes over you, perhaps bearing the scent of the pines that lie ahead. Nearly coincident with the change of vegetation is a change in the rocks and soils underfoot. As you climb higher, light-colored granitic boulders and soil replace the dark brown, crumbly metasedimentary rocks you saw earlier. Although the younger granitic rock doesn't crop out below, you may remember seeing granitic boulders down in the bed of Trabuco Canyon. These resistant blocks, originally weathered out of the granitic mass above, were swept downhill during flash floods.

At 3.3 miles from the Trabuco Canyon roadhead, the Horsethief Trail joins Main Divide Road in a sparse grove of Coulter pines. Turn right and follow the road east, then south, for an easy, meandering, viewful 2.5 miles. On the left, you will soon pass the East Horsethief Trail. During prehistoric times, the entire Horsethief Trail route was an important transmountain route from the coast to the inland valleys.

At 5.8 miles, amid a patch of Coulter pines and incense cedars, you come to Los Pinos Saddle. At the northwest corner of a large, cleared area in the saddle itself, find the old roadbed (Trabuco Canyon Trail) angling downward along the shady slopes of Trabuco Canyon's main fork. Be careful not to take the Los Pinos Trail, which is just to the left but climbs. Thick stands of live oak and bigcone Douglas-fir keep this part of the trail dark and gloomy during fall and winter and delightfully cool at other times. Trailside flowering currant and ceanothus shrubs brighten things up in the spring.

One mile below the saddle, the trail veers left, crosses a divide, and begins descending along a tributary of Trabuco Canyon. You walk by thickets of California bay (bay laurel), which exude an enigmatically pleasant, pungent scent. After crossing the tributary ravine twice, the trail clings to a dry and sunny south-facing slope. Down below, in an almost inaccessible section of the ravine, you may hear water trickling and tumbling over boulders half-hidden under tangles of brush and trees. Before long, you arrive back at the junction of the Horsethief Trail in shady Trabuco Canyon and continue down to the trailhead.

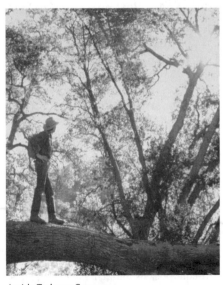

Inside Trabuco Canyon

trip 15.17 Bell Peak

Distance	4 miles (out-and-back)
Hiking Time	2 hours
Elevation Gain	1,300'
Difficulty	Moderately strenuous
Trail Use	Cyclists, dogs
Best Times	November–April
Agency	CNF: TD
Recommended Map	*Cleveland National Forest Visitor Map*

DIRECTIONS From Interstate 5, exit east on Alicia Parkway. At a T-junction in 5.5 miles, turn right on Santa Margarita Parkway. In 2.7 miles, turn left on Plano Trabuco. In 0.3 mile, turn right on Robinson Ranch Road. In 1.1 miles, park on the side of the road by a small park just above the intersection of Robinson Ranch and Vista.

United States Geological Survey maps show an unnamed trail leading partway up the ridge between Bell and Trabuco Canyons, but the Cleveland National Forest does not list this trail among their system trails. Mountain bikers call this route Bell Ridge, have extended the trail all the way to Los Pinos Peak, and have erected a flagpole on Bell Peak, the first peaklet along the ridge. This is a hike for the adventurous.

From the park, an OC Parks post marks the Bell View Trail. This is the lesser-used upper end of the long trail that begins in Caspers Wilderness Park. Follow the trail, a wide rocky fire road, for 0.5 mile up an S-turn. The sage scrub is rich in prickly pear cactus, which produces beautiful flowers in the spring. The orange parasite growing on the sage scrub is witches hair. At the top of the S, an unsigned use trail departs on the right, making an extremely steep shortcut up to the toe of Bell Ridge. It has confusing unmarked junctions, so our recommended route stays on the main Bell View Trail as it plunges down into a canyon. The Bell View Trail forks on the canyon floor; stay right and climb steeply onto the next ridge.

At the crest of the hill (0.9 mile from the start), meet the Bell Ridge Trail, an unsigned but well-used path on the right. Take this trail as it climbs steeply east up to Bell Ridge. As you gain the ridge in 0.5 mile, you may notice an unmarked trail on the right that is the top of the shortcut mentioned earlier. Shortly beyond, a short spur on the right leads to a viewpoint with great views over southern Orange County. In the drainage to the east, you may notice a dam forming a small pond dating back to the ranching days.

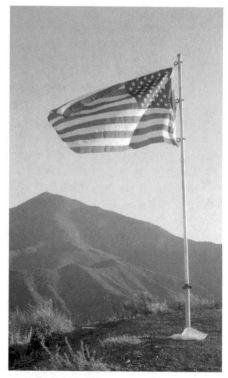

Santiago Peak from Bell Peak

Our trip continues northeast up Bell Ridge. You may see a use trail on the left side dropping into Trabuco Canyon. In 0.6 mile, reach the first prominent bump on the ridge, Bell Peak. Cyclists have erected a flag and placed a register on the peak.

VARIATION ————————————————————————

If you are looking for a long, strenuous hike with almost guaranteed solitude, continue up Bell Ridge all the way to Los Pinos Peak. The peak is 7 miles from the trailhead, with 4,100 feet of elevation gain on the ascent and 1,000 feet more on the return. Although it's not shown on maps, gonzo mountain bikers are keeping it in good condition. In the spring, this trail has terrific wildflowers, including bush monkeyflower, lupine, bush poppy, yerba santa, purple nightshade, deerweed, and virgin's bower. Wild pea and spiky cucumber vines curl through the dense chaparral. The trail passes over or around several bumps along the ridge.

After the last major hump (Peak 4066), as you descend toward a notch, you may see a use trail on the left descending toward Yaeger Mesa (see Trip 15.15). Make a steep final ascent to Los Pinos along a trail closely lined with poison oak. When it ends at an unsigned junction with the Los Pinos Trail, turn right and walk 200 feet to the peak, or left to reach Main Divide Road.

---

trip 15.18 East Horsethief Trail

see map on pages 166–167

Distance	9 miles (out-and-back)
Hiking Time	4½ hours
Elevation Gain	2,600'
Difficulty	Moderately strenuous
Trail Use	Cyclists, dogs
Best Times	November–April
Agency	CNF: TD
Recommended Map	*Cleveland National Forest Visitor Map*

DIRECTIONS From Interstate 15, exit southwest on Lake Street. In 2.4 miles, turn right onto Mountain Street, and proceed 0.5 mile to the end of the pavement, where you can find parking in the residential neighborhood.

Although the East Horsethief Trail appeared in the first edition of this guide, it was omitted from subsequent editions because of access issues. Most of the trail is in the Cleveland National Forest, but a 160-acre parcel at the base had blocked public access until it was acquired by the Western Riverside County Regional Conservation Authority in 2007–09 through the Multiple Species Habitat Conservation Plan. The steep, eroded trail receives only light maintenance, but it is thankfully open again to visitors seeking a wild experience. This is a highly varied and interesting hike with wildflowers, dense chaparral, and panoramic views from the Main Divide.

This trail has been used by Native Americans for at least 500 years. Horsethief Canyon was one of several canyons in the Santa Ana Mountains used as a hideout by bandits in the mid-19th century. Later, open pit mining for clay and coal came to the Alberhill District below the canyon mouth, and Pacific Clay continues to excavate entire hills to make bricks for Southern California's enormous housing industry.

From the end of the pavement, continue along the dirt road, which bends right

45 degrees to head northeast. Don't get lured onto one of the smaller side roads. In 0.3 mile, reach a gate on the left signed for Riverside County Wildlife Conservation Area. It is possible to park here, taking care not to block the gate, but broken glass on a 2014 scouting trip indicates that vehicles sometimes get vandalized here—take your valuables with you.

Pass through the gate and then through a yellow gate shortly beyond to enter a lovely canyon lined with oaks, sycamores, and eucalyptus. Walk past the foundation of a cabin, then watch for the path to turn right, cross the creek, and climb steeply up the slope to join a low ridge.

When you meet the trail on the ridge, 0.3 mile from the gate, turn left and follow the long ridge west between Horsethief and Rice Canyons to the crest of the Santa Ana Mountains. The path, steep and rutted in places, is lined with sage scrub and chaparral, including thick-leaf yerba santa, California sagebrush, chamise, scrub oak, buckwheat, yerba santa, and whipple yucca. As you climb higher, manzanita joins the mix. In the spring, watch for wildflowers, including bush poppy, prickly phlox, scarlet monkeyflower, purple nightshade, and Indian paintbrush. The first trees on the ridge are a trio of scraggly bigcone Douglas-firs, and near the crest you will encounter Coulter pines.

The trail unassumingly ends at a pipe fence on the Main Divide Road, 3.6 miles north of paved Long Canyon Road. Retrace your steps, or, for a much longer walk, join another of the many paths crisscrossing the Santa Ana Mountains.

San Jacinto Peak views

chapter 16

Santa Ana Mountains: Ortega Corridor

From San Juan Capistrano to Lake Elsinore, Highway 74 (Ortega Highway) stretches like a snake over the midsection of the Santa Ana Mountains. Leisurely rising from the west through San Juan Canyon to the oak-dotted crest, then descending the east escarpment via sharp curves, the road gives casual drivers their only glimpse of the interior of the Santa Anas.

The highway commemorates José Francisco Ortega, sergeant and scout in the Gaspar de Portolà party, which in 1769 passed through Orange County's coastal hills while heading up the California coast. The present roadway, completed in 1933, follows a turn-of-the-century wagon track, which in turn evolved from the route of a centuries-old Juaneno Indian trail. The highway's rustic character remains, much to the delight of the unhurried sightseer but not the growing numbers of frustrated commuters who race along it daily to and from employment centers in southern Orange County.

The US Forest Service recognizes Ortega Highway as an important recreational corridor. They have constructed campground facilities and developed several trailheads. But few roads penetrate the backcountry areas, and foot trails are the usual way of getting around.

Dayhiking (along with mountain biking and horseback riding) and car camping are popular in the Ortega Corridor. Overnight backpacking is allowed south of the highway, but only within San Mateo Canyon Wilderness (see Chapter 17 for complete coverage of this area). A wilderness permit is required for overnight trips.

Roadside camping facilities are found at Caspers Wilderness Park (Chapter 13) and in several areas within the national forest. The US Forest Service's El Cariso Campground along Ortega Highway can get considerable traffic noise. Delightful, secluded, first-come-first-served Blue Jay Campground rests high in the remote Potrero Los Pinos area, north of Ortega Highway. Its neighbor, Falcon Group Camp, is for large groups with reservations. These campgrounds are usually open from May until November and possibly during the off-season.

The drive up Ortega Highway is an enjoyable prelude to a day's hiking activities. Starting from the San Juan Capistrano side, the highway runs through outlying suburban development, rolling hills still used for grazing, and the rugged foothills of Caspers Wilderness Park. Past Caspers, you come to San Juan Fire Station and the national-forest boundary. On ahead, Ortega Highway winds along the precipitous south wall of San Juan Canyon, passing Upper San Juan Campground (closed indefinitely). A major trailhead is next to the Ortega Candy Store, 0.7 mile past Upper San Juan Campground. From here, trails lead north into the Potrero Los Pinos area and south into San Mateo Canyon Wilderness.

After another 2.5 miles, Ortega Highway levels out in a pleasant oak woodland (Potrero El Cariso). Long Canyon Road, intersecting on the left (west), climbs higher to another oak-dotted area (Potrero Los Pinos) and Blue Jay Campground. A little more than a mile past Long Canyon Road, Ortega Highway passes the El Cariso ranger station and visitor center (open

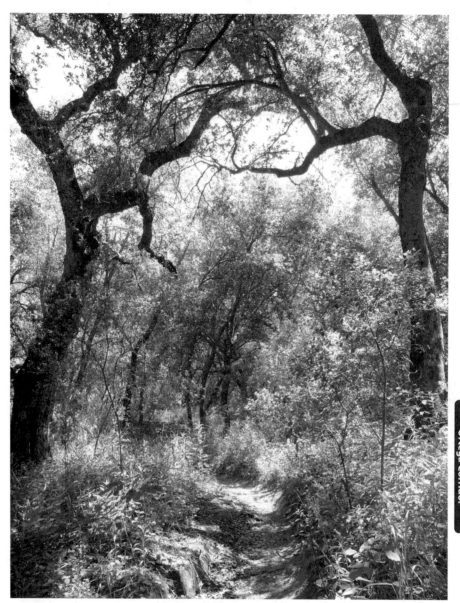

San Juan Trail

daily, offers maps and information) and El Cariso Campground.

Just east of that, Main Divide Road crosses Ortega Highway, providing access to areas along the Main Divide of the Santa Ana Mountains to the north and to the Elsinore Mountains to the south. A little farther on, Ortega Highway begins its abrupt descent to Lake Elsinore. Wending your way through the community of Lake Elsinore, you can pick up Interstate 15, which takes you back to Orange County if you use I-15 north and take the Riverside Freeway (Highway 91) west at Corona.

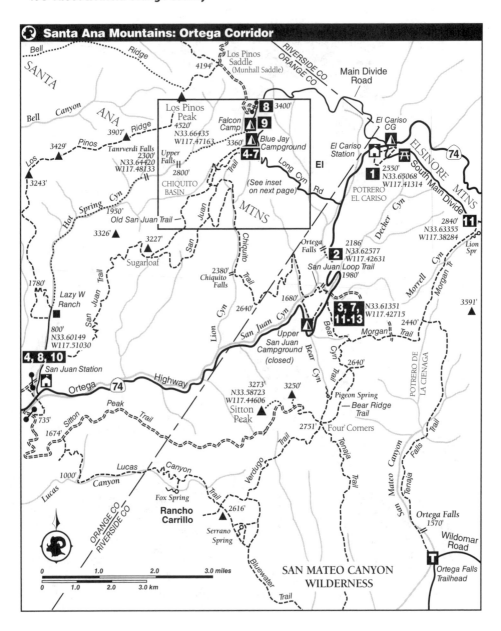

Santa Ana Mountains: Ortega Corridor

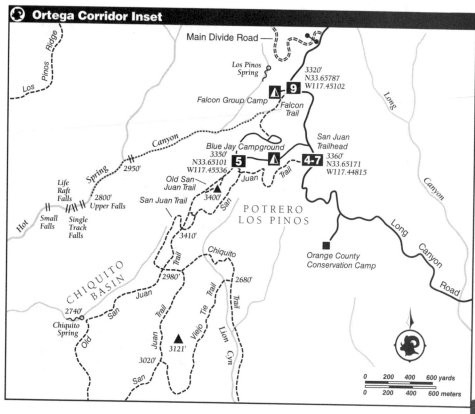

Ortega Corridor Inset

Main Divide Road

Los Pinos Spring

3320'
N33.65787
W117.45102

Falcon Group Camp

Falcon Trail

Los Pinos Ridge

Canyon

Blue Jay Campground
3350'
N33.65101
W117.45536

San Juan Trailhead
3360'
N33.65171
W117.44815

Spring

2950'

Juan Trail

Life Raft Falls

2800'
Upper Falls

Old San Juan Trail

San Juan Trail

3400'

San

POTRERO
LOS PINOS

Long

Canyon

Hot

Small Falls

Single Track Falls

3410'

Chiquito

Orange County
Conservation Camp

Long Canyon Road

CHIQUITO BASIN

2980'

2680'

Juan

Trail

Viejo Tie Trail

Lion Cyn

2740'

Chiquito Spring

San

Old

Juan Trail

3121'

3020'

San

Trail

0   200   400   600 yards
0   200   400   600 meters

---

trip 16.1   **El Cariso Nature Trail**

Distance	1.5 miles (loop)
Hiking Time	1 hour
Elevation Gain	200'
Difficulty	Easy
Trail Use	Dogs, good for kids
Best Times	All year
Agency	CNF: TD

DIRECTIONS Park at the El Cariso Visitor Center, on the south side of Ortega Highway near mile marker 74 RIV 6.50, 23 miles east of Interstate 5 at San Juan Capistrano and 6 miles west of Lake Elsinore.

If you're unfamiliar with the natural history of the Santa Ana Mountains, stop first at El Cariso Visitor Center along Ortega Highway. Inside the small center (open on weekends), you'll find some small but instructive exhibits on the local flora, fauna, and geology. To learn even more, walk the El Cariso Nature Trail, which begins just behind the visitor center.

The opportunity to become familiar with common varieties of native shrubs is the real value of taking this short walk. You'll see examples of chamise, buckwheat, manzanita, scrub oak, sugar bush, and three types of sage. In spring, monkeyflower, blue-eyed grass, nightshade, and other vividly hued annual flowers compete for attention, while the blooms of wild peonies nod circumspectly close to the ground. Amid the tangled branches of the shrubs look for the spiny, green poisonous fruits of the wild cucumber.

At the start of the trail, miner's lettuce (in winter and spring) coats the shady ground almost like a manicured lawn. You pass briefly under some oaks, then the trail begins winding moderately upward on a chaparral- and sage-covered slope. The view to the west is of rolling country dotted with small houses on large lots (the area around El Cariso is a patchwork of national forest and private lands).

Soon the trail levels out and turns east to circle a hilltop, passing an old mine shaft. Then it descends slightly to cross South Main Divide Road. Continue diagonally across the road, and pick up the less distinct trail. After meandering through a grove of "Penny Pines" (Coulter pines), plus some oak and cypress trees, cross the road again near a firefighter's memorial, and follow the trail above the El Cariso South Picnic Area back to the visitor center.

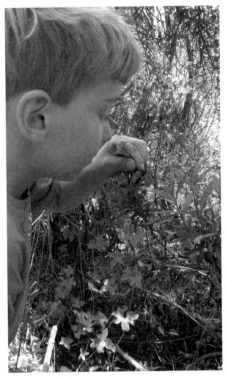

Monkeyflower

---

trip 16.2 Ortega Falls

see map on p. 198

Distance	0.5 mile (out-and-back)
Hiking Time	1 hour
Elevation Gain	200'
Difficulty	Moderate
Trail Use	Dogs, good for kids
Best Times	December–May
Agency	CNF: TD

DIRECTIONS Park at a wide unmarked turnout on the west side of Ortega Highway near mile marker 74 RIV 4.4, 21 miles east of Interstate 5 at San Juan Capistrano and about 8 miles west of Lake Elsinore.

Often dry or merely trickling, Ortega Falls can come to life for days or even weeks following any significant winter storm. During the unusually wet years of 1998 and 2005, when the region received double or more the average amount of precipitation, these falls managed to put on an impressive show until May or June.

The hike to the falls is almost trivially short but not quite a piece of cake, particularly for small kids. Try to pick the best of the unmarked use trails descending through brush and boulders and down a steep draw to the boulder-choked streambed of Long Canyon, which is an upper tributary of San Juan canyon and creek.

You turn upstream and make your way, preferably on the right bank, over sand, matted-down vegetation, and rocks. When the water is high, it may be easier to wade in a couple of spots rather than to boulder-hop. Beyond a series of smaller cascades, you arrive at the foot of the main waterfall, which drops about 35 feet over a blocky granitic outcrop. Rock climbers sometimes practice on these sheer rock faces, and it's obvious and unfortunate that spray paint vandals also visit this site from time to time.

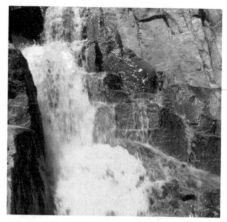

Ortega Falls

trip 16.3 San Juan Loop Trail

Distance	2.1 miles (loop)
Hiking Time	1 hour
Elevation Gain	350'
Difficulty	Easy
Trail Use	Cyclists, equestrians, dogs, good for kids
Best Times	October–June
Agency	CNF: TD
Recommended Map	*Cleveland National Forest Visitor Map*

see map on p. 198

DIRECTIONS Park at the San Juan Loop and Bear Canyon Trailhead opposite the Candy Store on Ortega Highway at mile marker 74 RIV 2.8, 19.5 miles east of Interstate 5 at San Juan Capistrano and about 10 miles west of Lake Elsinore.

If you've no more time to spare than an hour while cruising the Ortega Highway, at least stop and try the San Juan Loop Trail (not to be confused with the much longer San Juan Trail, Trip 16.4). Sights include a small waterfall along San Juan Creek, excellent wildflower displays in the spring, and some of the finest oak woodland in the Santa Anas.

Park in the large trailhead parking lot directly across from the Ortega Candy Store. From the east end of the lot, pick up the well-worn path leading north, slightly uphill, along the slope overlooking the highway. After curving left and dropping a little, the trail threads the side of a narrow gorge resounding (in the wet season at least) with falling water. A spur trail leads down toward the lip of the falls; from there, you can hop over to a reflecting pool and maybe settle into the polished granite for a moment's quiet meditation. A gnarled juniper clings sentinel-like to a bouldered slope overlooking the pool, far from its usual habitat on desert slopes 50 or more miles north and east.

From the falls area, you descend on easy switchbacks through the chaparral and reach, after more than a half-mile, an oak-dotted flat along San Juan Creek. Soon

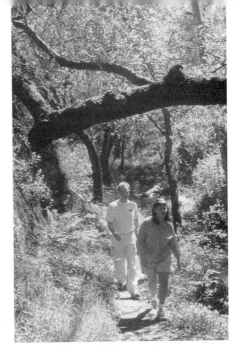

the mysterious Chiquito Trail branches north to cross the creek. The loop trail bears left (south) to follow Bear Canyon beside Ortega Highway. For a delightful few minutes as you walk here, the sky's brilliance is muted by the arching limbs of centuries-old live oaks, and the soft ground on the trailside is aglow with the seasonal greens, browns, and reds of ferns, poison oak leaves, and wild grasses.

After touching briefly upon the outermost campsites of Upper San Juan Campground, the trail veers sharply left to gain an open slope. It may be easy to lose the trail here because of various side paths worn down by campers and confused hikers. Continue for another 0.5 mile across this sunstruck slope more or less parallel to Ortega Highway, and arrive back at the parking lot.

San Juan Loop Trail

---

trip 16.4 San Juan Trail

see maps on pages 198–199

Distance	11.5 miles (one-way)
Hiking Time	5 hours
Elevation Gain/Loss	550'/3,100'
Difficulty	Moderately strenuous
Trail Use	Cyclists, equestrians, dogs
Best Times	November–May
Agency	CNF: TD
Recommended Map	*Cleveland National Forest Visitor Map*

DIRECTIONS This trip requires a car shuttle. To leave a vehicle at the west end: From the Ortega Highway 12.5 miles east of Interstate 5 at mile marker 074 ORA 12.50, turn north on Hot Spring Canyon Road. Continue 0.8 mile north to the San Juan Loop Trailhead. To reach the east end: Return to the Ortega Highway and continue 9.2 miles, then turn left onto Long Canyon Road at mile marker 74 RIV 5.2. Proceed 2.5 miles to the upper end of the San Juan Trail, which lies just short of the entrance to Blue Jay Campground.

With gentle grades most of the way, the San Juan Trail is tailor-made for a leisurely saunter from the Main Divide of the Santa Anas to the lower foothills. In recent years, the trail has received a lot more use from mountain bikers. Because the trail runs largely along dry ridgelines exposed to the sun, avoid hot days unless you're willing to carry a lot of water and to sweat copiously. Clear winter days bring out the best in the scenery. On some occasions, the view takes in much of the southern Orange County coastline and Santa Catalina and San Clemente Islands. Due to an elevation change of about 2,500 feet, most of the spring wildflowers common to the chaparral and sage scrub plant communities can be seen somewhere sometime along this trail.

This description traces the newer version of the San Juan Trail, originally an American

Indian trail but now built to modern standards with switchbacks where needed. You may take shortcuts using older and more direct sections of the trail (shown on the Ortega Corridor inset map, page 199) if you want to save a little time, but the numerous trail junctions may be poorly marked, so refer carefully to your map.

The San Juan Trail has appeared on several top 10 lists for mountain biking in North America. On a pleasant weekend morning, you can expect dozens of serious cyclists with bulging calves to pedal past you up to the highly technical trail and then bomb down it. They tend to be courteous trail-users, but if you're uncomfortable sharing the trail with bikers, pick a different trail in the area.

Begin at the roadside trailhead and parking area 100 yards south of the entrance to Blue Jay Campground. From here, the San Juan Trail winds west and south around the heads of two shady canyons, just below the level of the campground. Beware of unsigned spurs leading north to the campground and to the old trail. After about 1 mile, the trail starts descending along a sunny, sage-carpeted slope. At 1.5 miles, the new trail (the one you're on) crosses the old trail, a steep, rocky roadbed, and plunges into the deep shade of a ravine. For a time, live oaks keep the sun's rays at bay.

After rounding a single switchback and descending farther, you reach, in a sunny, sage-dotted clearing at 2 miles, a second crossing of the old trail, which from here leads to Chiquito Basin and then back up to join the new trail again just below Sugarloaf Peak. Keep straight and come to a junction, 2.1 miles, with the Chiquito Trail. Stay right here.

Continue south along the base of a hillside, through some tall and dense chaparral. Climbing slightly into a more sparsely vegetated zone, you arrive, at 2.7 miles (3.020 feet), at another junction, where the San Juan Trail bends right to cross the top of a gentle divide, and the Viejo Tie Trail, on the left, goes along the hillside.

Stay on the San Juan Trail, which now bears south-southwest through more chaparral. Reaching some oaks in a ravine bottom (3.9 miles), the trail zigzags a couple of times through grass and poison oak and crosses an intermittent stream. Enjoy the shade: This is the last grove of trees until you come to the end of the trail in Hot Spring Canyon.

On the far side of the ravine, the trail swings south of a peaklet (2,966 feet), and

Bee on buckwheat

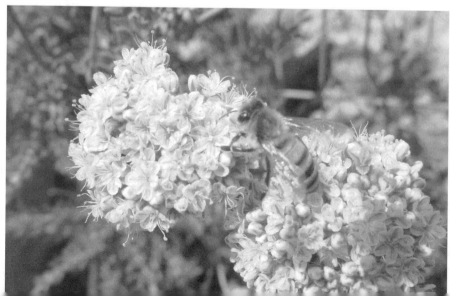

then climbs moderately toward a flat area (5 miles) just south of Sugarloaf, where the old trail, a rutted firebreak at this point, comes in from the right. You can tackle the short but tough climb to Sugarloaf's summit from near here, over big granitic boulders and through brush. The best place to start is 150 yards up the old San Juan Trail on the east side of the peak, where you can find a surprisingly good use trail climbing through the chaparral and squeezing through a granite slot before reaching the peak.

After dropping down along the west slope of Sugarloaf, you come to a saddle overlooking Hot Spring Canyon to the north. In the distant north, look for the flat-topped, antenna-crowded summit of Santiago Peak.

The gradual descent continues, largely on or near the spine of a ridge offering nice views of other ridges and canyons in every direction. Far below to the south, the gray blacktop of Ortega Highway resembles a giant snake propelling itself through the sycamores in San Juan Canyon. The trail now is hewn into friable metasedimentary rock, the same kind of metamorphosed sea floor sediment typically found in Silverado and Trabuco Canyons to the north.

At 8.5 miles, several switchbacks take you safely down a crumbling slope. East of them, look for a sharply folded anticline (bend) in the rock strata. To the west, you can spot other switchbacks on an earlier version of the trail. At 9.5 miles, you cross a saddle into Hot Spring Canyon. A final set of zigzags takes you down into the lower San Juan Trailhead, where the trail intersects the road coming up from San Juan Fire Station.

trip 16.5 Chiquito Basin

Distance	3 miles (out-and-back)
Hiking Time	2 hours
Elevation Gain	700'
Difficulty	Moderate
Trail Use	Cyclists, equestrians, dogs, good for kids
Best Times	All year
Agency	CNF: TD
Recommended Map	*Cleveland National Forest Visitor Map*

see maps on pages 198–199

DIRECTIONS At a point on Ortega Highway 21.7 miles east of Interstate 5 at San Juan Capistrano (and about 7 miles west of Lake Elsinore), turn west on Long Canyon Road at mile marker 74 RIV 5.2. Proceed 2.5 miles to Blue Jay Campground, on the left.

If you want to spot wildlife, take the hike to Chiquito Basin early in the day. One morning, in the soft wet ground along the way, Jerry discovered fresh tracks of a deer and a mountain lion, both apparently moving along at a running gait. With an earlier start, he might have witnessed a terrific chase. It might bear repeating that in this remote corner of Orange County, as well as in the parklands of the lower foothills, mountain lions are occasionally spotted, and they have very occasionally attacked hikers and mountain bikers. To stay as safe as possible, travel in groups and don't let kids stray.

Start hiking from the west edge of Blue Jay Campground, 0.5 mile west of the entrance, and take the Old San Juan Trail, which is the most direct route to Chiquito Basin. If the campground is closed (as it is in winter), park outside the gate, and pick up the new San Juan Trail skirting the campground (see Trip 16.4), or simply walk through the campground to reach the beginning of the old trail at the campground's west end.

The wide, rocky path of the old San Juan Trail leads southwest along the ridgeline. You may see one or more unmarked spurs on the left shortcutting down to the New San Juan Trail. The trail forks near the top of a bump on the right, with the left side going over the bump and the right side contouring around before they rejoin. Beyond, your path pitches downhill. At 0.5 mile and again at 0.8 mile, the new San Juan Trail, with its gentler but longer grade, crosses the old one. Keep straight to save time. Between these two crossings, white sage uniformly carpets the slopes on both sides of the old trail; in springtime, its dull, grayish foliage is upstaged by Indian paintbrush, a plant thought to be parasitic on the roots of sage.

Continue downhill through a meadow and over a footbridge into the large oak-rimmed meadow informally called Chiquito Basin, a great place for birdwatching, picnicking, or loafing. Beware that the meadow is full of foxtail barley, which has a nasty tendency to catch in your socks. Worse yet, the stickers can work their way into your dog's eyes, causing blindness.

In the ravine northwest of the meadow is Chiquito Spring, named by early Cleveland National Forest ranger Kenneth Munhall, who stopped there one warm afternoon in 1927 with his horse, Chiquito. The spring is bedecked with giant chain ferns and poison oak vines and buzzes with insects. The use trail to it has faded to nothing, and searching for the spring involves wading through poison oak. On the poison oak–infested slope north of it, you can find at least half a dozen morteros, Indian grinding holes worn into the granitic bedrock.

Return the same way, or if the spirit moves you, explore further. From the edge of Chiquito Basin, the old San Juan Trail veers south and climbs 300 vertical feet up a steep, oak-shaded slope to reach an open ridgetop offering a fine view of the basin and its surroundings. The old trail then turns southwest along this ridgeline and connects with the new San Juan Trail at the base of Sugarloaf Peak. From here, you might loop back to Blue Jay Campground by following the twists and turns of the new trail, if you have time.

Chiquito Basin

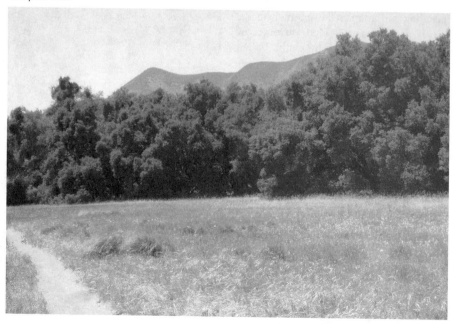

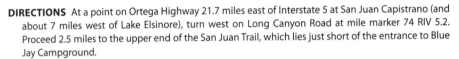

trip 16.6   **Viejo Tie Loop**

Distance	7 miles (loop)
Hiking Time	3 hours
Elevation Gain	1,000'
Difficulty	Moderate
Trail Use	Cyclists, equestrians, dogs
Best Times	November–June
Agency	CNF: TD
Recommended Map	*Cleveland National Forest Visitor Map*

see maps on pages 198–199

DIRECTIONS   At a point on Ortega Highway 21.7 miles east of Interstate 5 at San Juan Capistrano (and about 7 miles west of Lake Elsinore), turn west on Long Canyon Road at mile marker 74 RIV 5.2. Proceed 2.5 miles to the upper end of the San Juan Trail, which lies just short of the entrance to Blue Jay Campground.

In Orange County, the most dependable and lavish displays of springtime flowering take place in the chaparral plant community. Beginning with the longer days and warmer soil temperatures of March and ending with the onset of heat and drought in May or June, the higher mountains are alive with the color and fragrance of blooming plants large and small.

This hike takes you into stands of mature chaparral, dotted here and there with live oak trees. Aside from the common white-blooming ceanothus, you may discover more than a dozen kinds of wildflowers, including red monkeyflower, nightshade, prickly phlox, aster, golden yarrow, cow parsnip, wild pea, wild hyacinth, Indian pink, and mariposa lily.

Begin as in Trip 16.4 by taking the new San Juan Trail for 2.7 miles, then bear left on the unsigned Viejo Tie Trail. After swinging left around the brow of a ridge, you descend northward through tall chaparral to reach the oak-shaded bed of Lion Canyon. On the far bank, you come to the Chiquito Trail (1.2 miles). Turn left, climb 300 vertical feet and 0.6 mile back to the San Juan Trail (crossing the creekbed again), and return the way you came.

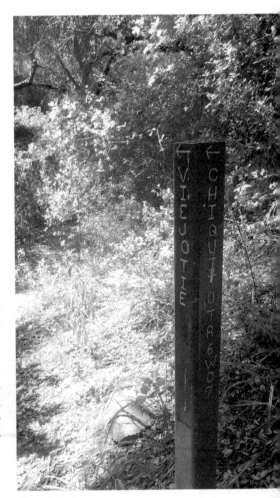

Viejo Tie Trail

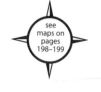

see maps on pages 198–199

trip 16.7 Chiquito Trail

Distance	9 miles (one-way)
Hiking Time	5 hours
Elevation Gain/Loss	900'/2,300'
Difficulty	Moderately strenuous
Trail Use	Cyclists, equestrians, dogs
Best Times	November–May
Agency	CNF: TD
Recommended Map	*Cleveland National Forest Visitor Map*

DIRECTIONS This trip requires a car shuttle. Leave a vehicle at the San Juan Loop and Bear Canyon Trailhead (south end) opposite the Candy Store on Ortega Highway at mile marker 074 RIV 2.8, 19.5 miles east of Interstate 5 and 10 miles west of Lake Elsinore. To reach the north end (the starting point), continue northeast on the Ortega Highway, then turn west on Long Canyon Road at mile marker 74 RIV 5.2. Proceed 2.5 miles to the upper end of the San Juan Trail, which lies just short of the entrance to Blue Jay Campground.

Like the San Juan Trail, the Chiquito Trail is best explored from end to end, preferably in the downhill direction. Along the way, you'll enjoy cool passages through canyon bottoms but also endure (if the weather is warm) a seemingly endless traverse across a sun-blasted slope. This lightly maintained trail is lined for miles with poison oak, so wear pants and long sleeves.

Completed in 1974, the Chiquito Trail is easy to follow, yet it can be an ankle-twister. In some places, sharp rocks have eroded out of the decomposed granite bed of the trail—watch your step.

Begin at the upper terminus of the San Juan Trail (see Trip 16.4) and descend, using the easy switchbacks, to the Chiquito Trail junction, 2.1 miles. Turn left (east) and descend into Lion Canyon, which has water about half the year. At 2.7 miles, pass a junction with the Viejo Tie Trail.

The next couple of miles down-canyon are delightful, with patchy shade provided by large oaks—the survivors of wildfires—and young sycamores. On the banks of the creek, you'll find poison oak, wild blackberry, toyon, barberry, and ceanothus. Profuse displays of monkeyflower brighten the scene in April. The red monkeyflower and the sticky (yellow) monkeyflower may have hybridized here: The spectrum of monkeyflower colors includes orange, pink, and magenta, as well as the usual scarlet and light yellow hues.

At 4.3 miles, the trail makes an abrupt bend to the left and begins a long traverse across the ridge to the east. Just below this bend is Chiquito Falls, where the stream drops about 15 feet over an outcrop of granite. Impressive only after heavy rains, the site is pleasant anytime for a picnic.

Rising through scrubby chaparral and granitic boulders, the trail works around to a south-facing slope. The din of traffic from Ortega Highway less than one beeline mile away is enough to convince you the end is near, but instead, the trail curves northeast and crookedly descends for another 2.6 miles to an unnamed tributary of San Juan Canyon. To occupy yourself on the way down, look for hawks and golden eagles riding the thermals and squirrels or lizards scurrying around at ground level.

Upon reaching the bottom of the unnamed canyon, the trail turns south to follow an intermittent watercourse, similar to the creek in Lion Canyon. After another 0.8 mile, you come to San Juan Canyon and the San Juan Loop Trail. Go either right or left around the loop to reach the large trailhead parking lot opposite the Candy Store.

trip 16.8   Los Pinos Ridge

Distance	10 miles (one-way)
Hiking Time	7 hours
Elevation Gain/Loss	2,500'/5,200'
Difficulty	Strenuous
Trail Use	Cyclists, dogs
Best Times	November–April
Agency	CNF: TD
Recommended Map	*Cleveland National Forest Visitor Map*
Permit	Call for permission from Lazy W Ranch

see map on p. 198

DIRECTIONS This trip requires a car or bicycle shuttle. Leave a vehicle at the San Juan Trailhead, the west end. From the San Juan Fire Station on Highway 74 at mile marker 74 ORA 12.50 (12.5 miles east of Interstate 5), turn north on Hot Spring Canyon Road. Proceed 0.8 mile to the San Juan Trailhead.

Then, to reach the top of the hike, return to Highway 74, and drive east for 9.2 miles to mile marker 74 RIV 5.2, and turn west on Long Canyon Road. Follow this steep, narrow road 3.5 miles west and north to the Main Divide Road on the left. If you have a high-clearance, four-wheel-drive vehicle and the gate is open, you can drive 1.7 miles up the road to Los Pinos Saddle, shaving 800 feet of climbing off the trip.

If you are planning a bicycle shuttle, consider doing this trip in reverse, hiking up the ridge and mountain biking down the magnificent and technical San Juan Trail (see Trip 16.4). Only the most skilled bikers should attempt to ride Los Pinos Ridge.

Although plotted as a trail on US Forest Service and topographic maps, the Los Pinos ridge route had for decades received only irregular or no maintenance. Once a wide firebreak, it now serves as a through-way only for wildlife and a few adventurous humans, including a cadre of hard-core mountain bikers who have been trimming back the brush. Clinging religiously to the undulating ridgeline, the route is tiring with its many uphills and absurdly steep downhills. Although the trail was in good condition when I walked it in 2014, prospective hikers should be ready to do battle with brush; wear tough trousers and sturdy shoes. Rattlesnakes may be present in warm weather; proceed slowly and cautiously through areas where you can't see the ground.

The hike's greatest reward is the fine views west and south to the Pacific Ocean and the islands, east past Lake Elsinore to the highest summits of the Peninsular Ranges, and down into the V-shaped upper gorges of Hot Springs and Bell Canyons.

The Los Pinos Trail is designated by the Forest Service as "landlocked," which means that there is no public access at its lower end. *If you plan to hike this route all the way through, as I describe here, you'll need permission to pass through the Lazy W Ranch church camp (call 949-728-0141 in advance) at the lower end of the trail.* Parking is limited and probably unavailable at the church camp itself.

From the north end (starting point), trudge up the steep road 1.7 miles to Los Pinos Saddle (aka Munhall Saddle), where the Trabuco Canyon Trail joins Main Divide Road. Step over a metal fence, and follow the wide firebreak very steeply up the ridge to the southwest. The crumbly metasedimentary rock on the slope is a foretaste of what you will have to contend with in the miles ahead. Chamise, bush poppy, ceanothus, manzanita, and scattered Coulter pines keep a low profile along the ridge, allowing clear vistas in nearly every direction.

Just before the peak, beware of an unsigned, unofficial trail on the right descending the ridge between Trabuco and Bell Canyons; stay on the main trail heading south. Nearby surveyor's bench marks identify Los Pinos Peak, the fourth highest named peak in the Santa Ana Mountains. (The three highest peaks—Santiago, Modjeska, and Trabuco—are on the Main Divide.) The true summit (elevation more than 4,520 feet) lies a little to the northeast of the bench marks. The fantastically weathered outcrops are a small exposure of the Santiago Peak Volcanics formation in this area. As the Farallon Plate subducted beneath the edge of North America during the Jurassic age, the crust melted and produced volcanoes that spread lava over the older Bedford Formation.

Beyond Los Pinos Peak, the trail drops south and west to a saddle and then undulates over a series of high points. Over the next 3.2 miles, make sure you stay on the well-defined ridge between Hot Springs and Bell Canyons. Scattered bigcone Douglas-firs struggle up the north-facing slopes, where the sun's drying effects are allayed. Coastal fog or haze sometimes fills the canyon bottoms. With the relief between ridgetop and canyon bottoms a somewhat sheer 2,000 feet, you seem perched between two yawning abysses.

Just past Peak 3429, the trail turns south to follow the ridge between Cold Spring Canyon and a tributary of Hot Spring Canyon. In another 2.9 miles, reach a faint junction marked with a cairn at the end of the last hill on Los Pinos Ridge. A lesser-used trail switchbacks east down to the upper end of the church camp, but your well-defined trail switchbacks south down the ridge to a prominent saddle before turning east to reach the trailhead in 0.8 mile. Descend a dirt road through the camp past an archery range and cabins to meet the paved Hot Spring Canyon Road in 0.2 mile near the registration office. Turn right and walk down the paved road for 0.5 mile to the San Juan Trailhead where your getaway vehicle awaits.

Los Pinos Ridge

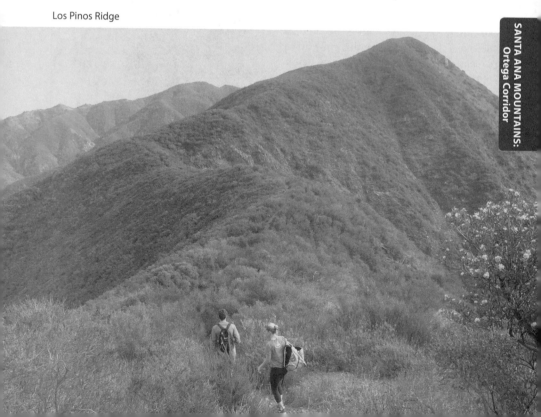

trip 16.9   Upper Hot Spring Canyon

Distance	3 miles (out-and-back)
Hiking Time	2½ hours
Elevation Gain	450'
Difficulty	Moderately strenuous
Trail Use	Hiking only
Best Times	December–May
Agency	CNF: TD

DIRECTIONS At a point on Ortega Highway 21.7 miles east of Interstate 5 at San Juan Capistrano (and about 7 miles west of Lake Elsinore), turn west on Long Canyon Road at mile marker 74 RIV 5.2. Proceed 2.5 miles to Falcon Campground (on the left), and park at a clearing outside the campground.

Silent, except for the gentle gurgle of water over stone, upper Hot Spring Canyon is an easy-to-reach retreat not far from the popular campgrounds in the Potrero Los Pinos area. Boulder-hopping and mild bushwhacking take you to an interesting area of small waterfalls and dark, limpid pools.

Walk along the road into Falcon Group Camp for 60 yards, and turn left onto the signed Falcon Trail that connects to Blue Jay Campground. In 0.1 mile, when the trail crosses a shallow gully, veer right at an unsigned junction onto a use trail that descends the gully. Follow this gully downstream, dodging brush along the way. Beware of the plentiful poison oak. You soon join a bigger gully at the head of Hot Spring Canyon carrying water from Los Pinos Spring, which lies a short distance upstream. Memorize or mark this junction for the trip back.

A narrow, lightly beaten path goes downcanyon along grassy benches and across crumbly metasedimentary rock, crossing the creek several times. The canyon ahead trends consistently southwest, despite a few bends. You're following the Los Pinos Fault, an inactive fault running perpendicular to the Elsinore Fault and other faults responsible for the recent (in a geological sense) uplift of the Santa Ana Mountains.

Just before you reach the junction of a major, wet canyon to the north (2,950 feet), there's a small waterfall and a grotto with two shallow pools. On the rocks, ferns, mosses, and live-forever (a type of succulent descriptively known as "lady fingers") add to the charm. A cluster of alders grows nearby; they are found in increasing numbers downstream, all the way to San Juan Canyon.

After another 0.4 mile, the canyon bottom makes a bend to the right and drops abruptly. All but experienced climbers should stop here and go no farther. Intrepid climbers may want to try (very

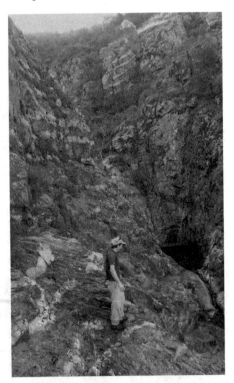

Hot Spring Canyon

cautiously) working their way over the loose metamorphic rock ahead to get a glimpse of a hidden 25-foot waterfall and a deep pool. Below it, the water shoots down a slot through polished granite. (**Note:** *The rock in this area is very loose and unstable. Standard rock-climbing techniques are of little value.*)

VARIATION

Farther progress down-canyon toward the big falls (read on—Trip 16.10) is possible only by long and nasty traverses over the canyon walls to either side or with technical canyon-eering gear, including two 60-meter ropes. Poison oak is unavoidable in places.

trip 16.10   Lower Hot Spring Canyon

Distance	10 miles (out-and-back to falls)	
Hiking Time	10 hours	
Elevation Gain	1,600'	
Difficulty	Strenuous	
Trail Use	Hiking only	
Best Times	December–March	
Agency	CNF: TD	
Permit	Call for permission from Lazy W Ranch	

see map on p. 198

DIRECTIONS At a point on Ortega Highway 12.5 miles east of Interstate 5 at San Juan Capistrano at mile marker 74 ORA 12.50, turn north on Hot Spring Canyon Road. Continue 0.8 mile north to the San Juan Trailhead.

This is a trip of superlatives—arguably the most beautiful canyon hike in the Santa Ana Mountains, and arduous to boot. Your goal is a magnificent 140-foot waterfall, one of Southern California's highest. This is also a deceptively difficult hike—in fact, it's the most strenuous, and objectively the most hazardous, of all the trips in this book. (**Note:** *A portion of this route unavoidably passes through an inholding in the national forest—the Lazy W Ranch, a church camp. You must ask for permission in advance to hike through the property by calling 949-728-0141.*)

Being in excellent physical condition, having considerable experience in cross-country travel over rugged terrain, and possessing good judgment do not automatically guarantee that you'll be able to reach the falls and return without mishap. You must be cautious, patient, and determined too. Hazards include slippery rocks (some concealed by leaf litter), prickly vegetation, and forests of poison oak. Pants, a long-sleeved shirt, and sturdy boots are musts. Line your pack with a trash bag to keep your gear dry as you wade chest-deep pools. Trekking poles will help you keep your footing on the slick terrain.

Several factors determine the appropriate time of year to take this trip. Autumn leaves put on a great show during November and December, but if the rains are late, there won't be much water cascading over the falls or flowing down the creek. Wildflowers and new leaves in early spring add to the canyon's beauty, but by then, the ubiquitous poison oak bushes and vines are sporting fresh, virulent leaves, and rattlesnakes are emerging from their winter burrows. Most years, fair-weather days in January and February are good as long as you start early enough in the morning to take advantage of the limited daylight; however, you may need a wetsuit in the creek.

Parking is not allowed at the church camp and is very limited near the camp's entrance, so leave your car at the west end trailhead for the San Juan Trail, 0.8 mile north of Ortega Highway. Walk 0.6 mile north to the church camp entrance, then continue another 0.3 mile past several buildings. Stay close to the Hot Spring Canyon streambed, and continue up an old roadbed flanked on both sides by huge, spreading coast live oak trees.

By 1.5 miles (from your car), the route deteriorates to little more than a game trail. The creek bubbles alongside, with scattered sycamores and alders growing from the granite-bouldered banks. At 2 miles, the canyon makes a decided turn to the northeast. From this point on, dark brownish and grayish metamorphic rocks gradually replace the granite, and the canyon becomes considerably narrower. Progress is slowed by a factor of two or three. You will likely find that it is better to rock-hop and slosh through the creek while dodging nettles and alder branches than to battle thickets of willow, sage, wild blackberry, and poison oak on the banks. In the winter and spring, you will inevitably get wet. Here and there, the creek may disappear under porous sands for brief stretches.

Although amphibians are in severe decline across Southern California, Hot Spring Canyon is one of the best places to find them, especially in the spring. More often than not, one or more bright orange California newts will be lazily swimming in

Rappelling Tanrverdi Falls

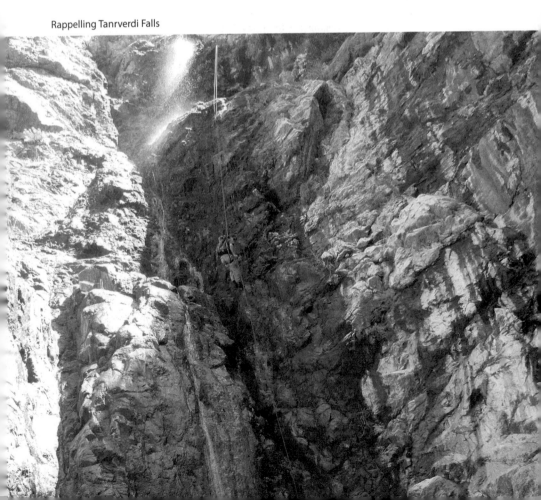

a pool. During spring mating season, you'll often see a pair *in flagrante*, sometimes with another male hoping to get in on the action! The spotted gray frogs are California tree frogs, though you could be forgiven for calling them rock frogs instead. Like chameleons, they change color to camouflage themselves and are so effective that you may only notice them when they move.

At 3.4 miles (1,620 feet), the creek slides over a series of granite slabs and collects in limpid pools almost perennially shaded by an overhanging south wall. Fallen sycamore, oak, and alder leaves dimple the water's mirrored surface. On the north bank, a smooth granite slab, perfect for lounging, catches early afternoon winter sunlight; it's a soothing place to rest on your return down-canyon if you have time. Just beyond, the canyon broadens, and a usually wet tributary, draining Chiquito Basin, comes in on the right. At 4.1 miles (1,950 feet), another usually wet tributary joins on the left; a 70-foot waterfall with a scant flow lies immediately up this tributary from the main canyon.

By now, it should be possible to glimpse, just 200 yards ahead, the top of a sheer headwall. From the lip, water plunges an estimated 140 feet down Tanrverdi Falls. Some boulder-hopping will get you to the base of a much smaller fall (a moss-covered 20-footer) below the big one, but further progress directly up-canyon is possible only with some dicey hand-and-toe climbing, and two more falls block access to the base of the big one.

To reach the base of the main falls, you can try backtracking a little and scrambling up the steep, broken slope to the south. As you do so, look for a raptor's aerie on a banded cliff wall to the north.

The top of the main falls can be reached by making long traverses either right or left; from there, it's possible, with great effort, to continue up-canyon toward the upper series of falls described in Trip 16.9.

trip 16.11 Morgan Trail

Distance	5 miles (one-way)
Hiking Time	2½ hours
Elevation Gain/Loss	300'/1,300'
Difficulty	Moderate
Trail Use	Backpacking, equestrians, dogs, good for kids
Best Times	October–May
Agency	CNF: TD
Recommended Map	USFS *San Mateo Canyon Wilderness*
Permit	Wilderness permit required for overnight trips

see map on p. 198

DIRECTIONS This trip requires a car shuttle. The trip ends at the San Juan Loop and Bear Canyon Trailhead parking lot at mile 74 RIV 2.8, opposite the Ortega Oaks Candy Store on Ortega Highway, 19.5 miles east of Interstate 5. Leave a car there, and then to reach the east end (the starting point), continue east on Highway 74 for 3.5 miles (0.2 mile east of mile marker 74 RIV 6.50). Then turn right on South Main Divide Road, and drive 2.6 miles to the signed Morgan Trailhead on the right.

As I (Jerry) rambled down the Morgan Trail one crisp autumn morning before dawn, the crackling of oak leaves underfoot played counterpoint to the drone of a hundred crickets singing in unison. Dozens of cold, blue stars sparkled overhead, while moonbeams, caught in a tangled aerial net of limbs and branches, painted the ground shades of black, gray, and silvery white. These simple kinds of sensations, jelled together, added up to a powerful, almost mystical experience.

The Morgan Trail crosses the northern edge of San Mateo Canyon Wilderness, one of coastal Southern California's newest national-forest wilderness areas and possibly its last. You can camp overnight along portions of the trail within the wilderness boundary, but don't forget the required wilderness camping permit (see the introduction to Chapter 17 for details). This description assumes you are going to hike the trail one-way north to south, the predominantly downhill direction.

On the trail, you quickly drop through scrub oak and chamise, mixed with the occasional black sage, sugar bush, laurel sumac, and yucca. In 0.2 mile, reach a trail register where day hikers must sign in (in lieu of a formal wilderness permit). Join the promenade of live oaks in Morrell Canyon. Willows and a few sycamores hug the canyon bottom, where water flows during the wet season. Going only this far is rewarding in itself if you have little time.

In another 0.7 mile, reach the signed wilderness boundary, where the best campsites of the trip may be found. Just beyond, the trail cuts left (south) across the creek and rises to higher and sunnier terrain. Soon you're back on chaparral-covered slopes, dotted with granitic boulders.

In another 1.1 miles, pass the Tenaja Falls Trail on the left at a signed junction.

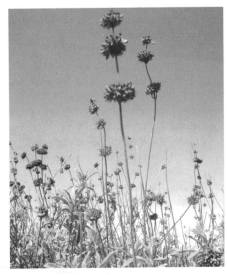

Black sage

The next segment passes west along the perimeter of private lands in Potrero de la Cienaga and Round Potrero. Watch for unsigned horse trails, and cross two dirt roads. At 3 miles, cross the last dirt road, continue west in thick chaparral, and then begin a crooked descent into some oak woods. In 1.1 miles, turn right at a signed junction onto the Bear Canyon Trail (4 miles). Continue another 0.9 mile downhill through tunnel-like chaparral and boulders to the Bear Canyon Trailhead adjacent to the Candy Store.

trip 16.12 **Sitton Peak**

see map on p. 198

Distance	9.5 miles (out-and-back)
Hiking Time	5 hours
Elevation Gain	2,150'
Difficulty	Moderately strenuous
Trail Use	Backpacking, dogs
Best Times	October–May
Agency	CNF: TD
Recommended Map	USFS *San Mateo Canyon Wilderness*
Permit	Wilderness permit required for overnight trips

DIRECTIONS Park at the San Juan Loop and Bear Canyon Trailhead opposite the Ortega Oaks Candy Store on Ortega Highway at mile 74 RIV 2.8, 19.5 miles east of Interstate 5 at San Juan Capistrano and 8.9 miles west of Lake Elsinore.

From below, Sitton Peak looks unimposing—a mere bump on a rambling ridge—despite its distinction as one of the highest points in the Santa Ana Mountains south of Ortega Highway. On the summit, though, the feeling is decidedly "top of the world." When an east or north wind blows, cleansing the sky of water vapor and air pollution, vistas may extend 50 miles or more in every direction.

The hike to the summit is always peaceful because it passes through lands included in San Mateo Canyon Wilderness. Trail camping is allowed within the wilderness area, provided you obtain the necessary free permit from the US Forest Service (see the introduction to Chapter 16).

Begin by taking the Bear Canyon Trail south from the Candy Store. Before long you pass into San Mateo Canyon Wilderness, where mountain bikes and other mechanized transport is banned. After 1 mile of moderate ascent, you come to a trail junction in the midst of a small oak woodland. Go right (as the Morgan Trail forks left), and begin climbing more steeply along a chaparral-clothed slope.

At 2 miles, you reach a summit, and then you descend slightly to a trail junction. You can either turn right on an old truck trail that carries the name Bear Canyon Trail or continue straight across on the newer, narrower Bear Ridge Trail (Bear Canyon Loop Trail on some maps). Both lead to Four Corners, originally a four-way meeting of fire roads and now a junction of five trails. The older route is more scenic, as it follows a brushy draw flanked by blue-flowering ceanothus, and visits Pigeon Spring, with an old watering trough and the last bit of shade you may find on the way to the peak.

At Four Corners, swing right on the wide path climbing northwest, a disused section of the Sitton Peak Road. After a steady ascent of about 300 vertical feet, you reach a flat area (4 miles) just below a boulder-studded ridge, with a 3,250-foot high point, to the north. Easily climbed, the ridge summit offers a view somewhat similar to that seen from Sitton Peak. The flat area by the road (just inside the wilderness boundary) makes a good overnight campsite for those who backpack in.

On the summit of Sitton Peak

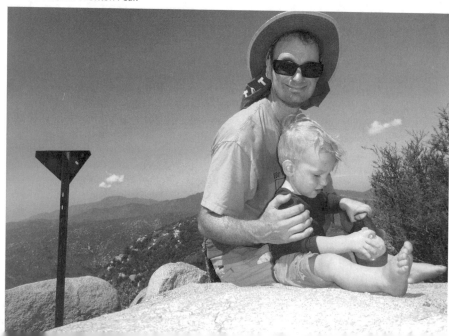

Beyond the flat area, the road descends another 0.5 mile to a saddle just below Sitton Peak. From this saddle, you leave the road and follow a steep climbers' trail up through scattered manzanita and chamise on the east slope of the peak.

The view from the top is especially impressive to the west. Here the foothills and western canyons of the Santa Anas merge with the creeping suburbs of southern Orange County. Beyond lies the flat, blue ocean punctuated by the profile of Santa Catalina Island. Some 2,000 feet below, toylike cars on the highway make their way down the sinuous course of San Juan Canyon.

see map on p. 198

trip 16.13   Lucas Canyon

Distance	14.4 or 19.5 miles (one-way)
Hiking Time	7 or 10 hours
Elevation Gain/Loss	2,200'/3,400'
Difficulty	Strenuous
Trail Use	Backpacking, equestrians, dogs
Best Times	November–May
Agency	CNF: TD
Recommended Map	USFS *San Mateo Canyon Wilderness*
Permit	Wilderness permit required for overnight trips

DIRECTIONS This trip requires a car shuttle. First, you must leave a vehicle at the Juaneno Trailhead (the west end) in Caspers Wilderness Park. From Interstate 5 in San Juan Capistrano, take Highway 74 east for 7.6 miles to Caspers Wilderness Park on the left at mile marker 74 ORA 7.50. Pay your entry fee, and follow the park road 0.4 mile. Then make a right into the San Juan Meadow group area, and head to the Juaneno Trail parking area at the north end of the group area.

From there, to reach the east end (your starting point), return to Highway 74. Proceed 5 miles east to the San Juan Fire Station and then 7 more miles east to the San Juan Loop and Bear Canyon Trailhead opposite the Candy Store.

Under construction for years, primarily through the efforts of volunteer workers, the Lucas Canyon Trail was finally completed in 1992. Its opening inaugurated the first legal access to the San Mateo Canyon Wilderness trail system from the west. Shortly thereafter, in October 1993, virtually all of the vegetation traversed by the trail was incinerated to ash and blackened twigs when flames swept through. Chaparral regenerates rapidly, and you must look carefully to find evidence of the burn.

Lucas Canyon has been called Orange County's "Mother Lode"—an overstated reference to the placer-mining activity that took place here in the late 1800s. If you see old mining debris in the canyon, remember that it is considered historical and therefore must be left as is.

Note: In previous editions, this trip was a 14.4-mile hike from the Bear Canyon Trailhead to the San Juan Fire Station. The last segment is in the Caspers Wilderness Park, which presently forbids hikers to hop their gate to reach the Ortega Highway near the fire station. Instead, hikers must continue through Caspers for 5 miles to a trailhead in the main park, such as the Juaneno Trailhead, bringing this trip up to a grueling 19-mile undertaking. Caspers Wilderness Park is considering establishing open-access days when hikers can exit near the fire station. Check with Caspers (not the US Forest Service) for current information.

Begin, as in Trip 16.12, by following the Bear Canyon Trail south to the Four Corners trail junction, 3.2 miles. From there, take the Verdugo Trail (former Verdugo Truck Trail) southwest across dry, chaparral-coated hillsides. At 5.8 miles, the Bluewater Trail intersects on the left. Keep straight and bend right (west) through a shady oak woodland to the next trail junction (6.4 miles), just north of a rounded 2,616-foot hill. Here, turn right, pass through a fence, and head north on the Lucas Canyon Trail.

The trail meanders along the headwaters of Lucas Creek. To the south, you may spot some houses on the nearby ridgeline; they are part of the Rancho Carrillo development, an inholding in the wilderness area. In 1 mile, these signs of civilization disappear, and a signed spur on the left leads 0.1 mile to Fox Spring. The trail now plunges down steep switchbacks into deep Lucas Canyon, and you cross the stream on the bottom of the gorge at 8.7 miles. Follow the south side for 0.4 mile, and watch for the foundation of a cabin just before crossing back to the north side. For the next 1.2 miles, the trail sticks close to the stream, which flows about half the year, and you may see evidence hereabouts of past gold mining.

At 10.3 miles, the trail leaves the stream, bending northward along a small tributary and climbing steeply toward the ridge above. At 11.7 miles, you strike that ridge and turn right on an old truck trail, which brings you to Sitton Peak Trail (an abandoned fire road) at 12.1 miles. Turn left there, and pass through a gate in 0.2 mile to exit Cleveland National Forest and enter Caspers Wilderness Park. Make a winding 1.6-mile descent on the maintained dirt road to Ortega Highway.

Just before the highway gate, turn right onto an obscure trail that briefly parallels San Juan Creek before turning north and passing beneath the highway to reach a dirt road in 0.2 mile. Turning right on the dirt road leads 0.3 mile northeast to a parking area and locked gate, and the San Juan Fire Station is just south of it via Hot Spring Canyon Road. It was the former end of the Lucas Canyon hike.

Unfortunately, Caspers Wilderness Park strictly forbids hikers from jumping the gate. Unless you are here on an open access day when the gate is unlocked, you now face a 5.4-mile hike to the park's main entrance. Instead of turning right on the dirt road, stay on the trail that crosses the road and curves west. Immediately before climbing a hill, watch for palms and other lush vegetation on your left marking San Juan Hot Springs.

Continue west on the San Juan Creek Trail into the main section of Caspers. Surmount the low hill, and drop into the shady mouth of Cold Spring Canyon, where you pass a trail leading up the canyon. Abruptly climb and descend to cross the steep ridge pressing up against the highway, and pass a junction with the Oso Trail. Your path now becomes a wide, dull boundary road paralleling the noisy highway. In 1.7 miles from the hot springs, pass the Badger Pass Trail. In another 0.2 mile, you can veer right onto the slightly longer but much more interesting Juaneno Trail that weaves along the dry wash, approaches the dramatic cliffs, and meanders through groves of oak and sycamore for 3.1 miles to the Juaneno Trailhead, where your getaway vehicle awaits.

chapter 17

Santa Ana Mountains: San Mateo Canyon Wilderness

Down along the creek, a warm breeze carries the scent of sage and blooming chaparral. There are no sounds but the distant drone of bees, the soft music of water coursing down polished rock, and your own footsteps. A fat gopher snake lounging by the creek stiffens at your approach. Tiny fish dart about in the stream eddies, while a pond turtle launches itself from a rock shelf, deftly slicing through the surface of a crystalline pool. You might as well be a thousand miles away from civilization.

This is the world of San Mateo Canyon, the heart of one of California's few coastal wilderness areas, the 62-square-mile San Mateo Canyon Wilderness. Carved out of the southernmost third of the Cleveland National Forest's Trabuco District, this charming but rugged area lies within 30 airline miles of 6 million people. Only 10 miles away are the expanding edges of three of the nation's fastest-growing suburban regions: southern Orange County, southwestern Riverside County, and northern San Diego County.

San Mateo Canyon seems close according to the map, but getting there may prove problematic. Some access roads receive little maintenance and may become impassable in wet weather. Exploring the inner sanctum of the wilderness can be both physically taxing and mentally stimulating; trails may melt into the scenery, and you can lose track of your location. But these difficulties are exactly what shields the area from casual users. If you're willing to put up with them, this is your paradise.

Prepare to make a long day of it, or pack in enough equipment to stay a night or two along the trail. Unlike many national-forest wilderness areas in California, which require permits for both day and overnight trips, this one requires a permit only for overnight trips (backpacking). Camping regulations emphasize the importance of fire control. Campfires are never allowed within the wilderness, though backpacking stoves are permitted if they are used within areas cleared of flammable vegetation. Mountain bikes are also always prohibited, in accordance with a general prohibition of mechanical conveyances—even wheeled carts—in all federal wilderness areas.

Wilderness camping permits can be obtained at the El Cariso Visitor Center on Ortega Highway and at any Cleveland National Forest fire or ranger station. Since many of the ranger and fire stations keep irregular hours during the rainy months, it may be best to apply well in advance by mail or phone with the Trabuco Ranger District office in Corona (see Appendix 4). The Corona office is also your best source for information about national-forest road conditions.

Three primary entrance points have been designated for San Mateo Canyon Wilderness. The northern two are the San Juan Loop Trail Trailhead, across from the Candy Store on Ortega Highway, and the Morgan Trailhead, on Killen Trail, or South Main Divide Road. The Chapter 16, Ortega Corridor map, page 198, shows these entrances best.

The primary entrance to the southern half of the wilderness is the Tenaja Trailhead, accessible via Wildomar in southwestern Riverside County. From most parts of

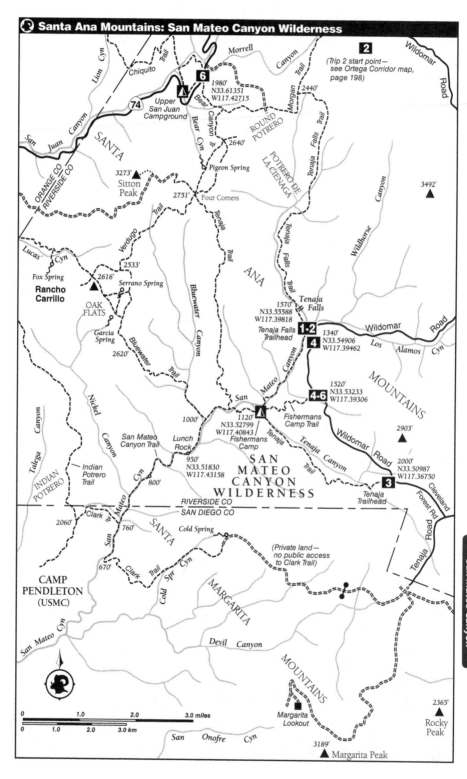

Santa Ana Mountains: San Mateo Canyon Wilderness

Lion Cyn
Chiquito Trail
Morrell
Canyon
Canyon Trail

2
(Trip 2 start point—
see Ortega Corridor map,
page 198)

Wildomar Road

6
1980'
N33.61351
W117.42715

Morgan
2440'

74
Upper
San Juan
Campground

Bear Canyon Tr
Bear Cyn

San Juan Canyon

ROUND
POTRERO

SANTA

2640'

Tenaja Falls Trail

Pigeon Spring

POTRERO DE LA CIENAGA

3492'

3273'
Sitton
Peak

2751'
Four Corners

Tenaja Trail

Tenaja Falls Trail

Wildhorse Canyon

ANA

Lucas Cyn
Fox Spring
**Rancho
Carrillo**

2533'

2616'
Serrano Spring

OAK
FLATS

Garcia
Spring

2620'

Verdugo Trail

Bluewater Canyon

Bluewater Trail

Tenaja Trail

1570'
N33.55588
W117.39818

Tenaja
Falls

Wildomar
Road

Tenaja Falls
Trailhead

1-2

4
1340'
N33.54906
W117.39462

Los Alamos Cyn

Nickel Canyon

Talega Canyon

INDIAN
POTRERO

Indian
Potrero
Trail

San Mateo
Canyon Trail

Bluewater Cyn

1000'

Lunch
Rock

950'
N33.51830
W117.43158

San

San Mateo Canyon

Mateo Canyon

San

1120'
N33.52799
W117.40843
Fishermans
Camp

4-6
1520'
N33.53233
W117.39306

Fishermans
Camp Trail

Tenaja Canyon

Tenaja Trail

MOUNTAINS

Wildomar Road

2903'

2000'
N33.50987
W117.36750

Cleveland Road

Forest Rd

3
Tenaja
Trailhead

**SAN
MATEO
CANYON
WILDERNESS**

RIVERSIDE CO
SAN DIEGO CO

2060'
Clark Tr

San Mateo Cyn

760'
Clark Trail

670'
Cold Spr

Cold Spring

SANTA

MARGARITA

(Private land—
no public access
to Clark Trail)

Tenaja Road

**CAMP
PENDLETON
(USMC)**

San Mateo Cyn

Devil Canyon

MOUNTAINS

2365'
▲ Rocky
Peak

0   1.0   2.0   3.0 miles
0 1.0 2.0 3.0 km

San Onofre Cyn

Margarita
Lookout

3189'
▲ Margarita Peak

Orange County, it takes 80 or 90 minutes to get there. Drive south on Interstate 15 from Corona, and exit at Clinton Keith Road. Proceed 6 miles south on Clinton Keith Road (passing through the Santa Rosa Plateau Ecological Reserve), and curve sharply right where the road becomes Tenaja Road. After 1.7 more miles, make a right turn to remain on Tenaja Road. Continue west on Tenaja Road for another 4.2 miles, then go right on the paved, one-lane Cleveland Forest Road. Proceed another mile to the Tenaja Trailhead parking area.

Heading north from the Tenaja Trailhead by car, you can follow the narrow, paved Wildomar Road, which replaces the former dirt road called Tenaja Truck Trail on older maps, down to secondary trailheads (basically turnouts or small parking lots) at Fishermans Camp Trail (for Trips 17.4–17.6) and at Tenaja Falls Trail. Beyond the Tenaja Falls Trailhead, Wildomar Road,

paved the rest of the way, reaches the Wildomar Off-Road Vehicle Area, and continues north to Ortega Highway as South Main Divide Road. Note that Wildomar Road, particularly between Wildomar ORV area and Tenaja Trailhead, is subject to vehicle closure due to wet weather in winter or hazardous fire conditions in summer.

The US Forest Service has published an up-to-date (2003) topographic map of San Mateo Canyon Wilderness (with the neighboring Agua Tibia Wilderness in Riverside and San Diego Counties on the reverse side). Although the contour interval on this map is 80 feet—less detailed than the 40-foot contours on the US Geological Survey 7.5-minute topo maps—and some of the trail alignments are only approximately shown, this is the best map to have for any exploration of San Mateo Canyon Wilderness and adjoining national-forest areas south of Ortega Highway.

San Mateo Canyon Wilderness

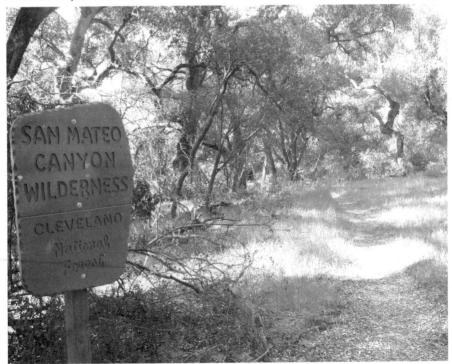

trip 17.1 Tenaja Falls

Distance	1.4 miles (out-and-back)
Hiking Time	1 hour
Elevation Gain	300'
Difficulty	Easy
Trail Use	Backpacking, equestrians, dogs, good for kids
Best Times	December–June
Agency	CNF: TD
Recommended Map	USFS *San Mateo Canyon Wilderness*
Permit	Wilderness permit required for overnight trips

see map on p. 219

DIRECTIONS Exit Interstate 15 at Clinton Keith Road in Wildomar. Proceed 5.2 miles south on Clinton Keith Road (passing into the Santa Rosa Plateau Ecological Reserve), and curve sharply right where the road becomes Tenaja Road. After 1.7 more miles, make a right turn to remain on Tenaja Road. Continue west on Tenaja Road for another 4.2 miles, then go right on the one-lane, paved Cleveland Forest Road. Proceed another mile to the Tenaja Trailhead. Continue another 4.3 miles north on the narrow pavement of Wildomar Road to the Tenaja Falls Trail parking area on the left.

Alternately, from Highway 74 (0.2 mile east of mile marker 74 RIV 6.50), follow the narrow and winding South Main Divide (Wildomar Road) south for 15.9 miles.

With five tiers and a total drop of about 150 feet, Tenaja Falls is the most interesting natural feature in San Mateo Canyon Wilderness. In late winter and spring, water coursing down the polished rock produces a kind of soothing music not widely heard in this somewhat dry corner of the Santa Ana Mountains.

Sign in at the self-registration box just down the trail, then head down to San

Upper tier, Tenaja Falls

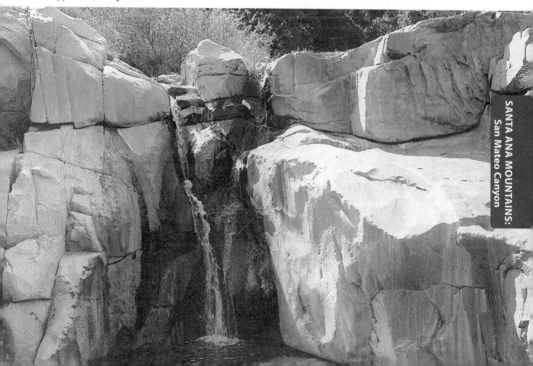

Mateo Creek and cross it on a concrete ford of an old roadbed. You may have to make a delicate rock-hop or wade through an ankle-deep froggy stagnant pool. Make certain you cross the creek first. If you bear right too soon, you will be following another stream going through Los Alamos Canyon—an easy mistake.

Continue north on the steadily rising former fire road. A spur on the right in 0.1 mile leads to a fine campsite under the oaks (beware of poison oak). Along the main trail, you'll soon be treated to a distant view of the falls. After 0.7 mile, the trail passes near the upper lip of the falls, where a few large oaks provide welcome shade at another good campsite.

Close exploration of the falls requires rock climbing skills and extreme caution; serious accidents occur here regularly. The flow of water has worn the granitic rock almost glassy smooth. Don't be lured into dangerous situations. A somewhat safer way of approaching the lower falls is to scramble over the roughly textured rocks well away from the water. You could also backtrack down the road and then scramble down the slope into the brush-choked creekbed down near the base of the falls.

trip 17.2 Tenaja Falls Traverse

Distance	8 miles (one-way)
Hiking Time	4 hours
Elevation Gain/Loss	600'/2,100'
Difficulty	Moderately strenuous
Trail Use	Backpacking, equestrians, dogs
Best Times	November–May
Agency	CNF: TD
Recommended Map	USFS *San Mateo Canyon Wilderness*
Permit	Wilderness permit required for overnight trips

see map on p. 219

DIRECTIONS This trip requires a car or vigorous bicycle shuttle. First, you must leave a vehicle at the Tenaja Falls Trailhead (the south end). At a point on Ortega Highway 0.2 mile east of mile marker 74 RIV 6.50 and the El Cariso Visitor Center (23 miles east of Interstate 5), drive 15.9 miles south on South Main Divide Road (Forest Road 6S07, formerly Killen Trail, eventually Wildomar Road) to the signed Tenaja Falls Trailhead on the right.

To reach the north end (the starting point) from there, retrace your path northward for 13.3 miles to the signed Morgan Trailhead.

This one-way traverse from the Morgan Trailhead on the South Main Divide down to the Tenaja Falls Trailhead in San Mateo Canyon lets you see plenty of gorgeous springtime scenery—without repeating any steps. You can set up a car shuttle arrangement or have someone drop you off at the start and later pick you up at the finish. Or, if you have access to only one car, you might think of a way to use a bicycle (that you could leave at the start or end point) to turn this trek into a hybrid hike and bike loop. Bikes are not allowed on the hiking route itself, but they are well suited to traveling the 13 miles of mostly narrow, thinly paved Wildomar Road connecting the start and finish points.

From Morgan Trailhead, you begin with a short descent through chaparral on the Morgan Trail. Dayhikers should sign in at the self-registration box. Soon, you enter the boundary of San Mateo Canyon Wilderness and plunge into the dark, upper reaches of Morrell Canyon. It is loaded with magnificent live oaks, the ever-hardy survivors of periodic wildfires. The trail crosses

Morrell Canyon's small creek at 1.1 miles, then rises back into the sunny chaparral.

At 2.2 miles, Tenaja Falls Trail branches left. Heading east, you cross a wooded ravine and steadily and crookedly rise on rocky, chaparral-clad slopes. Later you turn south on those slopes, still climbing, and skirt the boundary of a parcel of private land lying within both the national forest and the wilderness area. Most of this private inholding covers the flat, grassy valley named Potrero de la Cienega (translation: "Pasture of the Marsh"), which sheds its water into upper San Mateo Canyon.

Your climbing ends at a high point just above the 2,800-foot contour, some 400 feet above the potrero's flat floor. You then descend south into its southeastern corner. At 4.3 miles, you join a disused dirt road, which continues going south around its east edge. In the next mile, there are plenty of potential backpacking campsites amid scattered live oaks.

The old road curls west around the inholding and then, starting at 5.5 miles, assumes a descending course south down the left side of V-shaped upper San Mateo Canyon. You can often hear water cascading down the canyon bottom, which is virtually impossible to reach due to dense chaparral growth.

By 7 miles, you're right alongside the canyon bottom, and you benefit from the soothing sound of rushing water and the sheltering shade of streamside oaks. At 7.5 miles, you cross San Mateo Canyon's creek on an old concrete ford just above Tenaja Falls, switching over to the canyon's west side. After rapidly descending on the popular southernmost leg of Tenaja Falls Trail, there's only one more creek crossing to contend with, plus a short climb up to the Tenaja Falls Trailhead.

Tenaja Falls

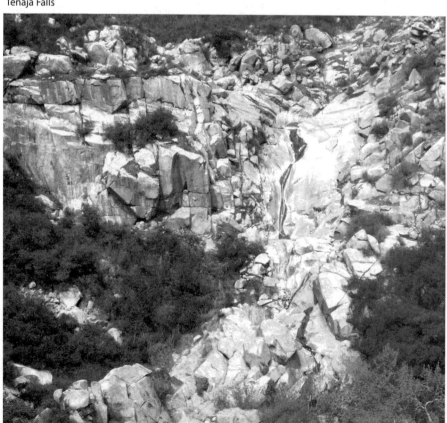

trip 17.3 Tenaja Canyon

Distance	7 miles (out-and-back to Fishermans Camp)
Hiking Time	3½ hours
Elevation Gain	1,300'
Difficulty	Moderately strenuous
Trail Use	Backpacking, equestrians, dogs, good for kids
Best Times	November–May
Agency	CNF: TD
Recommended Map	USFS *San Mateo Canyon Wilderness*
Permit	Wilderness permit required for overnight trips

see map on p. 219

DIRECTIONS Exit Interstate 15 at Clinton Keith Road in Wildomar. Proceed 5.2 miles south on Clinton Keith Road (passing into the Santa Rosa Plateau Ecological Reserve), and curve sharply right where the road becomes Tenaja Road. After 1.7 more miles, make a right turn to remain on Tenaja Road. Continue west on Tenaja Road for another 4.2 miles, then go right on the one-lane, paved Cleveland Forest Road. Proceed another mile to the Tenaja Trailhead.

Alternately, from Highway 74 (0.2 mile east of mile marker 74 RIV 6.50), follow the narrow and winding South Main Divide (Wildomar Road) south for 20.2 miles.

As the gloom of a late afternoon descended upon the deeply cut, linear furrow of Tenaja Canyon on one particular scouting trip, dozens of orange-bellied newts waddled determinedly uphill and across the trail, oblivious to my footfalls. The cute faces and beady eyes of these little amphibians mirrored a mindless desire I (Jerry) could not fathom: sex in a bower of leaf litter and ferns? A bellyful of succulent tree-dwelling insects, ripe for the taking?

The south segment of the Tenaja Trail follows Tenaja Canyon down to its confluence with San Mateo Canyon. The route takes you down and later all the way back up, so remember that if the day is warm or you feel fatigued, you can reverse your course at any time. *Tenaja* is Spanish for "bowl," and you may note that the canyon was named for its natural stone basins that collect water.

Sign in at the self-registration box, and head downhill on the trail going west. A few minutes' descent takes you to the shady bowels of V-shaped Tenaja Canyon, where huge coast live oaks and pale-barked sycamores frame a limpid, rock-dimpled seasonal stream. Mostly the trail ahead meanders alongside the stream, but for the canyon's middle stretch, it carves its way across the chaparral-blanketed south wall, 200–400 feet above the canyon bottom.

After 3.7 miles of general descent, you reach Fishermans Camp, a former drive-in campground once accessible by many miles of bad road. The site, distinguished by its parklike setting amid a live oak grove, now serves as a fine wilderness campsite for an overnight backpack trip (requires a wilderness permit). The name of the place

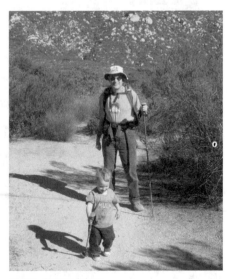

Tenaja Canyon hikers

hints at the fishing opportunities afforded by nearby San Mateo Canyon creek during and after the rainy season. A native species of steelhead trout was discovered in this drainage in 2002, surprising experts who thought that steelhead might be extinct south of Los Angeles County.

At Fishermans Camp, three other trails diverge. Fishermans Camp Trail (an abandoned roadcut) travels east uphill to Old Tenaja Road. The San Mateo Trail, a narrow footpath, continues northeast up San Mateo Canyon to the Tenaja Falls Trailhead. To the west, the San Mateo Trail heads down San Mateo Canyon and connects with the northern segment of the Tenaja Trail, which goes to Four Corners and Bear Canyon Trail.

---

trip 17.4   ### Fishermans Camp Loop

see map on p. 219

Distance	5 miles (loop)
Hiking Time	2½ hours
Elevation Gain	550'
Difficulty	Moderate
Trail Use	Backpacking, equestrians, dogs, good for kids
Best Times	November–May
Agency	CNF: TD
Recommended Map	USFS *San Mateo Canyon Wilderness*
Permit	Wilderness permit required for overnight trips

DIRECTIONS Exit Interstate 15 at Clinton Keith Road in Wildomar. Proceed 5.2 miles south on Clinton Keith Road (passing into the Santa Rosa Plateau Ecological Reserve), and curve sharply right where the road becomes Tenaja Road. After 1.7 more miles, make a right turn to remain on Tenaja Road. Continue west on Tenaja Road for another 4.2 miles, then go right on the one-lane, paved Cleveland Forest Road.

Proceed 3.7 miles north on the narrow pavement of Wildomar Road to reach the small parking turnout for Fishermans Camp Trail on the left. You will walk back along the road to your vehicle at the end of the trip, but you could avoid this road walk by putting a bicycle or second car at the Tenaja Falls Trailhead, 1.5 miles farther north.

After a good rain, upper San Mateo Canyon brims with cold, sparkling water. If you come on a sunny winter day, you can often enjoy a couple hours of very comfortable, almost summerlike temperatures. By midafternoon, low sunlight floods the canyon, and you may be tempted to slide into one of the shallow pools for a quick cooling off.

From the parking turnout, an old road, reverted to a hiking trail called Fishermans Camp Trail, descends to the abandoned Fishermans Camp, a former drive-in campground, 1.5 miles away. At the bottom of the grade, pass a junction with the San Mateo Canyon Trail, ford shallow Tenaja Creek, and reach Fishermans Camp. The camp lies at the mouth of Tenaja Canyon, whose linear alignment is associated with a rift called the Tenaja Fault.

Beautifully shaded by oaks and sycamores, Fishermans Camp is an idyllic and practical setting for a trail camp. Campstoves can be used in one of the large bare patches amid the knee-high grass (remember, though, campfires are prohibited). In winter and spring, water in Tenaja Canyon's stream trickles by on its way to the bottom of San Mateo Canyon, just 300 yards north.

A restful pause at this seductive spot is alone worth the trip, but there's more to see ahead. Return to the San Mateo Canyon Trail, which leads north toward boulder-strewn, vegetation-choked San Mateo Canyon. There

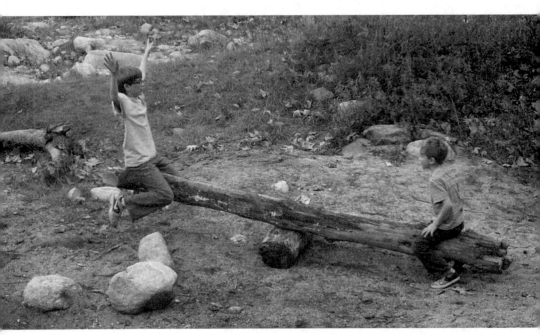

Fishermans Camp

you will cross the creek and swing north to follow the canyon upstream along the canyon's west side. You curve around the mouth of a prominent side canyon, and then go across a grassy bench.

After a second creek crossing, the trail splits. The High Trail stays right, while the Creekside Trail veers left, fords the creek twice more, and rejoins in 0.5 mile. Unless the water is very high, the Creekside Trail is recommended. Several shallow pools, set amid colorful metamorphic slabs in the canyon bottom, may tempt you into trying a cooling dip. Spring wildflowers include bush lupine, snapdragon penstemon, monkeyflowers of various hues, owl's clover, paintbrush, and wild morning glory. Yuccas send up their candlelike flower stalks along the hillsides.

After the trails rejoin, the trail sticks to the east bank until, 1.9 miles from Fishermans Camp, you cut right and arrive at the Tenaja Falls Trailhead along Wildomar Road. Close the loop by walking 1.5 miles on the road back to your car.

trip 17.5 San Mateo Canyon

see map on p. 219

Distance	8 miles (out-and-back to Lunch Rock)
Hiking Time	4 hours
Elevation Gain	1,100'
Difficulty	Moderately strenuous
Trail Use	Backpacking, equestrians, dogs
Best Times	November–May
Agency	CNF: TD
Recommended Map	USFS *San Mateo Canyon Wilderness*
Permit	Wilderness permit required for overnight trips

DIRECTIONS Exit Interstate 15 at Clinton Keith Road in Wildomar. Proceed 5.2 miles south on Clinton Keith Road (passing into the Santa Rosa Plateau Ecological Reserve), and curve sharply right where the road becomes Tenaja Road. After 1.7 more miles, make a right turn to remain on Tenaja Road. Continue west on Tenaja Road for another 4.2 miles, then go right on the one-lane, paved Cleveland Forest Road. Proceed 3.7 miles north on the narrow pavement of Wildomar Road to reach the small parking turnout for Fishermans Camp Trail on the left.

Alternately, from Highway 74 (0.2 mile east of mile marker 74 RIV 6.50), follow the narrow and winding South Main Divide (Wildomar Road) south for 17.4 miles.

With no roads and sometimes only the barest hint of a trail in view, San Mateo Canyon's inner depths are the essence of wilderness. The sky above is the bluest of blues, and the air is alive with moist, woodsy odors. The canyon walls resonate with gurgling water. Papery sycamore leaves chafe on the wind, and birds flit noisily about, staking out territory in brush and treetops. Under the shade of live oaks, American Indian morteros pock a granite slab. In the stream below, pond turtles hitching rides on the current careen from rock to rock. A gopher snake on the bank slithers through dry grass in search of a small, furry meal. Only the passing of high-flying aircraft gives evidence of the outside world a few miles away.

Following the canyon may be a bit problematic. You'll be tracing the latest incarnation of the San Mateo Canyon Trail, originally constructed before the turn of the century. Trail maintenance is occasional. Floods routinely obliterate the trail where it passes close to the creekbed, and rapid regeneration of riparian vegetation and grasses tends to conceal what remains. Poison oak, nettles, and other irritating plants abound along the streambed, so wear pants in these areas. Beware of ticks, especially in the spring.

Begin, as in Trip 17.4, by descending to Fishermans Camp at the mouth of Tenaja Canyon. This is the site of one of several primitive fishing camps that lined San Mateo Canyon before World War II. During a series of wet winters in the 1930s, steelhead (sea-running rainbow trout) ran upstream to spawn in San Mateo Canyon's middle and upper reaches. More runs occurred in 1969, and again during the late 1990s.

From the western edge of the grassy, oak-bowered clearing at Fishermans Camp, find the foot trail through ceanothus and scrub oak that rises onto the south wall of San Mateo Canyon. This section avoids a narrow, vegetation-choked area about 200 feet below. After 0.4 mile, you round a bend and drop quickly down 10 switchbacks to the bottom of San Mateo Canyon. Cross to the north side of San Mateo Creek, where you will see a signed junction with the lightly used North Tenaja Trail leading up the ridge. Just beyond, watch for a fine campsite on the left overlooking a pool and sandy beach. As the canyon widens, the trail diverges from the stream a little and traverses an oak-dotted potrero ("pasture," or grassy area). At the mouth of the Bluewater Canyon, in 0.7 mile, the lightly used Bluewater Trail diverges up the canyon (see Trip 17.6).

Stay left and continue down San Mateo Canyon. Another 0.7 mile ahead, the canyon bottom narrows, and the water slides over car-sized boulders and gathers in languid pools (950 feet in elevation). About 50 square miles of watershed lie upstream of this point. The largest flat-topped rock, dubbed "Lunch Rock" by hikers, is a worthy destination. The trail now climbs high on the north slope above the rock, so backtrack east 0.1 mile, then pick a path down the canyon floor to Lunch Rock. The walls are overhanging, but those comfortable with scrambling can mantle up from an adjacent rock near a sycamore. Most people will want somebody to spot them on the descent.

You've come 3.5 miles from the starting point, probably the farthest you would want to venture in a single day. After sunning, swimming, eating, and a siesta, it's uphill all the way back.

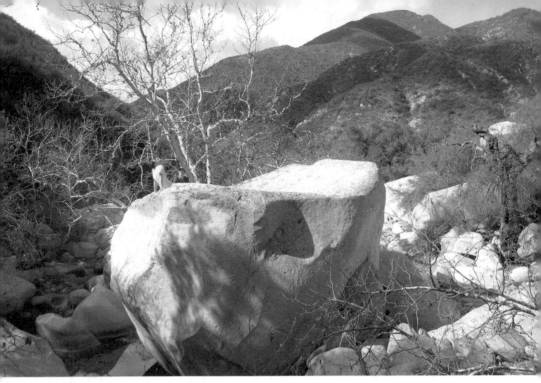

Lunch Rock

VARIATION

For backpackers, San Mateo Canyon offers a number of pleasant campsites. Dry, sandy benches abound along the wider parts of the canyon. Any such campsite could be used as a base camp for further dayhike explorations. And there's plenty to explore beyond Lunch Rock.

Down-canyon from Lunch Rock, travel may be impeded in places by big boulders and dense growths of cattails, wild grapevines, blackberry vines, stinging nettles, mulefat, and willow saplings. If the existing trail leads into impenetrable brush thickets, then try wading the creek. However, as of 2014, the trail had received maintenance for at least 1.5 miles beyond Lunch Rock. At the 800-foot contour (4.7 miles from Wildomar Road), there's a fine swimming hole, about 5 feet deep, set amid outcrops of dark gray metamorphic rock. The trail climbs high above this spot on the north wall to bypass a cliff band, so you'll have to walk down the canyon floor if you wish to visit. Near Nickel Canyon, at 5.3 miles, your speed may increase as you pick up the bed of an old mining road.

At 5.9 miles, you reach a junction with the west branch of the Clark Trail, more recently called the Indian Potrero Trail. A side trip up this trail (a gain of 1,300 feet in 1.3 miles) would take you to Indian Potrero, a bald area on the north ridge overlooking San Mateo Canyon. The other roads and trails to Indian Potrero come from access-restricted Camp Pendleton or from private lands having no public access.

For a mile farther, the trail continues down San Mateo Canyon along the bed of the old mining road, where you can spot evidence of the mining days—old rusted equipment and a tumbledown hut—in the shade of the oaks. Then comes Clark Trail rising on the left, a so-called landlocked route that has no exit on public land and receives scant maintenance. Beyond the Clark Trail junction lies a trail-less passage down through the most beautiful part of San Mateo Canyon, where the creek dances over sun-warmed granite and swirls through shallow pools. At a point 2 miles down from Clark Trail, the creek enters Camp Pendleton, where entry is prohibited.

trip 17.6　**Bluewater Traverse**

Distance	13 miles (one-way)
Hiking Time	7 hours
Elevation Gain/Loss	2,400'/2,900'
Difficulty	Strenuous
Trail Use	Backpacking, dogs
Best Times	November–May
Agency	CNF: TD
Recommended Map	USFS *San Mateo Canyon Wilderness*
Permit	Wilderness permit required for overnight trips

see map on p. 219

DIRECTIONS This trip requires a lengthy car shuttle. First, leave a vehicle at the small Fishermans Camp Trailhead (the south end): From Highway 74, 23 miles east of Interstate 5, follow South Main Divide Road 17.4 miles south to the Fishermans Camp Trailhead on the right. Then to reach the north end (your starting point) from there: Return to Highway 74, and go southwest 3.8 miles to the San Juan Loop and Bear Canyon Trailhead at mile 74 RIV 2.8, opposite the Ortega Oaks Candy Store.

From Ortega Highway to the north to Tenaja Road to the south, this route traverses the heart of the San Mateo Wilderness by way of old roads and primitive trails. Carry a full backpack, and plan to spend a night out in Oak Flats or San Mateo Canyon, or go light and make it a long day's outing. Without a doubt, March and April are the most rewarding times: knee-high grasses ripple across the potreros, chaparral blooms release their potent fragrances, and water trickles down the shady ravines. Depending on its state of maintenance, the Bluewater Trail may be quite overgrown by encroaching vegetation, so it would be wise to contact the US Forest Service before attempting this route.

From the Candy Store on Ortega Highway, pick up the Bear Canyon Trail. Day-hikers should be sure to complete the self-registration at the wilderness box near the trailhead. Hike south to Four Corners, at 3.2 miles. From Four Corners, two routes lead into San Mateo Canyon. On the left (southeast) is the north branch of the Tenaja Trail, which monotonously follows the spine of a treeless ridge all the way to the canyon. Our way, the Verdugo Trail straight ahead (southwest) is much more interesting.

For a mile or so, the Verdugo Trail winds along steep, brushy slopes offering

excellent views of the San Mateo Canyon drainage and the rounded Santa Margarita Mountains to the south. Passing over the shoulder of a ridge, the roadbed suddenly drops about 400 feet to cross an oak-shaded tributary of Bluewater Canyon (at 4.7 miles). Winding upward, then down

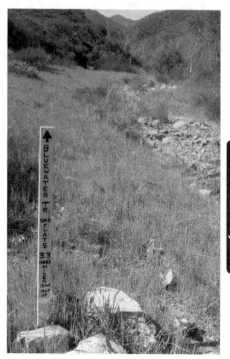

Bluewater Trail

again, you reach, around 5.5 miles, the edge of a pleasant woodland—several hundred rolling acres shaded by live oaks and tall chaparral. At 5.8 miles, bear left onto the Bluewater Trail, which follows the eastern edge of the Oak Flats area.

Oak Flats is one of the nicest back corners of the Trabuco District, containing a charming mixture of oak-rimmed potreros and deeply shaded ravines. Scottish highlander cattle graze on these meadows on account of a lease grandfathered into the wilderness. Meadow wildflowers include owl's clover, lupine, blue-eyed grass, and some nonnatives typically found in grazed areas: filaree and scarlet pimpernel.

A web of unsigned trails crosses the flats. A complete reconnaissance of the Oak Flats area might include a visit to nearby Peak 2616, overlooking the private Rancho Carrillo development in Verdugo Potrero (an area well within the overall outlines of, but excluded from, San Mateo Canyon Wilderness by a boundary that resembles a cherry stem). The coastline is only 13 air-miles away from here, and the wide, blue arc of the Pacific Ocean can be seen on most days.

During winter and spring, water trickles down the ravine containing Serrano and Garcia Springs and flows onward toward Nickel Canyon. If they purify it, backpackers camping overnight in the area can use it.

Beyond Oak Flats, the poor roadbed that has so far served as the Bluewater Trail veers left (southeast) and attains a nearly barren summit (at 7.5 miles). The Bluewater Trail (now a footpath) continues southeast, descending gradually toward Bluewater Canyon, 1,500 feet below. After a short, confusing stretch through a grassy area, the route pitches very sharply down a brushy ridgeline. Newer switchbacks do little to keep your feet from sliding; backpackers may at times feel safer sliding down on the seat of their pants! There's a short respite about halfway down, followed by even steeper switchbacks down to the bottom of the canyon (at 9 miles).

After the effort of the descent, the cold, bubbling stream in Bluewater Canyon is the hiker's equivalent of paradise. Small oaks and sycamores provide semishade. The Bluewater Trail, overgrown by small shrubs and grasses, continues downstream on the banks for 0.8 mile, crossing the creek repeatedly.

At the signed junction with the San Mateo Canyon Trail on a bench at Bluewater Canyon's mouth (at 9.8 miles), turn left and work your way east along the north side of San Mateo Canyon. The lightly used North Tenaja Trail forks north at a sign just before you cross San Mateo Creek (at 10.5 miles). If you want to loop back to Ortega Highway, this path up the long ridge is the expedient if tedious way to go. A fine campsite overlooking a pool and sandy creekside beach can be found just west of this junction.

Otherwise, pick up the series of switchbacks leading toward Fishermans Camp (at 11.5 miles). Go north across Tenaja Creek (usually a trickle), to a junction, where you go right onto Fishermans Camp Trail, an abandoned roadbed that climbs to Wildomar Road (at 13 miles).

chapter 18

Long-Distance Trails

Over the years, Orange County has developed an extensive system of regional trails and bikeways. Three of these trails are especially notable because they trace important watersheds from the foot of the Santa Ana Mountains to the Pacific Ocean: the Santa Ana River Trail, the Mountains to Sea Trail, and the Aliso Creek Trail.

These long-distance trails all pass various city and regional parks that serve as staging areas. You can expect to meet cyclists, joggers, and parents pushing baby strollers, as well as hikers tracing segments or the complete trails. Each of the descriptions in this section summarizes the trail's main attractions and key access points, and they're organized by mileage value and trailhead.

Santa Ana River Trail

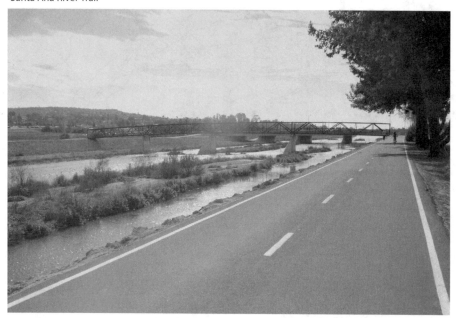

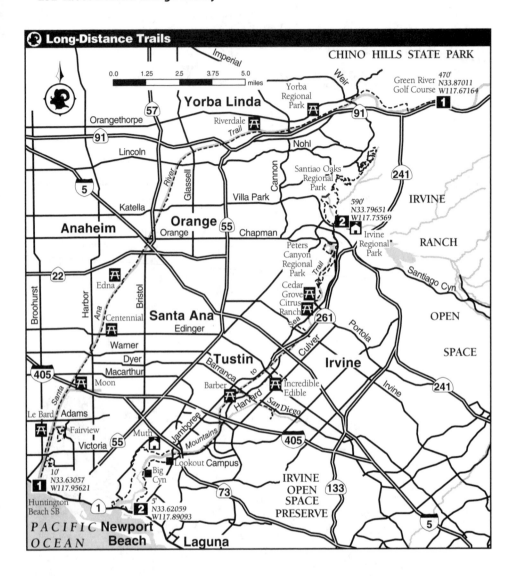

Santa Ana River Trail

Distance	Up to 29 miles (one-way)
Elevation Gain/Loss	100'/500'
Difficulty	Depends on length
Trail Use	Cyclists, equestrians, dogs
Best Times	All year
Agency	OC Parks

The Santa Ana River Trail is envisioned to run 110 miles from the river's headwaters between Big Bear Lake and the San Gorgonio Wilderness all the way down to the Pacific Ocean at Huntington Beach. At the time of this writing, two stretches in Riverside and San Bernardino County are still under development, but the 29-mile Orange County segment is paved all the way from the county line at Green River Golf Course to the sea. The nearly flat path receives heavy use by cyclists. Much of the route is paralleled by a dirt track that is more pleasant for hikers and equestrians. The upper portion in the Santa Ana Canyon is quite scenic and teems with bird life, while the lower portion is an austere and usually dry flood control channel. Major trailheads as you head from the Riverside County line toward the Pacific Ocean include:

29 GREEN RIVER ROAD

Exit the 91 Freeway at Green River Road, and go west 1 mile to find parking on the shoulder of the road near the golf-course entrance road. This area is under construction and may see changes. This attractive segment through the canyon has the only significant hills on the Orange County part of the trail.

At Gypsum Canyon Road by the Canyon RV park, follow the trail over the bridge to the north side of the canyon. The trail then parallels La Palma Avenue for 3 miles before rejoining the edge of the water course at Yorba Linda Boulevard. The next 1.5 miles run alongside Yorba Regional Park, with numerous family-oriented recreational opportunities.

21 YORBA LINDA REGIONAL STAGING LOT

Exit the 91 Freeway on Imperial. Go north one block across the river, and turn right on La Palma Avenue. Proceed 1 mile to the large and popular free gravel lot. This is a great place for families to begin a bike ride in Yorba Regional Park.

This stretch of the Santa Ana River Trail continues to be beautiful, pleasantly landscaped, and rich with waterfowl. Near Imperial Highway, the bikeway crosses from the north to the south side of the river on a bridge. There is a picnic area with an outhouse near the south side.

19 RIVERDALE PARK

Located at 4500 Riverdale Ave. in Anaheim, Riverdale Park has an outhouse, water, and a playground. West of here, the river trail passes under the 91 Freeway and then under the Metrolink tracks, where another trailside picnic area is located. As the river turns south, it sinks into the sand except during the rainy season. The area is quite industrial, and a homeless encampment may be found opposite Angel Stadium near the restrooms and picnic area by Katella Avenue and the 57 Freeway.

10.5 EDNA PARK

Located at 2140 W. Edna St. in Santa Ana at the south end of Riverview Golf Course, Edna Park has a playground, restrooms, a picnic area, and convenient staging for outings on the lower end of the river trail. Just south of the park, the trail crosses to the east side of the river.

7.5 CENTENNIAL PARK

Located at 3000 W. Edinger Ave. in Santa Ana, Centennial Park has all the usual amenities, along with a lake and sports fields. It is a notable site for bird-watching and draws osprey, cormorants, and American white pelicans. Bats hunt near the lake at dusk.

5 MOON PARK

Located at 3377 California St. in Costa Mesa, Moon Park is named for its unique cratered dome adjacent to a small playground.

3 FAIRVIEW PARK AND TALBERT NATURE PRESERVE

Located at 2525 Placentia Ave. in Costa Mesa, this park and preserve are covered in detail in Trip 1.2. The Santa Ana River Trail meets a bridge east over the Greenville-Banning Channel into Talbert Preserve and Fairview Park. Just south of here, another bridge leads west over the Santa Ana River to Le Bard Park. On the south side of Victoria Avenue, gates provide access to the two ends of South Talbert Preserve.

2.5 LE BARD PARK

Located at 20461 Craimer Lane in Huntington Beach, Le Bard Park is a major Little League Baseball facility. It also has a playground, restrooms, and plenty of parking (except on game days). Those planning a day at Huntington Beach can avoid the parking crunch by starting here and pedaling or jogging to the beach. The Le Bard Bridge takes self-propelled travelers across the river.

0 HUNTINGTON BEACH STATE PARK

Park along the Pacific Coast Highway (Highway 1) south of Brookhurst Street. The Santa Ana River flows under the PCH and empties into the Pacific, delimiting the boundary between Huntington and Newport Beaches. Huntington Beach State Park occupies the beach on the northwest side of the river mouth. A fenced plot of land by the mouth protects the Least Tern Reserve, where Southern California's largest breeding population of the endangered seabird can be found. The nearby Talbert Marsh is an unimposing but important wetland. Banning Ranch, near the river mouth on the east side, is one of the last parcels of undeveloped land along the river. Conservationists hope to acquire the land to connect it with Talbert Nature Preserve and create an Orange Coast River Park. Beachfront parking is costly.

Santa Ana River Trail

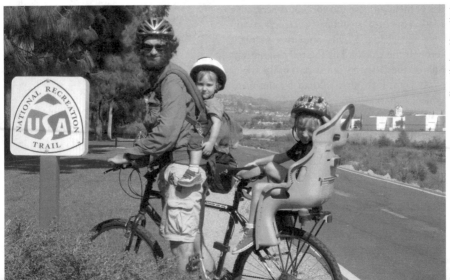

Photo: Abraham Money Harris

trip 18.2 Mountains to Sea Trail

Distance	Up to 18-plus miles (one-way)
Elevation Gain/Loss	100'/700'
Difficulty	Depends on length
Trail Use	Cyclists, equestrians, dogs
Best Times	All year
Agency	OC Parks
Permit	OC Parks parking fee required at Irvine Park and Peters Canyon Regional Park

see map on p. 232

The Mountains to Sea Trail stretches from Irvine Regional Park to Upper Newport Bay, loosely paralleling Jamboree Road south from the foothills of the Santa Ana Mountains through Peters Canyon and along San Diego Creek to the water. Whether you pick a segment or follow the entire trail, you'll be sure to encounter unexpectedly interesting sights along this urban trail. In 2006, the National Park Service designated this route a National Scenic Trail.

Strictly speaking, the trail begins in Weir Canyon, but this portion lies in the Irvine Ranch Open Space and is presently open only by docent-led tour. The next leg through Irvine Regional Park is unmarked. Therefore, the easiest places to pick up the trail are at the entrance to Irvine Regional Park or at Peters Canyon Regional Park.

The quality of signage along it is variable. Some segments are clearly marked as the Mountains to Sea Trail. Others are designated Peters Canyon Trail or San Diego Creek Trail. Most of the trail is asphalt, but the segment between Peters Canyon Regional Park and the Peters Creek Wash has a parallel dirt path favored by hikers and equestrians. The portion in Peters Canyon itself is gravel and dirt with occasional patches of soft sand.

18.4 IRVINE REGIONAL PARK

After passing the entrance gate (request a park map), veer right at the first junction, and then turn left into the first parking lot (Lot #7). Now on foot or bicycle, head back out of the park. The marked trail picks up southbound at the corner of Jamboree and Santiago Canyon Roads, with a paved bicycle path on the west and a dirt trail on the east side of Jamboree.

17.4 PETERS CANYON REGIONAL PARK

At the corner of Canyon View Avenue and Jamboree Road, a Mountains to Sea Trail sign marks the start of the segment through the park. Trailhead parking can be found just west at the main park entrance. Follow the main Peters Canyon Trail south past an overlook of Peters Canyon Reservoir and down the popular dirt trail through the canyon. At the small Lower Peters Canyon Reservoir, the trail veers west, then turns back south when it exits the park.

14.5 CEDAR GROVE PARK

The pleasantly landscaped trail has many gentle curves as it passes Cedar Grove Park, where the first free trailhead parking could be found near Pioneer Road.

14.1 CITRUS RANCH PARK

Trailhead parking at Citrus Ranch Park can be reached from Portola Parkway. The trail then dips under Jamboree Road.

13.3 VALENCIA PARK

Valencia Park has trailhead parking.

11.4 PETERS CANYON WASH

Cross the 261 Toll Road, then cross the bridge over Peters Canyon Wash, and make a 270-degree turn to join the paved trail alongside the wash. The sterile concrete channel soon gives way to a lush wetland favored by waterfowl. Cross under Interstate 5, and continue along the wash.

9.6 HARVARD SIDE PATH

The Peters Canyon Trail is presently closed between Como Channel and Edinger Avenue. If the gates are open, stay on the trail along Peters Canyon Wash. Otherwise, veer left onto the Como Channel Trail. Cross Harvard Avenue and the Metrolink/Amtrak tracks to reach the Incredible Edible Park, where you can join the Harvard Side Path leading southwest along Harvard Avenue. This path has a paved bike trail and dirt equestrian trail, but it tediously crosses city streets at unprotected intersections.

7.8 SAN DIEGO CREEK TRAIL

After crossing Barranca Parkway, turn right onto the San Diego Creek Trail, which serves double purpose as the Mountains to Sea Trail here. Follow it west, then cross a bridge to the south side of the creek, where you reach Colonel Bill Barber Community Park. The San Diego Creek Trail now leads southwest paralleling the creek.

2.9 BACK BAY LOOKOUT

The paved path along San Diego Creek passes under the 405 Freeway, near the San Joaquin Marsh and William Mason Regional Park, and alongside the University of California–Irvine. After passing under the 73 Toll Road near Bonita Creek Park, your path also crosses under Jamboree Road where San Diego Creek opens into Upper Newport Bay. You may see mullet jumping from the water; at sunset, bats emerge from their homes under the bridge. Your path joins the Back Bay Loop Trail, veers left to parallel Jamboree, then veers right along Eastbluff Drive. Soon reach Back Bay Lookout, where you may peer through a telescope to watch waterfowl in the estuary.

1.2 BIG CANYON

Drop down onto Back Bay Drive, which is one-way northbound for cars but used heavily in both directions by joggers and cyclists. Curve along the east rim of the wetlands to reach a small parking area with an interpretive kiosk at the mouth of Big Canyon. The canyon has a small network of trails with good opportunities to view wildlife.

0 BACK BAY SCIENCE CENTER

The final leg of the Mountains to Sea Trail continues along Back Bay Drive to a signed trailhead at the Back Bay Science Center in the Upper Newport Bay Ecological Reserve. There is limited parking outside the center and more on the shoulder of the road farther south. The center is only open for scheduled events.

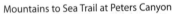

Mountains to Sea Trail at Peters Canyon

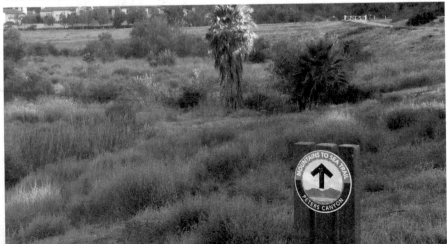

trip 18.3 Aliso Creek Trail

Distance	Up to 13 miles (one-way)
Elevation Gain/Loss	50'/800'
Difficulty	Depends on length
Trail Use	Cyclists, equestrians, dogs
Best Times	All year
Agency	OC Parks
Permit	OC Parks parking fee required at AWCWP

see map on next page

The Aliso Creek Trail, designated a National Recreation Trail in 2012, is another long-distance urban trail through Orange County. It follows Aliso (Spanish for "alder") Creek from its seasonal headwaters at the foot of the Santa Ana Mountains down to Aliso and Wood Canyons Wilderness Park, where the trail ends at a private property boundary just before reaching the Pacific Ocean.

The mostly paved trail is especially popular with cyclists, who can ride up and back from the bottom, and with locals who walk segments in their neighborhood, but this trip, requiring a car shuttle, offers a one-way tour from top to bottom. Kids on bicycles will particularly enjoy the series of parks along the way. If you want to go the full distance, leave one vehicle at Aliso and Wood Wilderness Park at the corner of Awma Road and Alicia Parkway. Then head up Alicia Parkway, Muirlands Boulevard, and El Toro Road to your starting point at Cooks Corner or the El Toro Road Trailhead.

13.2 COOKS CORNER

Cooks Corner is a famous biker bar at the intersection of Santiago Canyon, Live Oak Canyon, and El Toro Roads. It bustles with an odd mix of Harleys, mountain bikes, and families; the food is so-so, but the location is terrific. Parking options are very limited near the start of the Aliso Creek Trail, and Cooks Corner parking is now signed customers only. If you want to park here, head for the fenced dirt area at the end of the lot.

From Cooks Corner, head south on El Toro Road for 100 yards to the signed start of the Aliso Creek Bikeway on the east side of the road opposite Ridgeline Road. It leads south for 0.2 mile to a tunnel under El Toro. The Live Oak Canyon Trail continues south on the east side, but the Aliso Creek Trail passes through the tunnel and heads south on the west side of El Toro.

12.7 MCFADDEN RANCH

The historic McFadden Ranch now serves as the ranger headquarters for Whiting Ranch Wilderness Park, although there is no easy access to the trails from here. The ranch house was built in 1915 by James McFadden for the ranch foreman.

11.5 EDISON TRAIL JUNCTION

The Edison Trail follows a powerline road back to Whiting Ranch.

10.9 EL TORO TRAILHEAD

This small trailhead on the north side of El Toro Road opposite Marguerite Parkway offers the first legal parking directly along the trail. Go early; it fills up on pleasant days.

8.8 SUNDOWNER PARK

This park offers a drinking fountain and parking.

7.5 CHERRY REST AREA

This small picnic area alongside Cherry Avenue has a drinking fountain.

6.8 HEROES SPORTS PARK

There are restrooms, a drinking fountain, and parking at the huge sports field. Beyond,

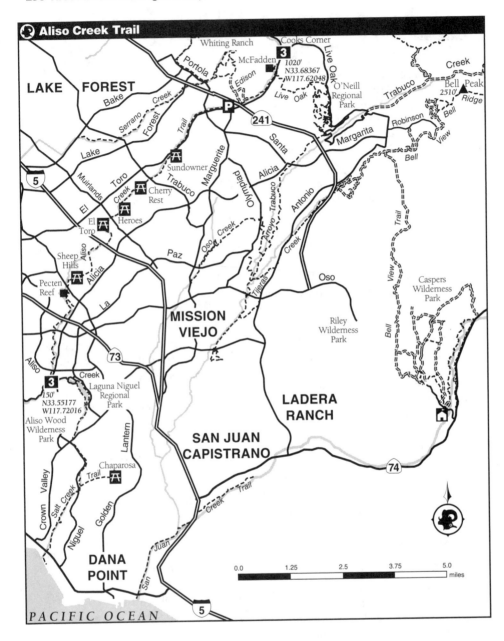

Aliso Creek Trail

pass beneath Amtrak tracks, and turn sharply to bypass a golf course.

6.0 EL TORO PARK

This park has water and parking on Larkwood Lane. Soon after, the trail passes beneath Interstate 5, leaves Aliso Creek, and parallels Paseo de Valencia and then Laguna Hills Drive.

3.5 SHEEP HILLS PARK

Rejoin Aliso Creek at Sheep Hills Park, which has water and streetside parking on Laguna Hills Drive.

3.2 PECTEN REEF TRAIL

After passing beneath Moulton Parkway, enter the northern reaches of Aliso and Woods Canyon Wilderness Park and watch for a sign for the Pecten Reef Trail on the right. This 0.5-mile loop passes sandstone embedded with enormous scallop fossils and rejoins the Aliso Creek Trail (see Trip 5.6). At another junction shortly beyond, be sure to veer right and cross Aliso Creek on a sturdy bridge.

0.0 ALISO AND WOODS CANYONS WILDERNESS PARK: AWMA TRAILHEAD

The major wilderness park staging area is a good place to end a trip. It is possible to continue down the Aliso Creek Trail through the park, but your path is eventually blocked by the private Aliso Creek Golf Course.

VARIATION

It is possible to extend this trip 7 miles to reach the Pacific Ocean at Salt Creek Beach. Because the Aliso Creek Trail is blocked ahead, the variation climbs out through Laguna Niguel Regional Park, briefly follows city streets, and then drops onto the Salt Creek Trail.

From the Awma Trailhead, return to Alicia Parkway and follow it south 0.1 mile to a crosswalk, where you can cross the parkway and then backtrack 100 feet to a gated access road into Laguna Niguel Regional Park. Follow this road past picnic grounds to a T-junction with a loop road. Go left, pass the park entrance road and a playground, and pick up a paved hiking and riding trail that climbs to the spillway of Sulphur Creek Reservoir.

The trail becomes dirt and follows the east side of the lake, a favorite area for birders, then crosses a bridge to a T-junction where pavement resumes. Turn left and head out the south end of the park, following the Sulphur Creek riparian corridor past a water-treatment facility. Continue on the main path as you pass Crown Valley Community Park and the Laguna Niguel YMCA, then cross a road in the park and soon end at Crown Valley Parkway.

Turn right and follow the busy road to the first traffic light, Niguel Road, where you turn left and take the sidewalk up a steep hill. At the second light (Marina Hills Drive), you can drop into a tunnel and join the Salt Creek Trail. Stay right (south) after the tunnel, and proceed south along a narrow corridor between Niguel Road and a subdivision. Pass a spur on the left from Chapparosa Park, then pass through a tunnel under Niguel Road, and continue along the marked trail through a restored canyon and past the Monarch Beach golf course to the trail's end at Salt Creek Beach (see Trip 6.1). If you go this far, you may wish to leave a getaway vehicle at the large beach parking lot on Ritz-Carlton Drive.

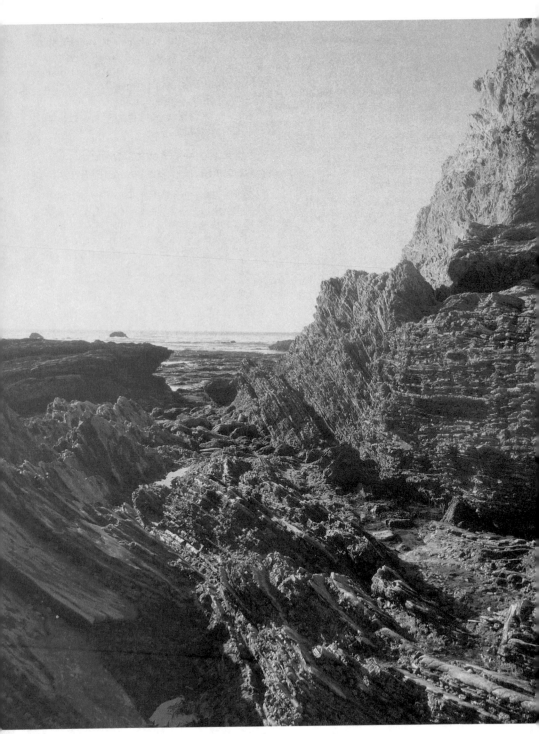

Treasure Cove, Crystal Cove State Park *(see Chapter 3)*

Best Hikes

Best Beach Hikes

TRIP 3.2: CRYSTAL COVE Walk the beach past tidepools, and return on the bluffs watching for whales.

TRIP 6.5: SAN ONOFRE STATE BEACH Here, the primeval Southern California coastline survives more or less intact.

Best Suburban Hikes

TRIP 3.4: EL MORO CANYON LOOP Ocean views and passages through dark, spooky oak groves.

TRIP 4.2: LAUREL CANYON LOOP A still-wild coastal canyon with oaks, sycamores, and a seasonal waterfall.

TRIP 8.1: OAK CANYON NATURE CENTER An agreeable patch of wilderness amid the wilds of suburban Anaheim.

TRIP 9.1: BORREGO AND RED ROCK CANYONS Shady canyons and eroded sandstone cliffs.

Best Mountain Hikes

TRIP 15.12: HOLY JIM FALLS An intimate canyon setting highlighted by a picturesque little waterfall.

TRIP 15.16: WEST HORSETHIEF TO TRABUCO CANYON LOOP From a shady canyon to a viewful summit ridge, and back down.

Best Canyon Hikes

TRIP 15.9: HARDING CANYON Narrow, rugged, sublime canyon graced with a crystal-clear winter-time stream.

TRIP 17.5: SAN MATEO CANYON Ramble among oaks, wildflowers, and pools along San Mateo Creek.

Best Waterfalls

TRIP 15.5: BLACK STAR CANYON FALLS Your effort to ascend the wild canyon is rewarded with a remarkable waterfall.

TRIP 16.10: LOWER HOT SPRING CANYON The water drops 140 feet—Orange County's tallest falls. This hike is remote, difficult, and inaccessible to the average hiker.

TRIP 17.1: TENAJA FALLS A multitiered cascade hewn in polished granite and an easy hike.

Best View Hikes

TRIP 3.3: EMERALD VISTA POINT Bird's-eye view of Orange County's coast and the offshore islands.

TRIP 5.2: SEAVIEW AND BADLANDS TRAIL Easy hike with breathtaking coastal views.

TRIP 11.1: BOMMER CANYON AND RIDGE LOOP: Highly varied scenery from canyons to coast to the interior.

TRIP 15.13: SANTIAGO PEAK The peak's 100-mile views encompass most of coastal Southern California.

Best Wildflowers

TRIP 14.5: LOS SANTOS TO TRANS PRESERVE LOOP Catch some of California's finest springtime displays of greenery and wildflowers in March or April.

TRIP 16.3: SAN JUAN LOOP TRAIL Wildflowers of the mountain meadows and chaparral.

TRIP 17.6: BLUEWATER TRAVERSE Wildflowers of the chaparral and potrero country.

Best Autumn Colors

TRIP 15.15: TRABUCO CANYON Tawny colors of willow, sycamore, and maple; best in December.

Best Bird- and Wildlife-Watching

TRIP 2.3: SAN JOAQUIN WILDLIFE SANCTUARY
Local as well as migrant bird life.

TRIP 13.2: BELL CANYON Frequented by deer, bobcats, and mountain lions.

TRIP 16.5: CHIQUITO BASIN A sunny, oak-rimmed valley; a natural pasture.

TRIPS 17.1–6: SAN MATEO CANYON Aquatic, oak woodland, and chaparral habitats attract a wide variety of reptiles, amphibians, birds, and mammals.

Best Mountain Biking and Running Trails

TRIP 3.3–5: CRYSTAL COVE BACKCOUNTRY AREA The entire backcountry part of the state park is mountain-bike friendly and has a variety of challenging fire roads and singletrack trails.

TRIP 4.3: EMERALD CANYON Ridgeline views plus an intimate canyon setting—this ride or run has it all.

TRIP 5.5: ALISO AND WOOD CANYONS One of the most popular spots for mountain biking in Orange County; not all trails are open to bikes.

TRIP 7.7: TELEGRAPH CANYON TRAVERSE Moderate grades; remarkably unspoiled yet close to the city's edge.

TRIP 7.8: GILMAN PEAK A short but challenging ascent on a graded roadway; excellent views at the top.

TRIP 8.4: ROBBERS PEAK All of the splendid trails above Santiago Oaks are worth riding.

TRIP 9.3: WHITING RANCH LOOP Moderate grades on mostly wide trails; a classic among mountain bikers.

TRIP 15.4: NORTH MAIN DIVIDE TRAVERSE Challenging trip up and over the northern crest of the Main Divide; delightful views.

TRIP 15.8: HARDING ROAD Long climb to the Main Divide just north of Old Saddleback. Return the same way, or continue along the Main Divide.

TRIP 15.14: INDIAN TRUCK TRAIL The most scenic ascent by road to the Main Divide from the east.

TRIP 16.4: SAN JUAN TRAIL A classic and demanding winding singletrack trail.

TRIP 18.1: SANTA ANA RIVER TRAIL Cross Orange County from the Santa Ana Mountains to Huntington Beach on a paved trail free of motor vehicles.

Recommended Reading

Allen, Robert L., *Wildflowers of Orange County and the Santa Ana Mountains,* Laguna Wilderness Press, 2013.

Arora, David, *Mushrooms Demystified,* 2nd edition, Ten Speed Press, 1986.

Bailey, H. P., *The Climate of Southern California,* University of California Press, 1966 (out of print).

Bakker, Elna, *An Island Called California,* 2nd edition, University of California Press, 1984.

California Coastal Commission, *California Coastal Access Guide,* 6th edition, University of California Press, 2003.

California Division of Mines and Geology, *Geologic Map of California—Santa Ana Sheet,* 1965.

Clark, Oscar F., Daniel Svehla, Greg Ballmer, and Arlee Montalvo, *Flora of the Santa Ana River and Environs,* Heyday Books, 2007.

Hogue, Charles L., *Insects of the Los Angeles Basin,* 2nd edition, Natural History Museum of Los Angeles County, 1993.

Mitchell, Patrick, *Santa Ana Mountains History, Habitat, and Hikes: On the Slopes of Old Saddleback and Beyond,* History Press, 2013.

National Geographic Society, *Field Guide to the Birds of North America,* 4th edition, 2002.

Peterson, P. Victor, *Native Trees of Southern California,* University of California Press, 1966.

Raven, Peter H., *Native Shrubs of Southern California,* University of California Press, 1974.

Rundel, Phillip W., and John R. Gustafson, *Introduction to the Plant Life of Southern California: Coast to Foothills,* University of California Press, 2005.

Schoenherr, Allan A., *A Natural History of Open Spaces in Orange County,* Laguna Wilderness Press, 2011.

Sharp, Robert P., *Coastal Southern California* (geology guide), Kendall/Hunt Publishing Company, 1978.

———, *Geology Field Guide to Southern California,* William C. Brown Co., 1972.

Stephenson, Terry E., *Shadows of Old Saddleback: Tales of the Santa Ana Mountains,* reprint of 1931 edition, Rasmussen Press, 1974.

Tway, Linda E., *Tidepools: Southern California: A Guide to 92 Locations from Point Conception to Mexico,* Wilderness Press, 2011.

Local Organizations

AMIGOS DE BOLSA CHICA (amigosdebolsachica.org) Activities associated with Bolsa Chica Ecological Reserve.

CHINO HILLS STATE PARK INTERPRETIVE ASSOCIATION (chinohillsstatepark.org) Activities associated with Chino Hills State Park.

HILLS FOR EVERYONE (hillsforeveryone.org) Advocates land acquisition for wildlife habitat and recreation in the Chino and Puente Hills area.

IRVINE RANCH CONSERVANCY (irconservancy.org) Stewards open space on the historic Irvine Ranch.

IRVINE RANCH NATURAL LANDMARKS (letsgooutside.org) Sign up for guided activities and open-access days in the Irvine Ranch Natural Landmarks.

NATURALIST FOR YOU (naturalist-for-you.org) Nonprofit agency organizes interpretive hikes and connects professional naturalists with youth groups and other organizations.

OC HIKING CLUB (oc-hiking.com) A Meetup group organizing hiking trips in Orange County and elsewhere.

SEA AND SAGE AUDUBON SOCIETY (seaandsageaudubon.org) Sponsors field trips and bird walks in Orange County's coastal wetlands and foothill canyons. Maintains an office at the San Joaquin Wildlife Sanctuary.

SIERRA CLUB ORANGE COUNTY GROUP (angeles.sierraclub.org/orange) Sponsors day hikes and camping trips throughout Orange County; advocates preservation of open spaces; plans and maintains trails in the Trabuco District of Cleveland National Forest.

Information Sources

The county and state parks and Cleveland National Forest generally have useful websites, most easily located by entering the park name into a search engine.

Cleveland National Forest

EL CARISO VISITOR INFORMATION OFFICE 951-678-3700, 32353 Ortega Hwy., Lake Elsinore, CA 92330

TRABUCO RANGER DISTRICT (CNF: TD) 951-736-1811, 1147 E. Sixth St., Corona, CA 92879

California State Parks

CRYSTAL COVE STATE PARK (CCSP) 949-494-3539

CHINO HILLS STATE PARK (CHSP) 951-780-6222

SAN CLEMENTE STATE BEACH (SCSB) 949-492-3156

SAN ONOFRE STATE BEACH (SOSB) 949-492-4872

Orange County Parks

ALISO AND WOOD CANYONS WILDERNESS PARK (AWCWP) 949-923-2200

CARBON CANYON REGIONAL PARK (CCRP) 714-973-3160

CASPERS WILDERNESS PARK (CWP) 949-923-2210

IRVINE RANCH OPEN SPACE (IROS) 714-973-6696

IRVINE REGIONAL PARK (IRP) 714-973-6835

LAGUNA COAST WILDERNESS PARK (LCWP) 949-923-2235

LAGUNA NIGUEL REGIONAL PARK (LNRP) 949-923-2240

O'NEILL REGIONAL PARK (ONRP) 949-923-2260

PETERS CANYON REGIONAL PARK (PCRP) 714-973-6611

RILEY WILDERNESS PARK (RWP) 949-923-2265

SALT CREEK BEACH PARK (SCBP) 949-923-2280

SANTIAGO OAKS REGIONAL PARK (SORP) 714-973-6620

TALBERT NATURE PRESERVE (TNP) 949-923-2250

UPPER NEWPORT BAY NATURE PRESERVE (UNBNP) 949-923-2290

WHITING RANCH WILDERNESS PARK (WRWP) 949-923-2245

Miscellaneous

BOLSA CHICA ECOLOGICAL RESERVE (BCER) 714-846-1114

CALIFORNIA DEPARTMENT OF FISH AND WILDLIFE (CDFW) 858-467-4209

CITY OF ANAHEIM 714-765-5191

CITY OF IRVINE: IRVINE OPEN SPACE PRESERVE (IOSP) 714-508-4757

CITY OF NEWPORT BEACH 949-644-3151

CITY OF SAN JUAN CAPISTRANO 949-493-5911

IRVINE RANCH WATER DISTRICT (IRWD) 949-261-7963

OAK CANYON NATURE CENTER (OCNC) 714-998-8380

OCEAN INSTITUTE, DANA POINT (OIDP) 949-496-2274

SANTA ROSA PLATEAU ECOLOGICAL RESERVE (SRPER) 951-677-6951

Map Sources

CLEVELAND NATIONAL FOREST See previous section and www.fs.usda.gov/main/cleveland/maps-pubs.

REI 714-505-0205, 2962 El Camino Real, Tustin, CA 92782; rei.com

INDEX

About the Authors

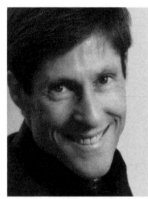

Photo: eabrownstudio.com

JERRY SCHAD (1949–2011) was Southern California's leading outdoors writer. His 16 guidebooks, including Wilderness Press's popular and comprehensive *Afoot & Afield* series, and his "Roam-O-Rama" column in the *San Diego Reader* helped thousands of hikers discover the region's diverse wild places. Jerry ran or hiked many thousands of miles of distinct trails throughout California, in the Southwest, and in Mexico. He was a sub-24-hour finisher of Northern California's 100-mile Western States Endurance Run, and he served in a leadership capacity for outdoor excursions around the world. He taught astronomy and physical science at San Diego Mesa College and chaired its physical-sciences department from 1999 until 2011. His sudden, untimely death from kidney cancer shocked and saddened the hiking community.

DAVID MONEY HARRIS is a professor of engineering at Harvey Mudd College. He is the author or coauthor of six hiking guidebooks and five engineering textbooks. David grew up rambling about the Desolation Wilderness as a toddler in his father's pack and later roamed the High Sierra as a Boy Scout. As a Sierra Club trip leader, he organized mountaineering trips throughout the Sierra Nevada. Since 1999, he has been exploring the mountains and deserts of Southern California. He lives with his wife and three sons in Upland, California, and delights in sharing his love of the outdoors with their boys.

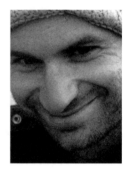